Published

Volume 21 in the Series
SAUNDERS
MONOGRAPHS
IN CLINICAL
RADIOLOGY

PLAIN FILM APPROACH TO ABDOMINAL CALCIFICATIONS

STEPHEN R. BAKER, M.D.

Associate Professor of Radiology
Albert Einstein College of Medicine
Co-Director of Radiology
Bronx Municipal Hospital Center
Bronx, New York

MILTON ELKIN, M.D.

Professor and Chairman
Department of Radiology
Albert Einstein College of Medicine
Bronx, New York

1983

W.B. SAUNDERS COMPANY
Philadelphia   London   Toronto   Mexico City   Rio de Janeiro   Sydney   Tokyo

W. B. Saunders Company: West Washington Square
                           Philadelphia, PA 19105

                           1 St. Anne's Road
                           Eastbourne, East Sussex BN21 3UN, England

                           1 Goldthorne Avenue
                           Toronto, Ontario M8Z 5T9, Canada

                           Apartado 26370—Cedro 512
                           Mexico 4, D.F., Mexico

                           Rua Coronel Cabrita, 8
                           Sao Cristovao Caixa Postal 21176
                           Rio de Janeiro, Brazil

                           9 Waltham Street
                           Artarmon, N.S.W. 2064, Australia

                           Ichibancho, Central Bldg., 22-1 Ichibancho
                           Chiyoda-Ku, Tokyo 102, Japan

Library of Congress Cataloging in Publication Data

Baker, Stephen R.
  Plain film approach to abdominal calcifications.

  (Saunders monographs in clinical radiology; v. 21)
  1. Abdomen—Radiography. 2. Abdomen—Calcification—
Diagnosis. I. Elkin, Milton, 1916–   II. Title.
III. Series. [DNLM: 1. Calcinosis—Radiography.
2. Calculi—Radiography. WI 900 B168p]
RC944.B34 1983   617'.55   82-42617
ISBN 0-7216-1498-1

Plain Film Approach to Abdominal Calcifications   ISBN 0-7216-1498-1

Last digit is the print number: 9   8   7   6   5   4   3   2   1

To my parents, Louis and Edith,
and to my wife Marjorie (S.R.B.).
In memory of my parents, Philip and Rose (M.E.).

CONTRIBUTORS

RICHARD A. ROSEN M.D.

Visiting Associate Professor of Radiology, Albert Einstein College of Medicine of Yeshiva University, Bronx, N.Y.; Director of Radiology, Woodhull Medical and Mental Health Center, Brooklyn, N.Y.; Attending Radiologist, Kings County Hospital Center, Brooklyn, N.Y.; Bronx Municipal Hospital Center, Bronx, N.Y. *Calcifications in Abdominal Lymph Nodes; Miscellaneous Abdominal Radiopacities*

CHUSILP CHARNSANGAVEJ, M.D.

Assistant Professor of Radiology, Albert Einstein College of Medicine of Yeshiva University, Bronx, N.Y.; Attending Radiologist, Bronx Municipal Hospital Center, Bronx, N.Y. *Calcification in Abdominal Arteries and Veins*

HARRIS COHEN, M.D.

Clinical Assistant Professor of Radiology, State University of New York—Downstate Medical Center, Brooklyn, N.Y.; Assistant Radiologist, Brookdale Hospital Medical Center, Brooklyn, N.Y. *Pediatric Abdominal Calcifications*

DUREE EATON, M.D.

Clinical Assistant Professor of Radiology, State University of New York—Downstate Medical Center, Brooklyn, N.Y.; Attending Radiologist and Physician-in-Charge of Pediatric Radiology, Brookdale Hospital Medical Center, Brooklyn, N.Y. *Pediatric Abdominal Calcifications*

PREFACE

Despite the development of improved imaging methods for the examination of the abdomen, such as computed tomography and ultrasonography, the scout radiograph remains the most important initial radiologic examination of the abdomen. With the availability of newer and more sophisticated techniques, it has become too commonplace to delay commitment to a diagnostic conclusion from the initial radiograph until additional studies have been completed. This is evident in the evaluation of calcifications.

In the characterization of discrete densities apparent on an abdominal radiograph, there are a number of important questions to be answered. Does the density represent calcification, ossification, ingested or injected radiopaque medication, metallic foreign body, or artifact? In what organ or tissue is the density located? Is it an incidental finding or a crucial indicator of disease? The authors contend that careful attention to the location, configuration, internal structure, and radiopacity of the density as seen on the scout radiograph often points to a single diagnosis or to a limited number of possibilities. Further workup, if needed, can then be strictly planned to reach specific determinations while avoiding unrewarding additional examinations.

The spectrum of abdominal radiodensities is spread from the common and easily recognizable to the rare and bizarre. Calcifications can be faint or dense, linear or conglomerate, minute or massive, mottled or homogeneous, spicular or smooth. Consideration of these and other factors, such as position and mobility, allows a grouping of diagnostic possibilities. The first chapter of this monograph presents, in detail, a system of differentiation that can be applied to any abdominal opacity.

Chapters 2 to 6 are devoted to abdominal calcifications in particular regions or organs. The emphasis is on plain film analysis, with comprehensive, but not encyclopedic, discussions and illustrations. Then come chapters on calcifications in vessels, lymph nodes, and the abdominal wall. The final chapter considers distinctive radiodensities found in the pediatric abdomen. Tables of differential diagnoses are included in the text and detailed bibliographies are provided for the interested reader.

While the subject of abdominal calcification is of particular interest to the radiologist, the emphasis on diagnosis from simple, routine radiographic examinations should be helpful to physicians in other clinical disciplines and also to medical students in their initiation to the orderly process of sifting available evidence to reach a clinical diagnosis.

The acquisition of materials for this book required the generosity and cooperation of many individuals. Radiographs were provided by contributors from numerous institutions on four continents, and to all of them we express our heartfelt gratitude.

Mr. Louis Mendez deserves special thanks for his diligence, skill, and cheerfulness in preparing the illustrations. Without him this book could not have been produced. Thanks also to Nancy Marchese, Gloria Cioffi, Sandy Ferrari, Ellen Massaro, Harriet McCready, and Rosanne Ditizio, who patiently and expertly typed endless drafts and rewrites. And, of course, we owe an incalculable debt to our families who gracefully put up with our absences and distractions during the gestation of this work.

STEPHEN R. BAKER, M.D.
MILTON ELKIN, M.D.

CONTENTS

Chapter 1

EVALUATION OF ABDOMINAL CALCIFICATIONS

Stephen R. Baker, M.D.

The analysis of abdominal calcifications and other radiopacities on plain radiographs is often a diagnostic challenge. Occasionally, historical information will be of value; at times, physical examination will contribute important clues. Laboratory data such as the presence of microscopic hematuria will sometimes be helpful. Yet, very frequently the appearance of the opacity is unexpected. Since the plain film is, in most cases, the first radiologic examination of the abdomen, there is often no further information available to the radiologist. Hence, the decision whether to proceed with further workup rests on an evaluation of the nature of the calcification.

While the literature abounds in short articles and case reports describing specific entities, little has been written about a systematic assessment of abdominal radiopacities. Careful attention to morphology, location, and mobility can narrow the diagnostic possibilities considerably. In most instances, the position and pattern of the calcification can be fairly well established even before contrast studies are performed. An analysis of the details of the appearance of the density and awareness of its relationship to other structures can often reveal its identity on plain films.

The purpose of this introductory chapter is to consider important distinguishing features of the appearance, position, and mobility of abdominal calcifications. Following a discussion of the basic physiological principles of calcification, the focus will be directed to a scheme for categorizing calcifications according to a set of readily observable morphological characteristics.

PHYSIOLOGY

Before proceeding with an analysis of the differentiating radiographic features of abdominal calcification, it is helpful to consider the physiological influences that promote the deposition of calcium. Precipitation of calcium salts may occur within hollow viscera and tubes, or in the walls of vessels and solid organs. Alterations in both local and general conditions lead to calcification.

Elevations in serum calcium and serum phosphorus predispose to the laying down of calcium salts. When there is also increased tissue alkalinity the process is accelerated. Metastatic calcification refers to calcium deposition in otherwise normal organs subjected to hypercalcemia and alkalosis. In the abdomen, the kidney and stomach are most affected. However, usually the extent of calcification is insufficient to be detected on plain films and this form of calcification is rarely encountered. A notable exception is renal tubular acidosis, where calcification may be visualized in the parenchyma of the kidney. Hyperparathyroidism, renal failure, hypervitaminosis D, and the various causes of bone destruction are often associated with metastatic calcification.[1]

Dystrophic calcification is the most common type of calcification involving solid structures in the abdomen. Serum calcium and phosphorus are usually normal with dystrophic calcification, but tissue damage and corresponding local alkalosis are thought to be responsible for calcium deposition. Histologic alterations may be caused by devitalization of tissue as a result of ischemia or necrosis.

1

Catabolism of lipids in fast-growing lesions can result in the formation of fatty acids, which may be avid binders of calcium. In some mucin-producing tumors, precipitation of calcium occurs because the glycoprotein produced by the tumor may be biochemically and functionally similar to the ground substance of ossifying cartilage.[2] Hyaline degeneration also appears to be a contributing factor in calcium deposition. It is not always possible to sort out the various factors that favor dystrophic calcification. Whether it be a fast-growing tumor, an infarct, scar, or involuting tissue, local tissue damage of one kind or another leads to calcification.

Bone formation in devitalized and degenerating tissue is rarer than dystrophic calcification but occurs occasionally, often with associated calcification and sometimes by itself. The same factors predisposing to dystrophic calcification also promote bone production as a metaplastic response in previously normal tissues. Abdominal scars, retroperitoneal neoplasms, ovarian tumors, and occasionally gastrointestinal malignancies may be bone formers. A less common type of calcium deposition, and one that is found primarily in ovarian serous cystadenocarcinomas, is psammomatous calcification. In dystrophic calcification, the deposition of calcium appears extracellularly. In psammomatous calcification, calcium is found intracellularly and occurs in growing tumor masses.[3]

Both local and systemic factors can regulate stone formation in the liquid medium occupying the lumen of conduits and hollow organs. Hypercalciuria increases the risk of renal, ureteral, and bladder stones. The gradient in intestinal pH from the duodenum to the ileum explains why calcified enteroliths are seen in the distal small bowel but are absent in the more acidic duodenum. Furthermore, local factors such as infection, debris formation, and stasis also promote the production of concretions. Stones can form in any obstructed lumen but their formation is accelerated if calcium concentration and pH are increased.

Much is still unknown about the mechanics and kinetics of calcium deposition. It is not clear how and at what rate damaged tissues take up calcium. In solid structures especially, these questions are largely unresolved. In most cases, however, calcification is a consequence of the interplay of recognizable local conditions and general factors.

MORPHOLOGY

The formulation of a classification of abdominal calcifications is difficult. The designated criteria of a particular group may be too general to be applied to a specific example or too detailed for practical implementation. Consequently, there has been no prior attempt to propose a comprehensive morphological classification of abdominal calcifications. Rather the emphasis has been on the demonstration of the uniqueness of a number of individual pathologic entities. For example, the term "staghorn," a vivid description of a renal calculus occupying the calyceal system, serves to differentiate the appearance of that stone from other abdominal radiodensities. However, only a very few calcifications are so easily identifiable.

Features of value for the classification of the morphology of calcifications include shape, border sharpness, marginal continuity, and internal architecture. An evaluation of these factors permits a grouping of abdominal calcification into four discrete morphological categories, each possessing a set of features peculiar to itself. The four categories are concretions, conduit wall calcification, cyst wall calcification, and solid mass calcification. In the following sections, this classification will be discussed in detail. Mention will also be made of potential pitfalls and notable exceptions.

Concretions (Table 1–1)

A concretion is a calcified mass formed in the lumen of a vessel or hollow viscus. Concretions can be faint or brightly calcified; the radiographic density depends on the size of the opacity and the amount of calcium per unit volume. While there are many sites in which concretions may form, the most common are the pelvic veins, the gallbladder, and the urinary tract (Table 1–2). Concretions can be formed by the precipitation of calcium salts, as in renal calculi, or by the deposition of calcium in pre-existing venous thrombi with the development of phleboliths. Prostatic calculi occur predominantly in the elderly while appendicoliths are usually encountered in younger patients. With some concretions, such as pancreatic stones, inflammation seems to play a role, but for others, such as

Table 1–1. Characteristics of Concretion Morphology

1. Sharp border
2. Smooth external margins
3. Continuous calcification of the perimeter
4. Geometric internal architecture
   a. Laminations
   b. Homogeneously dense
   c. Smooth rim
   d. Single central lucency
5. Confined within existing structures

Table 1–2. Abdominal Radiopacities Exhibiting a Concretion Morphology

Common
1. Phleboliths in pelvic veins
2. Renal, ureteral, and bladder calculi
3. Gallbladder stones
4. Prostatic calculi
5. Appendicoliths (fecaliths)
6. Pancreatic calculi

Uncommon
1. Urethral calculi
2. Choledocholithiasis
3. Phleboliths outside pelvis
   a. Gonadal veins
   b. Hemangiomata
4. Enteroliths in small bowel and large bowel
5. Stones in Meckel's diverticulum

enteroliths, the reasons for formation are more obscure. Hence, concretions do not share a common etiology.

Moreover, concretions do not have a common shape. Small stones tend to be round or oval (Fig. 1–1). Multiple gallstones are frequently faceted (Fig. 1–2), and multiple urinary stones, especially in a dilated system, may also be faceted on at least one side of their perimeter. Ureteral calculi are often angular but bladder calculi are usually smooth. Occasionally, specific diagnostic forms also occur, such as the star-shaped bladder calculus (Fig. 1–3).

Most stones exhibit a sharp, clearly defined external border, but on occasion, concretions may have irregular bulges (Fig. 1–4). Concretions are calcified throughout the entirety of their perimeter.

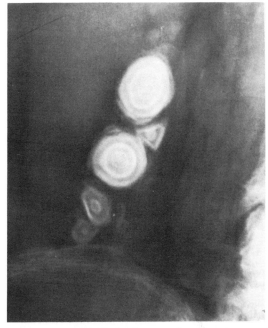

Figure 1–2. Calcified gallstones of varying shapes and sizes. Several of the stones are sharply faceted at points of interface with adjacent stones.

Almost always there are no discontinuities in the external margin. This is an important feature, especially if the interior of the concretion is lucent, because it helps to distinguish large stones from calcified cysts. If the outer ring of calcification is not complete, it is unlikely to be a stone.

The internal architecture of concretions is varied. They can be homogeneously dense, a pattern

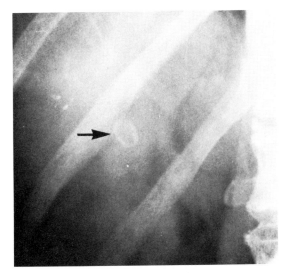

Figure 1–1. A single calcified gallstone (arrow).

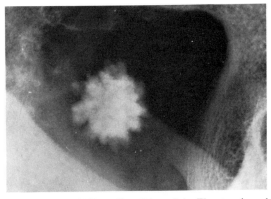

Figure 1–3. Oblique film of the pelvis. The star-shaped bladder calculus has symmetrically radiating projections giving it a characteristic appearance.

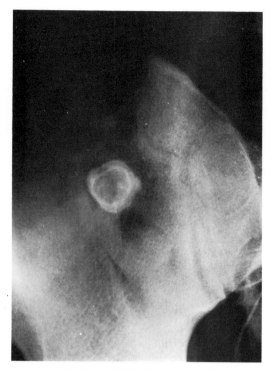

Figure 1–4. Appendicolith with a continuous margin of calcification and a small medial bulge of radiopacity.

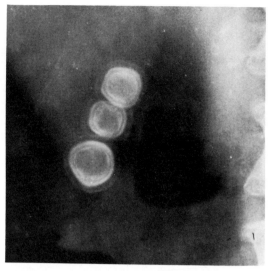

Figure 1–6. Three laminated gallstones. Note that the laminations are of varying density with the outer ring the most faint.

frequently encountered in urinary calculi (Fig. 1–5). They may have a central or slightly eccentric lucency, an appearance which is characteristic of many phleboliths. Multiple laminations indicate concretion morphology unequivocally. Alternating bands of encircling lucency may be found within a concretion (Fig. 1–6) or there may be a single lucent band close to the external rim (Fig. 1–7). Circumferential laminations are frequently encountered in gallstones, vesical calculi, and appendicoliths.

Each of the various internal patterns is quite distinctive. Laminations have a predictable parallel appearance. For the most part, central lucencies are single. When there is only a marginal rim of calcification, the width of the rim is continuous and usually of minimally varying thickness throughout the circumference. The inner pattern of stones is

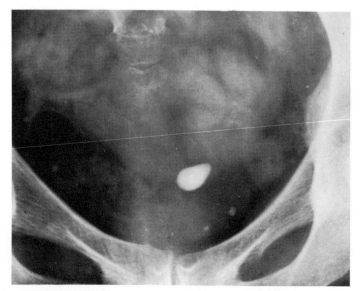

Figure 1–5. A stone in a ureterocele. Observe its homogeneous density and smooth contour.

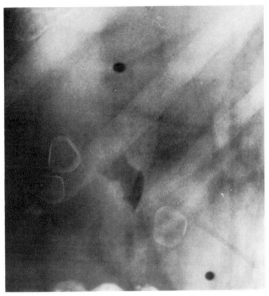

Figure 1–7. Two faceted stones in the gallbladder and another in the common bile duct. Calcification occupies only the margins of the calculi. While the calcification is faint, it is circumferential in all three stones.

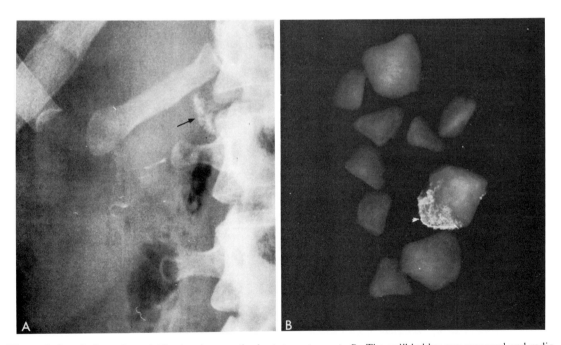

Figure 1–8. *A*, Irregular calcification in a cystic duct stone (arrow). *B*, The gallbladder was removed and radiographs of the stones were made. Note the dense calcification on only one side of the cystic duct stone (arrowhead) while the other calculi are only minimally calcified. (Courtesy of Dr. Ralph Goldin, Bronx, N.Y.)

hardly ever mottled, whorled, or patchy. Rarely, calcifications will deposit on only one surface of a stone, and on plain radiographs a streaky or amorphous focus of calcification will be seen (Fig. 1–8, *A* and *B*). These exceptions aside, the vast majority of stones will exhibit geometric outlines and continuous contours.

Stones form within the lumen of pre-existent structures. Unlike cysts or solid lesions, which are pathologic masses that distort or displace normal organs, stones tend to remain within vessels or hollow viscera. If multiple calcific densities appear to be arrayed in a line, this suggests a common location in a hollow tube (Fig. 1–9). Infrequently, concretions will be seen outside expected locations, such as gallstones in the ileum or colon, an appendicolith in the peritoneal cavity, or multiple phleboliths in a hemangioma (Fig. 1–10). Generally, however, concretions do not pass through vascular or visceral walls, and are seen in association with anatomic structures.

Conduit Wall Calcification (Table 1–3)

Conduits are hollow tubes through which fluids pass. In the abdomen, conduits include the biliary

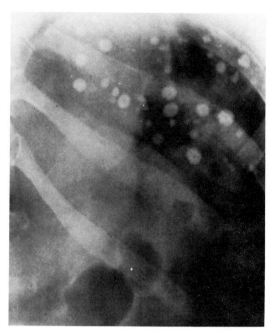

Figure 1–10. Multiple rounded concretions in the spleen. Some have central lucencies and most are greater than five mm. in diameter. These are calcified phleboliths in a splenic hemangioma.

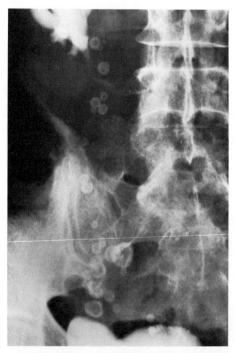

Figure 1–9. Multiple round densities adjacent to but outside the right ureter. All are phleboliths and the superior ones are in the right gonadal vein.

ductal system, the components of the urinary tract, pancreatic ducts, the vas deferens, and arteries and veins. The majority of conduit wall calcifications in the abdomen involve the aorta and its branches. The tubular appearance of conduits can easily be appreciated if the calcification is circumferential (Fig. 1–11). En face, a ringlike density will be seen (Fig. 1–12). Unlike concretions, discontinuities of the opaque ring are not unusual. Since calcifications in conduit walls are not uniform, unopacified and radiodense areas are irregularly arrayed along the course of a vessel (Fig. 1–13). However, calcification is confined only to the tubular walls. The presence of internal radiopacity suggests another morphologic category.

Because calcium deposition can occur throughout the circumference of a conduit, when the x-ray beam is directed perpendicular to the vessel, the margins presenting the greatest wall thickness will appear most densely calcified. Thus, in profile, conduit wall calcification appears as parallel tracks of increased density. Splenic artery calcification often appears as calcified tracks describing a serpiginous path (Fig. 1–14). Although less common, a branching pattern is also characteristic of vessel wall calcification. This can be seen at the bifurcation of the abdominal aorta and in intrarenal arterial calcification (Fig. 1–15). When a vessel of narrow caliber is densely calcified, a stringlike ap-

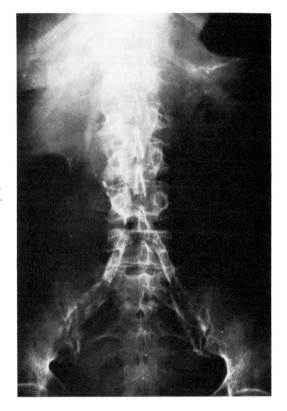

Figure 1–11. Tubular calcification characteristic of conduit morphology seen in both common iliac arteries and their branches.

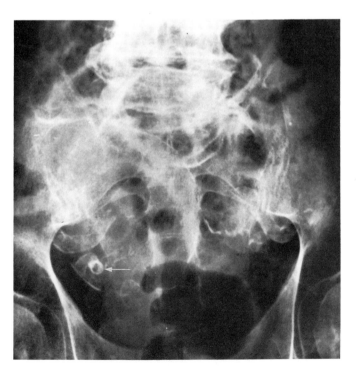

Figure 1–12. Calcification in pelvic arteries. Where a calcified vessel is seen en face it appears as a circle of radiopacity (arrow).

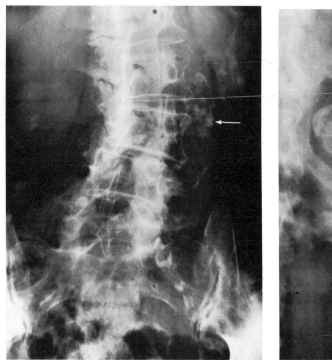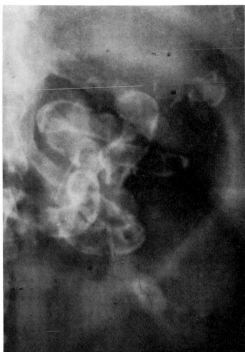

Figure 1–13   Figure 1–14

Figure 1–13.   Plaques of calcification (arrow) in the abdominal aorta. Dense calcification may be seen in localized areas even if the x-ray beam does not pass through them tangentially.

Figure 1–14.   Calcification in the walls of a markedly convoluted splenic artery. Note the maintenance of parallel tracks of calcification despite the tortuosity of the vessel.

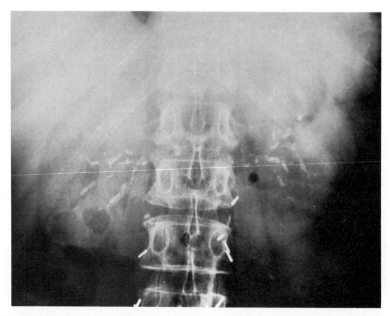

Figure 1–15.   Bilateral calcification of the main renal arteries and the branching intrarenal arteries.

Table 1–3. Radiographic Features of Conduit Calcification

1. Annular density en face
2. Tracklike parallel lines in profile
3. Thin vessel may have single line of calcification
4. Discontinuous calcification
5. Irregular margins of calcification
6. Borders may be indistinct
7. No internal calcification
8. Confined to anatomic structures
9. One wall calcification oriented along course of vessel

pearance will be noted (Fig. 1–16). In female pelves, horizontal, slightly undulating lines of density often represent uterine artery calcification.

However, conduit wall calcification is not always so obvious. When there is only a single fleck of calcification, differentiation from a small calculus or from cortical bone can be difficult. This is especially true when it occurs in the region of the renal pelvis. Often the question arises whether a linear density signifies calcification of the renal artery (Fig. 1–17, *A*) or the lateral margin of a vertebral transverse process (Fig. 1–17, *B*). Since calcification within the vessel wall is not homogeneous, the margins of a focal density may be irregular and the border may be indistinct. Also, conduit wall calcifications are found close to the expected location of a vessel. Hence, it would be very unusual for conduit calcifications to be located at the lateral margins of the liver or spleen or in other peripheral locations.

Cyst Wall Calcification (Table 1–4)

For this discussion, a cyst will be considered to be any abnormal fluid-filled mass. Included in this category are the epithelial-lined true cysts, pseudocysts which have a fibrous integument, and spherical and ovoid aneurysms. Although cysts are of various types with different histologic appearances and etiologies, they share, when calcified, common radiographic features that permit diagnosis on plain films. Of all the morphological categories, cyst wall calcification is the least variable and the easiest to recognize. Critical for cyst pattern recognition is the presence of a smooth curvilinear rim of calcification (Fig. 1–18). Very small cysts rarely calcify so that, when roentgenographically visible, cysts have a diameter larger than any nearby conduit. While arcuate linear radiopacities are seen in both conduits and cyst wall calcification, the calcific rim of a cyst usually has a larger diameter than that of a conduit. Yet, the calcific rim need not be complete. At times, only a portion of the wall may be radiodense (Fig. 1–19). This is in sharp distinction to concretions, where a complete rim of calcification is a hallmark. Moreover, since cysts usually have only one encircling wall, they are rarely laminated. An incompletely calcified single rim clearly indicates the presence of a cystic density, rather than a concretion.

Cysts are not always exquisitely round. They may be oval or compressed on one side and appear asymmetric (Fig. 1–20). The shape of a cyst depends in great measure on its location. Cysts can distort and displace organs or vessels, or they can be limited by adjacent solid structures. Most cysts present only with rim calcification. Occasionally there appears to be central calcification (Fig. 1–21), occurring when calcium deposition is so extensive that even surfaces which are not tangential to the x-ray beam are sufficiently dense to be visible. In such an instance, the "interior" of a heav-

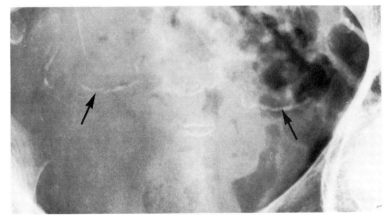

Figure 1–16. Bilateral uterine artery calcification (arrows). The lines of radiopacity represent calcification in these narrow vessels as they traverse the broad ligament.

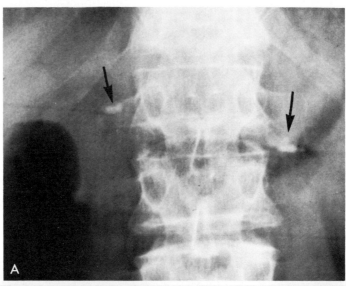

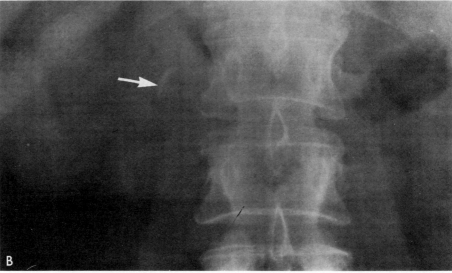

Figure 1–17. *A,* Bilateral focal renal artery calcification (arrows). Observe the horizontal orientation in the flecks of calcification in both arteries. *B,* A single linear density directed vertically cannot be a renal artery because of its orientation (arrow). In patients with bony demineralization, the ossified margin of a vertebral transverse process can be mistaken for arterial calcification.

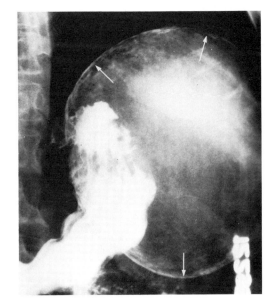

Figure 1–18. A large splenic cyst in a patient with barium in the stomach. The arrows point to its smooth outer margins.

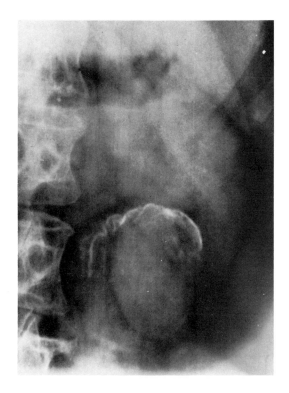

Figure 1–19. Calcified mesenteric cyst. Only a part of the cyst wall is calcified. Occasionally sections of a cyst wall may be noncurvilinear.

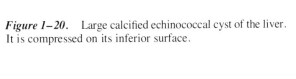

Figure 1–20. Large calcified echinococcal cyst of the liver. It is compressed on its inferior surface.

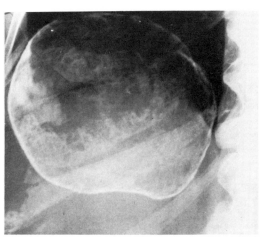

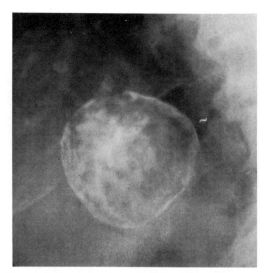

Figure 1–21. Heavily calcified hepatic echinococcal cyst with curvilinear opacities at the margin and poorly defined central calcification.

ily calcified cyst has an indistinct, smudgy appearance, less radiopaque than the wall.

Sometimes it is difficult to differentiate calcification in cyst walls from that in solid masses. The outer surface of a cyst is usually smooth, whereas the transition between the inner surface of a calcific rim and the liquid material contained within it may be indistinct and roughened. In solid mass calcification the outer margin of opacity is often ill-defined. In general, the calcific rim of cysts is well-demarcated and arcuate, while in solid densities, curvilinear calcification is usually irregular. However, occasionally leiomyoma of the uterus will have smooth linear calcification at its margin and may simulate cystic calcification.

The cystic pattern of calcification can be found anywhere in the abdomen. A peripheral density is unlikely to be a concretion or conduit. However, this restriction does not apply to cysts. The most common abnormalities with the radiographic appearance of the cystic type are aneurysms of the abdominal aorta and of the splenic artery, both seen frequently in the elderly. Aortic aneurysm is often associated with conduit calcification in the contiguous aorta and iliac vessels (Fig. 1–22). Splenic

Table 1–4. Radiographic Features of Cyst Calcification

1. Curvilinear calcification defining wall
2. Rim calcification may be discontinuous
3. Absence of laminations
4. Interior calcifications less dense than marginal calcifications
5. Cyst may occur anywhere in the abdomen

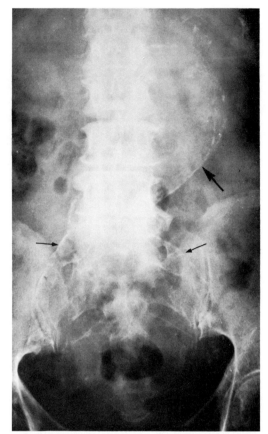

Figure 1–22. The curvilinear calcification (large arrow) is in the wall of an aortic aneurysm. Smaller arrows indicate calcification extending into the common iliac arteries.

artery aneurysms frequently occur in conjunction with calcification in adjacent portions of the splenic artery (Fig. 1–23). Cystic calcifications related to the genitourinary tract include renal cysts (about 5 percent calcify), renal artery and intrarenal aneurysms, echinococcal cysts, old perirenal hematomas, multicystic kidney (occasionally calcify in adults), parapelvic cysts, and adrenal cysts. On occasion, solid neoplasms (most often benign adenoma) of the kidney and adrenal show calcification simulating that of cyst walls. In North America calcified splenic and hepatic cysts are much less frequent than calcified renal cysts, whereas in other parts of the world (e.g., the Mediterranean Basin and the Middle East) calcified cysts of the spleen and liver are common because of the high incidence of echinococcus infestation. Retroperitoneal tumors such as pheochromocytomas may assume a cystic appearance. In the lower abdomen, calcified cysts are more rare. Some of the entities found in this location are calcified mesenteric cysts, calci-

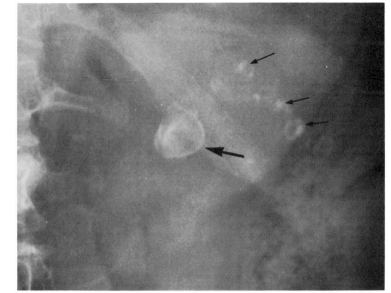

Figure 1–23. The large arrow points to a small splenic artery aneurysm. The smaller arrows are directed to calcifications in nondilated portions of the artery. Coincident conduit calcification elsewhere in this vessel makes splenic artery aneurysm a strong diagnostic consideration.

fied mucoceles of the appendix, and calcified benign cystic lesions in the ovary.

Solid Mass Calcification (Table 1–5)

The fourth category, solid mass calcification, is the most diverse in terms of radiologic appearance, yet in almost all cases can be identified by an irregular calcified border and a complex inner architecture. Solid masses may appear as mottled densi-

ties, with scattered radiolucencies within a calcified background. Calcified lymph nodes often present in this way (Fig. 1–24). A whorled pattern with incomplete bands and arcs of calcification around ill-defined lucent foci is frequently seen in uterine leiomyoma (Fig. 1–25). Irregular streaks and flecks of radiodensity may occupy the substance of a mass (Fig. 1–26). Another common pattern is flocculent calcification superimposed on a lucent background (Fig. 1–27). No matter how dissimilar the interior pattern, solid calcifications share this unifying fea-

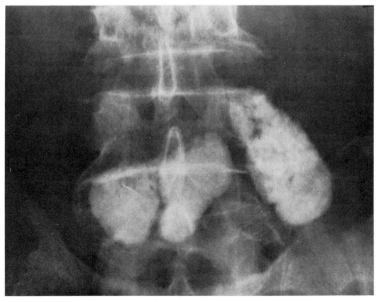

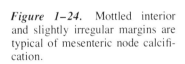

Figure 1–24. Mottled interior and slightly irregular margins are typical of mesenteric node calcification.

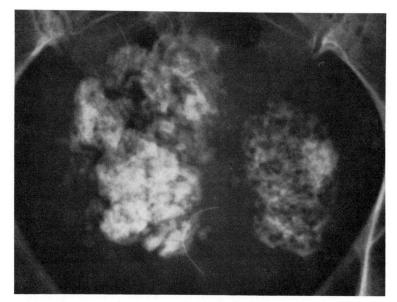

Figure 1–25. Two uterine leiomyomas in the pelvis show ill-defined calcification admixed with irregular lucencies.

Figure 1–26. A leiomyoma of the uterus. There is dense flocculation of calcium in the mass.

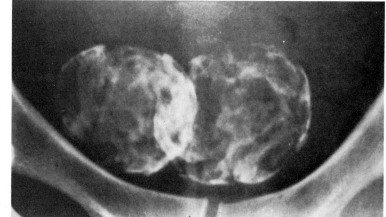

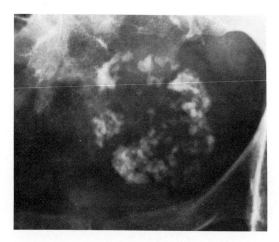

Figure 1–27. Two pelvic leiomyomas with both marginal curvilinear calcification and dense internal streaks and plaques.

Table 1–5. Features of Solid Calcification

1. Extensive interior calcification
2. Varied internal pattern
   a. Speckled
   b. Mottled
   c. Whorled
   d. Streaky
3. Ill-defined irregular external border
4. May occur anywhere in the abdomen
5. May be of any size

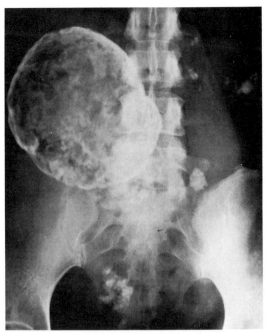

Figure 1–28. Multiple leiomyomas. Scattered foci of flocculent calcification in the pelvis and left upper quadrant. In the right upper quadrant there is a large calcific density resembling a cyst but the marginal calcification is slightly irregular and the interior is very radiodense.

ture: the inner architecture is nongeometric. There is no monotony or regularity in the distribution of calcium deposition detectable on plain films of the abdomen. In most instances, the interior calcification is more prominent than the marginal calcification. Frequently, the calcification does not extend to the edge of the mass, and the outer aspect of solid mass densities may be discontinuous, making the contours of calcium deposition irregular. At times, the mass contains separate islands of amorphous calcification (Fig. 1–28). Occasionally, the border of a solid mass is more densely calcified than the interior. While this appearance resembles cystic calcification, the margins are rarely smoothly curvilinear; rather they may appear crenated or slightly angulated.

Like cysts, solid masses can appear anywhere in the abdomen. They may be central or peripheral, adjacent to or within organs, in the retroperitoneal or intraperitoneal spaces. Most common are calcified mesenteric lymph nodes, which can occur anywhere along a broad arc extending from the left upper quadrant to the right lower quadrant of the abdomen along the course of the small bowel mesentery. They can be multiple and of varied sizes. Tuberculous infection has been invoked as the cause of these calcifications, but in the majority there is no other evidence of intra-abdominal granulomatous infection.

In women, the most frequent calcified solid mass in the pelvis is uterine leiomyoma. They are often multiple and may attain great size. They need not be confined to the pelvis, but can be seen almost anywhere in the abdomen. Usually, leiomyomas have a whorled type of calcification, but occasionally a prominent bordering rim of calcification may be seen. Solid mass calcification can occur in renal malignancies, adenomas, and hamartomas. Tuberculous and chronic abscesses in the kidney may also calcify. Calcification in the substance of the spleen is uncommon and pancreatic mass calcifications are very rare. More frequent, but still distinctly uncommon, are calcified metastatic deposits in the liver. Benign and primary malignant hepatic neoplasms with calcified foci are rare, as

are tumors in the hollow organs of the genitourinary tract. Occasionally, adrenal adenomas or carcinomas may present as a calcified mass. Uncommonly, other solid retroperitoneal tumors are calcified.

Psammomatous calcification is a type of solid calcification that is so distinctive that it merits separate consideration. Psammoma bodies are small calcified concretions that occur intracellularly within the substance of ovarian serous cystadenocarcinomas. Because individual calcifications are microscopic, they cannot be appreciated as distinct entities on a radiograph. Only masses of psammoma bodies, if sufficiently calcified and numerous, can be detected. When faint, psammomatous calcification is seen as a poorly localized, finely granular pattern. However, when dense, the calcification may be so intense that other structures will be obliterated if they are overlain by the mass. Psammomatous calcification appears as a cloudlike conglomeration without internal lucency or distinct borders (Fig. 1–29). It may occur in the primary lesion or in metastatic deposits in the peritoneal cavity, the liver, and retroperitoneal lymph nodes. Carcinoma of the stomach, colon, gallbladder, or liver may present with amorphous calcification on

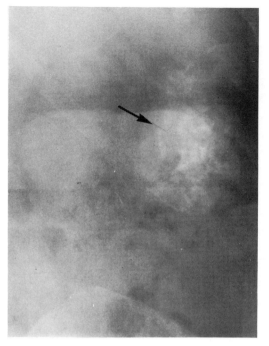

Figure 1–29. Psammomatous calcification. A film of the left lateral abdomen reveals a poorly defined area of increased density (arrow) representing an intraperitoneal metastasis from ovarian serous cystadenocarcinoma. Psammomatous calcification can easily be missed if not carefully looked for.

long thin strands of radiodensity oriented along a straight line or smooth arc. Parallel trabeculae are usually of equal width, as contrasted with the varying width and direction of solid mass calcifications. If a cortex which has a thickened rim with smooth external and internal margins can be recognized, the presence of bone is established (Fig. 1–30). Dermoid cysts in the ovary are common pelvic masses in young females. Many times calcified teeth are observable within the lesion (Fig. 1–31). Generally, there is no difficulty in differentiating between a calculus in the distal ureter and a tooth in a dermoid cyst. Sometimes, however, the two densities may resemble each other and proper identification can rest on the relationship of the calcification to an accompanying mass. Teeth are present within or at the margins of the dermoid cyst while stones will either be unassociated with a soft tissue mass or deviated away from it.

Occasionally there are calcifications with appearances reflecting the characteristics of more than one morphological type. Calcification in the wall of the gallbladder is not rare (Fig. 1–32); occasionally it may look like a single large gallstone. However, gallbladder wall calcification usually has a dense rim of variable width and may be discontinuously radiopaque, while large gallstones almost always calcify uninterruptedly throughout their perimeter. Sometimes it is not clear if a group of cal-

plain radiographs which is indistinguishable from psammomatous calcification. However, in these malignancies, the calcification is found in extracellular mucin formed by the tumor and also in sites of hemorrhage and necrosis.

Caveats

The classification of abdominal calcifications according to radiographic morphology can help in the analysis of an unknown opacity. However, there are several limitations that need to be emphasized. When a calcification is very small, it is difficult, if not impossible, to categorize. If it is too minute to have an inner pattern or definable contour, morphological analysis is not feasible. For example, a single fleck of calcification could represent a small stone, a segment of an artery, a section of the wall of a cyst, or a part of a solid lesion. Similarly, very faint calcification cannot be classified if no information about margins or center can be ascertained.

The distinction between solid mass calcification and ossification may sometimes be difficult. Ossified structures contain trabeculae, which appear as

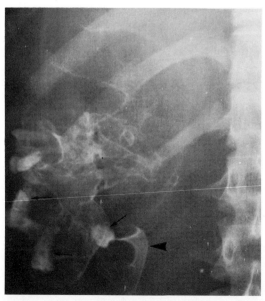

Figure 1–30. Retroperitoneal teratoma. Plain film of the abdomen reveals a complex density in the right midabdomen. Teeth are present (small arrows) along with bone (arrowhead). (Courtesy of Dr. C. Y. Park, Seoul, Korea.)

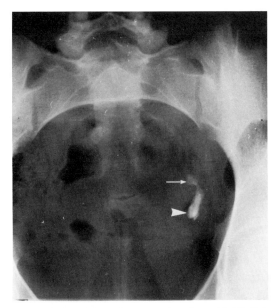

Figure 1–31. Teeth in an ovarian dermoid. Well-defined tooth in the left pelvis consists of crown (arrowhead) and root (small arrow).

cific densities consist of multiple stones or a large mass. Pancreatic stones are often dissimilar in size and configuration. They can appear to extend diffusely without evidence of placement within a closed space even though they are within pancreatic ducts (Fig. 1–33). In contrast, in a typical collection of gallstones, there is no confusion with solid mass calcification because the calculi are similar in size and shape and are seen to be clearly delineated within a hollow structure (Fig. 1–34). Some solid masses may have only marginal calcifications and thus may look exactly like cysts (Fig. 1–35). While these examples point out the possible pitfalls apparent in this classification scheme, in most cases it is still possible to ascribe a specific abdominal calcification to one of the four major categories with a reasonable measure of assurance.

LOCATION

Evaluation of morphology is the first step in the quest for the identity of an abdominal radiopacity. Diagnostic inferences can also be drawn from a consideration of the location of a calcification. Vascular calcifications occur in highly predictable positions. Other radiodensities may also be found in only a limited number of sites. Still others, such as lymph node calcification, can be seen in many abdominal locations. Thus, a knowledge of the common calcifications which occur in various re-

gions in the abdomen is helpful in determining the nature of the radiodensities seen on plain radiographs. In this discussion, the abdomen is divided into four quadrants with the upper quadrants located above a line drawn through the middle of the body of L3. Pelvic calcifications and calcifications that cross the midline are considered as separate categories.

Right Upper Quadrant

Most calcifications that occur in the right upper quadrant are related to either the gallbladder or the right kidney. Only 10 percent of gallstones calcify, but since the incidence of cholelithiasis is high, calcified gallstones are seen frequently. Often they are multiple, and occasionally they are laminated. Calcification of the gallbladder wall is seen infrequently, and choledochal or hepatic calcifications are distinctly uncommon. Renal and adrenal calcifications are often encountered in the right upper quadrant. Occasionally right renal artery calcification is noted, and, less often, calcification in renal

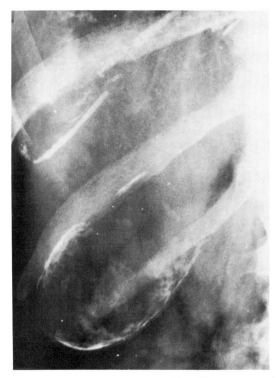

Figure 1–32. Calcified gallbladder. The presence of discontinuous linear calcifications describing an ovoid or pear-shaped mass is characteristic of the calcified gallbladder on plain films.

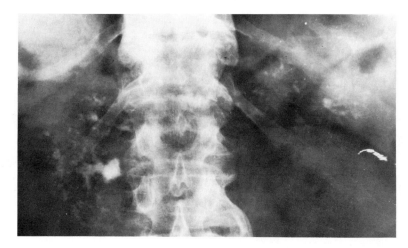

Figure 1–33. Diffuse pancreatic calcification. The intraductal calculi are of varying size, shape, and density.

Figure 1–34. Multiple gallstones. Innumerable stones of similar size. These closely packed calculi appear to be located within a single hollow viscus.

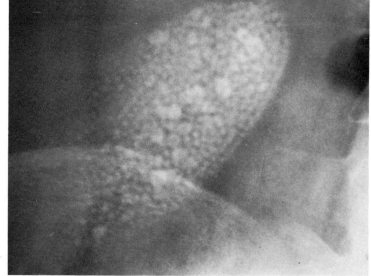

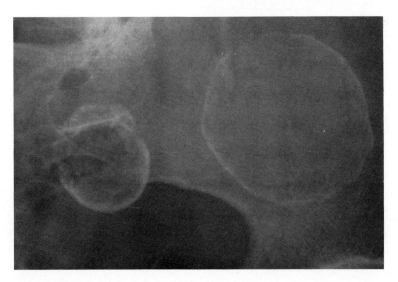

Figure 1–35. Two pelvic leiomyomas. The thin margin of calcification, the round configuration, and the minimal internal opacities make these solid lesions indistinguishable from calcified cysts on plain films.

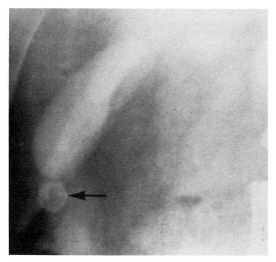

Figure 1–36. A plain film from an oral cholecysto-gram reveals a normal gallbladder and a calculus (arrow) adjacent to the fundus of the gallbladder. At operation a retrocecal appendix containing an appendicolith was found.

masses can be seen. Calcification in the parenchyma of the right adrenal gland and in cystic tumors of that organ occur less commonly. Also calcification may be confined to the pancreatic head and will be observed near the midline in the right upper quadrant. Appendicoliths in retrocecal appendices may present in the right upper quadrant, and may even abut on the gallbladder (Fig. 1–36).

Left Upper Quadrant

Renal and adrenal calcifications occur with equal incidence in both sides of the abdomen. Pancreatic

calculi can extend into the left upper quadrant, but other types of calcifications in the pancreas are rare. Splenic artery and aortic calcifications are frequent, and left renal artery calcification is occasionally encountered. Calcification of the substance of the spleen is uncommon, but is often observed in patients residing in the Ohio valley and other regions where histoplasmosis is endemic. Multiple punctate calcifications in the spleen, especially in patients from affected areas, suggest histoplasmosis infection, but they may also occur in tuberculosis.

Mesenteric lymph node calcification can be found in the left upper quadrant, but this is an unusual site for nodal calcifications. In both upper quadrants, costocartilage calcification may simulate intra-abdominal radiodensities. They may be annular like concretions (Fig. 1–37), have a tracklike appearance suggestive of conduit calcifications (Fig. 1–38), or they may be speckled and nodular like solid calcifications. Costocartilage calcifications move with the ribs in different projections and will change their location relative to the lumbar spine during respiration. Consequently, oblique as well as inspiratory and expiratory films are helpful in determining whether upper quadrant opacities are in the abdomen or attached to ribs.

Right Lower Quadrant

Ureteral calculi are common in the medial aspect of the right lower quadrant. This is also a favored location for calcified mesenteric nodes. Lymph nodes are generally larger than ureteral stones and have a mottled appearance. Appendicoliths are most often observed near the cecal gas shadow in the right lower quadrant. However, their

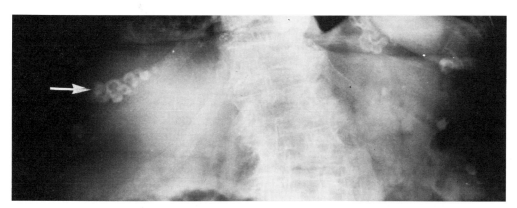

Figure 1–37. Bilateral costal cartilage calcifications. They conform to the shape of the anterior ribs. On the right, multiple costal calcifications resemble gallstones (arrow).

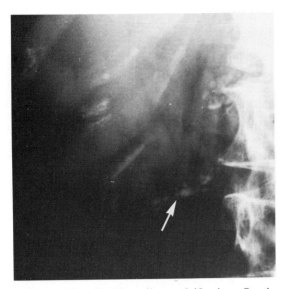

Figure 1–38. Costal cartilage calcification. On the right, the orientation and linear pattern (arrow) resemble those of vascular calcification in the right renal artery.

location is variable, depending on the position of the cecum and the length and direction of the appendix. Patients with enlarged livers may have calcified gallstones in gallbladders located in the right lower quadrant. Leiomyomas of the uterus may extend into this area as well.

Left Lower Quadrant

Among the abdominal regions, the left lower quadrant is least likely to contain calcific densities. Ureteral calculi may be located in the medial aspect of this region. Aortic calcification can be seen frequently in the left lower quadrant, as can calcifications in the common iliac arteries. Calcified aneurysms also extend into the area. Mesenteric nodes are seen in the left lower quadrant much less frequently than in the right lower quadrant. Leiomyomas in the uterus can also extend from the pelvis into the left lower quadrant. In general, aside from ureteral stones, vascular densities, and leiomyomas, left lower quadrant calcifications are unusual.

Calcifications That Cross the Midline

A number of calcifications cross the midline. In the upper quadrants, pancreatic calculi can be seen extending from the right of the lumbar spine to the splenic hilus. Aortic calcifications can occur on both sides of the lumbar vertebrae. The uncoiled, elongated aorta occasionally occupies a right paramedial location. Calcified tumors that grow out of the pelvis often cross the midline. A predominant member of this group is uterine leiomyoma.

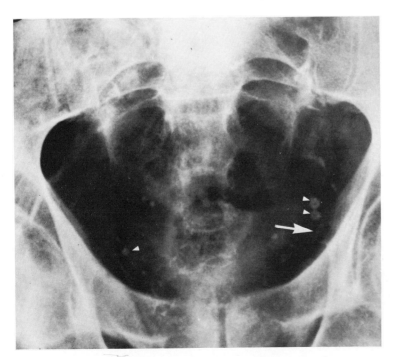

Figure 1–39. Multiple phleboliths on both sides of the pelvis (arrowheads). They extend obliquely inferiorly from just above the ischial spines (arrow).

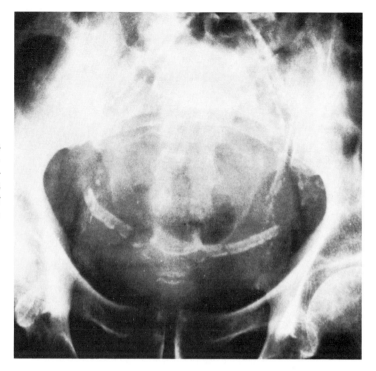

Figure 1–40. Bilateral vas deferens calcification. These conduit calcifications are similar to calcification in arteries but the course of the vas in the pelvis is more horizontal than that of the nearby internal pudendal and obturator arteries.

Pelvis

Phleboliths are by far the most common calcification in the pelvis. They can be seen at any site in the pelvis, but a characteristic location is just lateral to the lower part of the sacrum at or below the level of the ischial spine (Fig. 1–39). Phleboliths may be mistaken for distal ureteral calculi, but they can usually be differentiated by their central lucency and their curvilinear margins. Also, phleboliths are relatively fixed while ureteral calculi may move on successive films. In the elderly, arterial calcifications of the external iliac arteries and the proximal portion of the hypogastric arteries and their branches are often noted. Appendicoliths occasionally appear on the right side of the pelvis. In the center of the pelvis are found vesical calculi; these are often solitary, large, and laminated calcifications.

Prostatic calcifications most often appear as clusters of small fixed calculi in the midline at the level of the symphysis pubis. Occasionally, prostatic calculi may be large and multiple. In prostatic hypertrophy, the calcifications can extend above the symphysis. Calcifications in the walls of the vas deferens usually present as parallel lines of radiodensity coursing in either a horizontal or oblique direction from the midline just above the symphysis pubis (Fig. 1–40).

Calcifications in dermoid cysts can be seen in women of any age, but are primarily noted in young adults. A characteristic finding is a radiopacity in the form of a tooth which occurs within a relatively radiolucent and smoothly defined mass, located anywhere in the pelvis. Calcification in uterine leiomyomas, seen with increasing frequency after the fourth decade, most commonly presents with a mottled type of calcification, but infrequently a roughly curvilinear rim calcification is seen. Psammomatous calcification in the female pelvis strongly suggests serous cystadenocarcinoma of the ovary (Fig. 1–41). Occasionally, noncystic ovarian neoplasms show irregular calcification of the solid mass type.

MOBILITY

The movement of abdominal radiopacities, either during one examination or over a period of time, provides additional information and can lead to a plain film diagnosis. Gravity, respiration, peristaltic activity, and the growth of masses can all cause changes in the position of abdominal densities. An aid in the detection of calculi within a fluid medium is the recognition of layering in an upright position (Fig. 1–42). With the x-ray beam directed horizontally, stratification of freely moving calcified concretions in a liquid medium can be observed. This is most often noted with gallbladder stones and calculi in hydronephrotic sacs. Very striking is the layering in milk of calcium, also most

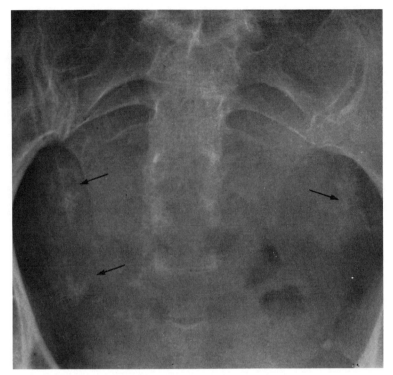

Figure 1–41. Multiple faint, poorly defined densities (arrows) in the pelvis in a patient with a pelvic mass and ascites. The densities represent psammomatous calcifications in serous cystadenocarcinoma.

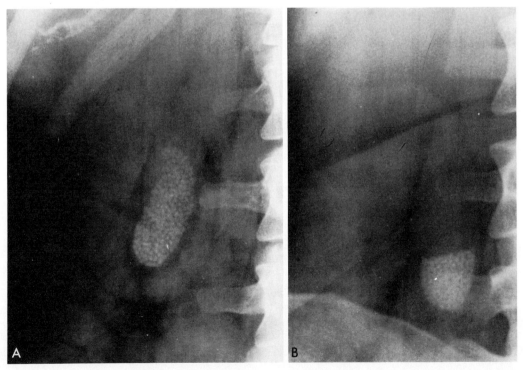

Figure 1–42. Supine *A* and upright *B* views of the abdomen in a patient with gallstones. Note the change in appearance when the patient is placed erect. The calculi sink to the fundus of the gallbladder.

common in the gallbladder, but milk of calcium may be found in other hollow structures in the abdomen.

Radiopacities that are free in the peritoneal cavity demonstrate great mobility. These are rare, but their marked change in position on sequential films permits recognition. Mesenteric calcifications also exhibit movement but to a lesser extent than free intraperitoneal densities. However, calcifications in fixed solid organs do not move. Calcifications within fluid-filled structures, such as the lumen of the gastrointestinal tract, the pelvicalyceal system or cysts, may also move.

Effect of Respiration

Alterations in position with respiration may help to distinguish retroperitoneal densities from intra-peritoneal masses. Retroperitoneal calcifications are usually fixed and do not change significantly with phase of respiration. Intraperitoneal calcifications, especially in the upper abdomen, may be displaced by the excursion of the diaphragm. Also, costal cartilage and soft tissue calcifications in the upper abdomen move with the ribs and thus will be at different locations in inspiration and expiration.

Effect of Peristalsis

The migration of urinary calculi on successive examinations is frequently observed. This is due to propulsion toward the bladder by ureteral contractions and the flow of urine. Similarly, peristaltic activity in the intestinal tract can cause movement of intraluminal densities (Fig. 1–43).

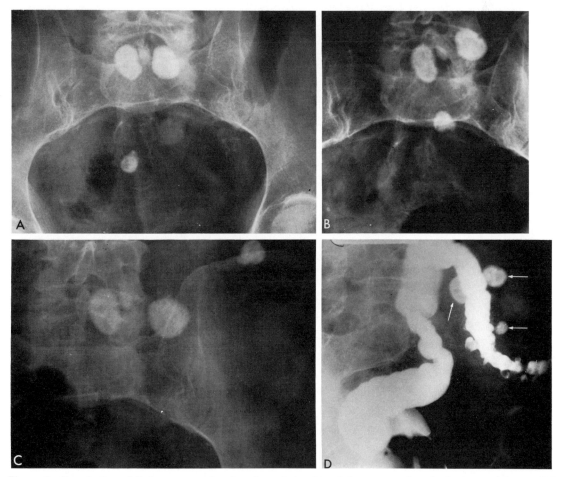

Figure 1–43. A, B, and C demonstrate the changing relationship of three concretions in the lower abdomen. B is three days after A, and C is three years later. Not only do the densities move in respect to fixed structures such as the sacrum, but the spatial relationships of each to the others also change. D is a film from a barium enema which reveals that all calculi are within diverticula in the sigmoid on a long mesentery (arrows). Peristalsis in the sigmoid continually changes the position of the stones.

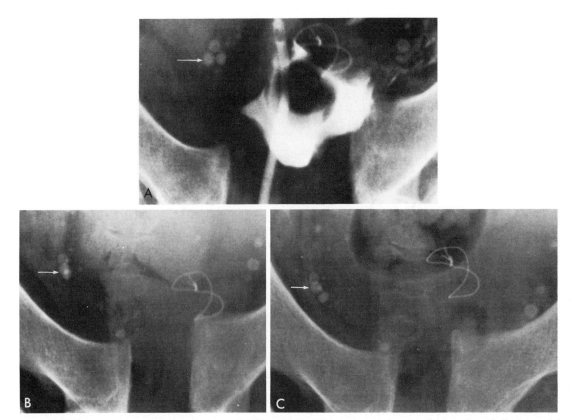

Figure 1–44. The phlebolith displacement sign. *A*, Three phleboliths (arrow) are displaced medially by a right pelvic hematoma, secondary to trauma. Note the diastasis of the symphysis pubis. In *B*, three weeks later, the hematoma is resolving and the phleboliths migrate laterally. Also, the phleboliths are now arrayed linearly. *C*, three weeks later the hematoma has fully resolved and the phleboliths have returned to their normal position.

Growth of Masses

The growth of calcium-containing masses can be evaluated by the change in position of calcification on serial radiographic studies. The size of aortic aneurysms can be ascertained by the separation of calcifications in the anterior wall of the vessel from the vertebral body on lateral films. Any increase in this distance suggests enlargement of the aneurysm. The growth of noncalcified masses may be evaluated by displacement of adjacent fixed calcific densities. Phleboliths will move very little in the pelvis, except when pushed by an adjacent mass. The "phlebolith displacement" sign is a neglected but a valuable aid in the detection of enlarging pelvic masses and cysts (Fig. 1–44).[4]

Finally, the mobility of abdominal calcification may be the result of processes not fully explainable by the effects of gravity, respiration, peristalsis, or local enlargement. Gallstone ileus is an intestinal obstruction caused by a gallbladder calculus that has eroded through the gallbladder wall usually to the duodenum and then progressed through the lumen of the small bowel only to be restricted by the caliber of the terminal ileum, or by narrowings in the large intestine. The initial observation of a right upper quadrant calculus and the later demonstration of the same calculus in the pelvis and left lower quadrant point to this possibility. The associated radiographic findings of air in the biliary tree and small bowel obstruction assure the diagnosis.

CONCLUSION

An abdominal calcification can often be identified after an evaluation of its morphology, location, and mobility. This approach is advantageous because it allows a determination to be made from the information provided from plain films alone. At the very least, close inspection of the characteristics of an abdominal radiodensity will narrow the diagnostic possibilities considerably and will direct further workup to the appropriate confirming studies. In the chapters that follow, specific radiographic entities will be discussed with reference to the analytical framework offered in this chapter.

REFERENCES

1. Hilbish TF, Bartter FC: Roentgen findings in abnormal deposition of calcium in tissues. Am J Roentgenol 87:1128–1129, 1962.

2. Kuturna P: A contribution to the problem of calcifications in malignant tumors: a case of late calcified retroperitoneal metastasis of an ovarian carcinoma. Neoplasma 11:633–642, 1964.

3. Widmann BF, Ostrum AW, Fried H: Practical aspects of calcification and ossification in the various body tissues. Radiology 30:598–609, 1938.

4. Steinbach HL: Identification of pelvic masses by phlebolith displacement. Am J Roentgenol 83:1063–1066, 1960.

Chapter 2

CALCIFICATION IN THE URINARY TRACT

Milton Elkin, M.D.

CONCRETIONS

Inasmuch as the urinary tract is a system of fluid-filled tubes subject to wide variations in pH and chemical content, it is not surprising that urinary calculi are common. Concretions can form in tubules within the renal parenchyma or more commonly in the larger lumina of the collecting systems. They can form in tubes of normal size and shape as well as in abnormal lumina.

In Normal Lumina

Among the factors predisposing to the formation of calculi, most important is hypercalcemia and hypercalciuria, as may be present with hyperparathyroidism, renal tubular acidosis, bone dissolution secondary to immobilization or widespread metastases, excessive ingestion and absorption of calcium from the gastrointestinal tract, and idiopathic hypercalciuria. Increased urinary excretion of oxalic acid promotes the formation of calcium oxalate stones. Uric acid stones are associated with hyperuricosemia and hyperuricosuria. Cystine stones result from hypercystinuria.

The pH of the urine is also important, alkaline urine promoting the precipitation of triple phosphate stones, and acid urine, uric acid stones. Stasis of the urine in an obstructed lumen or puddling in an abnormal lumen promotes the formation of stones. Urinary infections also predispose to calculi formation, probably related to changes in pH.

In the United States, urinary calculi consist most commonly of calcium oxalate. These are usually homogeneously dense and sharply outlined. Next in frequency are the triple phosphate stones (am-

monium, magnesium phosphate), less dense than calcium oxalate and occurring often in infected urine of alkaline pH. Uric acid stones, having the same radiodensity as surrounding soft tissue, cannot be visualized on the abdominal radiograph. Cystine, containing two atoms of sulfur, with its relatively high atomic number, is more radiodense than soft tissues, and thus cystine stones are visualized on abdominal radiographs as faint opacities.

Inasmuch as the growth and configuration of calculi are accommodated to the size and shape of the lumen, urinary concretions vary greatly in size and shape. Concretions in the collecting ducts are initially minute and rounded, later with growth assuming the linear shape of the duct, and then increasing in overall size with dilatation of the lumina and destruction of the enveloping tissues. In the large lumen of the urinary bladder a single calculus can reach very large size and maintain a spherical shape to conform to that of the bladder lumen (Fig. 2–1); or there may be multiple vesical calculi (Fig. 2–2), each maintaining a spherical shape or sometimes being faceted.

Sometimes specific shapes betray the nature of a calculus. The staghorn calculus, a triple phosphate stone, makes a cast of the pelvicalyceal system and is easily diagnosable on the abdominal radiograph (Fig. 2–3). On occasion a urinary calculus carries the distinctive shape of a calyx or of the renal pelvis in which it grew (Fig. 2–4). The triangular-shaped extruded necrotic papilla of renal papillary necrosis, when calcified, appears on the abdominal radiograph as a rim of calcific density, often with a shape distinctive enough to indicate the diagnosis. The stellate calculus occurs, for practical purposes, only in the urinary bladder, although it is by no means the most common shape for a vesical

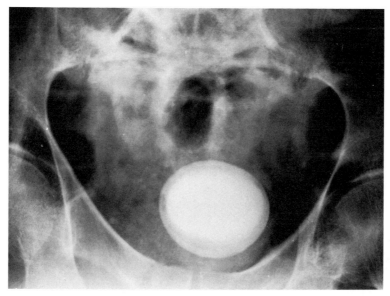

Figure 2–1. Large spherical vesical calculus. The dense center is most likely calcium oxalate and the less dense rim triple phosphate.

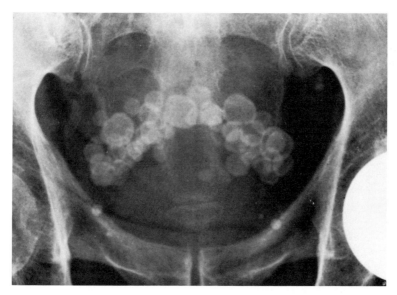

Figure 2–2. Multiple vesical calculi, the unusual configuration of the collection being due to an enlarged prostate.

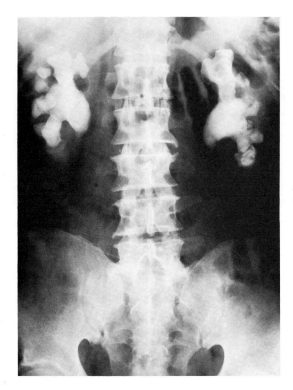

Figure 2–3. Bilateral staghorn calculi, of distinctive shape.

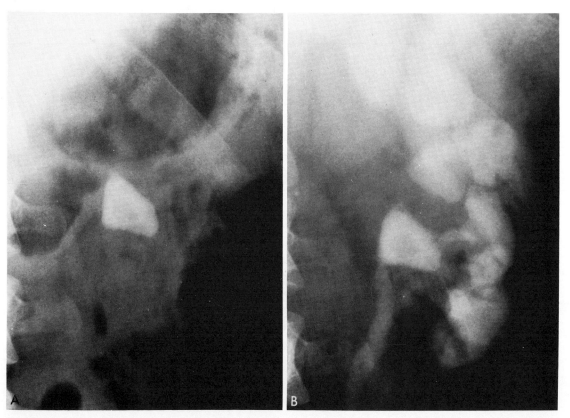

Figure 2–4. Triangular-shaped renal calculus, with a lucent center, the shape reflecting that of the renal pelvis in which the calculus formed. *A,* Scout radiograph. *B,* Intravenous urogram.

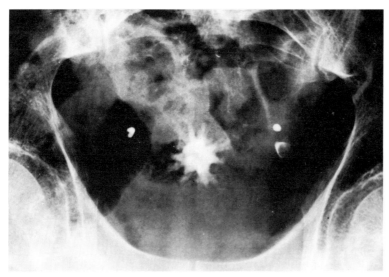

Figure 2–5. Stellate calculus in the urinary bladder. The three smaller opacities of metallic density represent barium in sigmoid diverticula.

calculus (Fig. 2–5). The dumbbell-shaped calculus occurs in the urinary bladder, with the waist of the dumbbell at the bladder outlet, the cephalad expanded portion at the bladder base, and the caudal expanded portion in the postprostatectomy urethral fossa (Fig. 2–6). A similarly shaped dumbbell calculus can form at the neck of a vesical diverticulum.

In Abnormal Lumina

Pyelogenic cyst (calyceal diverticulum), maintaining a communication with the pelvicalyceal system via a narrow isthmus, often contains concretions. There may be a single calculus occupying most of the lumen or there may be several small calculi (Fig. 2–7). Most distinctive is milk of cal-

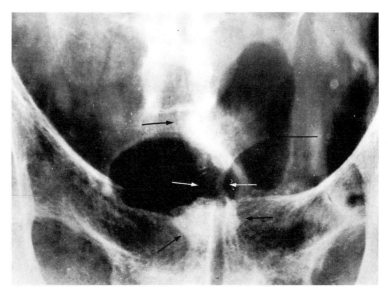

Figure 2–6. Dumbbell-shaped calculus at the bladder outlet. A 79-year-old man, who had had a prostatectomy in the past, now has hematuria. The white arrows point to the waist of the calculus and the black arrows to its expanded ends.

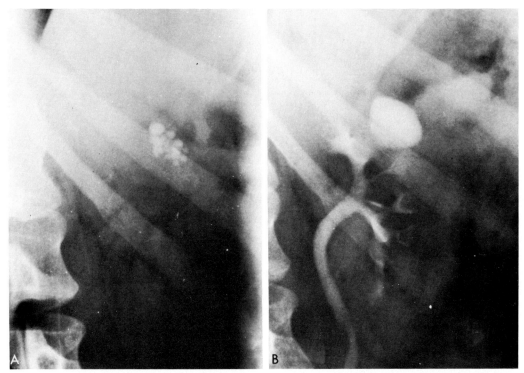

Figure 2–7. Calculi in a pyelogenic cyst. *A,* Scout radiograph shows a collection of concretions, in an oval configuration, at the upper pole of the left kidney. *B,* Urogram demonstrates that the calculi lie in a pyelogenic cyst.

cium, consisting of a colloidal suspension of calcific granules so small that they appear as a finely granular opaque cloud on the abdominal radiograph. The granules layer out dependently and are thus easily diagnosable by horizontal beam radiography with proper positioning of the patient (Fig. 2–8), the density maintaining a constant position within the kidney.[1] Reports of the chemical composition of the granules include calcium carbonate, calcium hydroxylapatite, calcium oxalate, calcium phosphate, and ammonium phosphate with calcium phosphate.[2]

Less commonly, concretions, including milk of calcium, occur in other types of renal cysts, communicating or noncommunicating, such as simple cyst or a cyst of the adult type polycystic kidney.[3] Similarly the cystic spaces of a hydrocalycosis (Fig. 2–9) or marked hydronephrosis, such as secondary to ureteropelvic junction obstruction, can contain calculi of various sizes, including milk of calcium.[2] In hydronephrosis and in large cysts there can be innumerable small calculi, usually spherical in shape and of uniform size, distinguishable on the abdominal radiograph as discrete concretions, referred to as seed calculi (Fig. 2–10). Milk of calcium has also been reported in the ureter.[4]

In medullary sponge kidney, the ectatic collecting ducts and associated small cysts communicating with these ducts form abnormal lumina in which concretions commonly form. Initially the calculi are small, rounded or sometimes linear in shape and located in the region of the pyramids; the appearance is that of a nephrocalcinosis, with the underlying anatomic abnormality becoming obvious on urography with demonstration of the dilated collecting ducts (Fig. 2–11). Later the concretions can become large and ulcerate into the pelvicalyceal system, obliterating the early distinctive plain film appearance.

Urinary tract diverticula, most frequently of the bladder and female urethra, are common sites for calculi formation. The urethral diverticula are often paired; a single concretion or collections of concretions on either side or both sides of the site of the urethra at the level of the symphysis pubis allow a diagnosis on the abdominal radiograph. Large urethral diverticula may contain seed calculi (Fig. 2–12). In a bladder diverticulum the concretion is most often single, projecting on the abdominal radiograph outside the limits of the soft-tissue density of the bladder (Fig. 2–13).

A calculus or calculi may form or lodge within

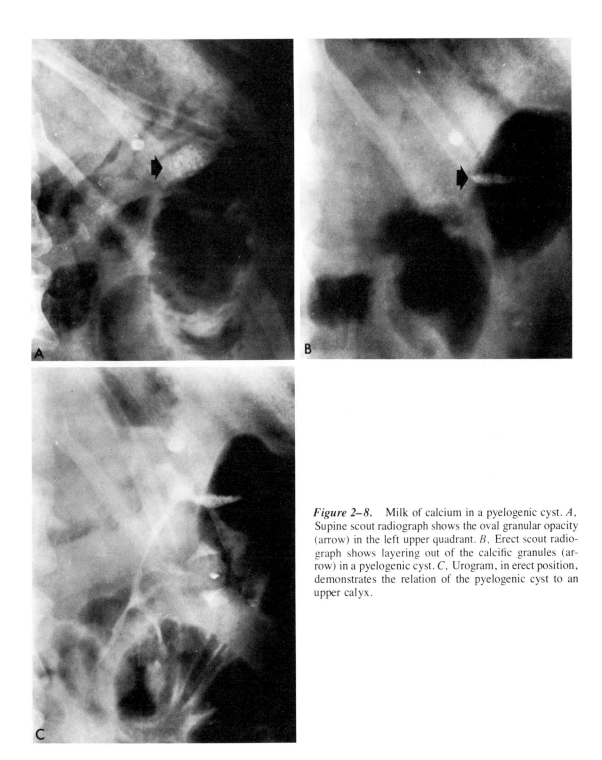

Figure 2–8. Milk of calcium in a pyelogenic cyst. *A*, Supine scout radiograph shows the oval granular opacity (arrow) in the left upper quadrant. *B*, Erect scout radiograph shows layering out of the calcific granules (arrow) in a pyelogenic cyst. *C*, Urogram, in erect position, demonstrates the relation of the pyelogenic cyst to an upper calyx.

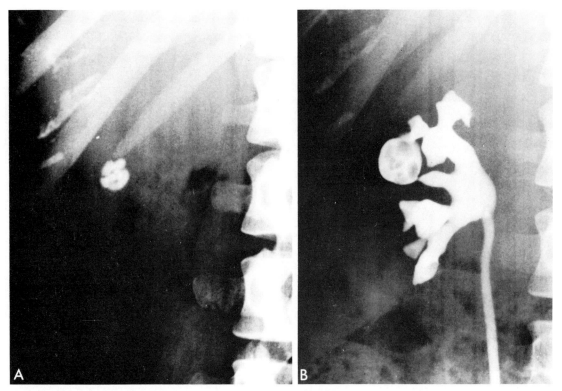

Figure 2–9. Multiple calculi in a hydrocalycosis. *A,* Scout radiograph shows multiple concretions in the right flank. *B,* Retrograde pyelogram demonstrates that the calculi are contained within a dilated calyx, secondary to stricture of the calyceal neck.

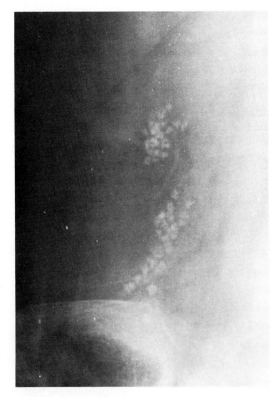

Figure 2–10. Seed calculi in a moderately dilated pelvicalyceal system of a 76-year-old woman with ureteropelvic junction obstruction.

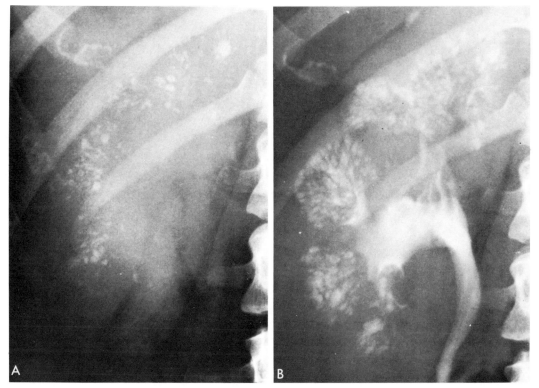

Figure 2–11. Medullary sponge kidney. *A,* Scout radiograph shows clusters of small calculi in the region of the renal pyramids. *B,* Urogram demonstrates that the calculi are in the pyramids, in association with streaks of contrast medium in dilated collecting ducts.

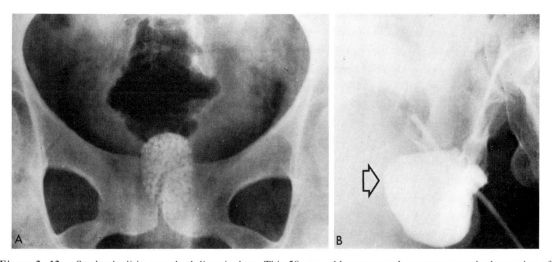

Figure 2–12. Seed calculi in a urethral diverticulum. This 58-year-old woman underwent transurethral resection of a bladder neoplasm one year ago, at which time the urethra was apparently injured. *A,* Scout radiograph shows many seed calculi overlying the symphysis pubis and collected in a smoothly oval configuration. *B,* Retrograde urethrogram shows the large urethral diverticulum (arrow).

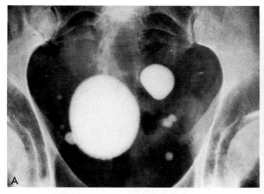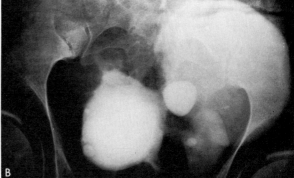

Figure 2–13. Calculus in the bladder and calculus in a vesical diverticulum. *A,* Scout radiograph shows two large dense concretions; both could be calculi in the bladder, but despite changes in the patient's position, such as decubitus projections, the calculi maintained a separation from each other. The other, smaller concretions are pelvic phleboliths. *B,* Cystogram demonstrates the larger dense calculus to be in the bladder and the other to be in a large vesical diverticulum, near the neck of the diverticulum. There is also a smaller diverticulum.

the lumen of a simple ureterocele, appearing as a single concretion (Fig. 2–14) or multiple concretions in the distal end of the ureter. If the calculus assumes the oval shape of the lumen of the ureterocele, diagnosis can be suggested from the plain film.

Except for their presence in diverticula, urethral calculi occur infrequently and then much more often in men than in women. The calculi, most often calcium oxalate, have been classified as primary, i.e., originating in the urethra, and secondary, i.e., having migrated to the urethra from elsewhere in the urinary tract (Fig. 2–15). The primary urethral calculus results from urinary stagnation and infection in a urethral recess, such as from prostatic and periurethral abscess or mucosal ulceration. A for-

eign body in the urethra could act as a nidus for the formation of a calculus. Over 90 percent of urethral calculi are of the secondary type.[5,6]

Nephrocalcinosis

Nephrocalcinosis refers to radiologically demonstrable diffuse small concretions in the renal parenchyma, either cortical or medullary in location, occuring initially in the cells of the tubules as well as in tubular basement membrane and tubular lumina; later, calcifications are also present in the interstitial tissues of the kidney, with focal scarring. Nephrolithiasis refers to calculi within the pelvicalyceal system. Patients with nephrocalcino-

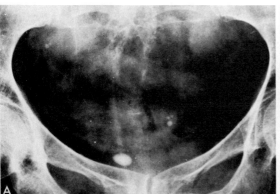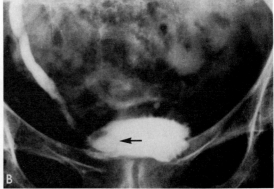

Figure 2–14. A 56-year-old woman with urinary infection. *A,* Scout radiograph shows an oval concretion just above the right pubic bone and at the right side of the soft tissue density of an emptied bladder. The smaller concretions are pelvic phleboliths. *B,* Urography shows the calculus to be in a simple ureterocele (arrow).

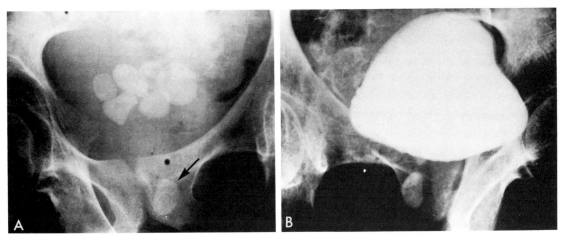

Figure 2–15. Urethral calculus and bladder calculi in a 27-year-old paraplegic man. *A,* Several round and faceted calculi in the urinary bladder, one of which (arrow), now in the region of the symphysis pubis, has passed into the urethra (a secondary urethral calculus). *B,* Urography shows the relationship of the urethral calculus to the bladder outlet.

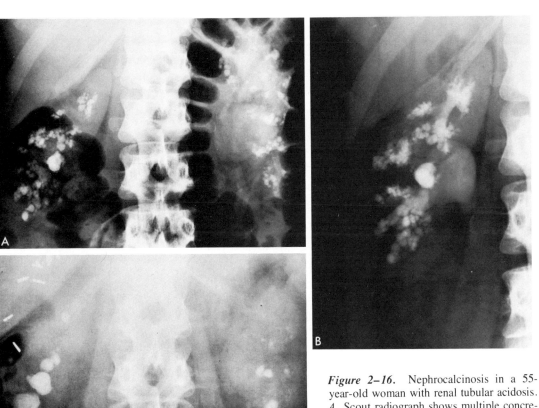

Figure 2–16. Nephrocalcinosis in a 55-year-old woman with renal tubular acidosis. *A,* Scout radiograph shows multiple concretions of varying sizes in both kidneys. *B,* Urogram (right kidney) demonstrates that the concretions occur in the pyramids. *C,* Six years later, there are fewer calculi in each kidney, many having been passed. The remaining calculi are larger than in *A.*

sis often also have nephrolithiasis, the underlying metabolic abnormalities favoring the formation of concretions in the pelvicalyceal system as well as in the parenchyma; also parenchymal calcifications can gain access to the pelvicalyceal system. Because of concentration of calcium in the pyramids, nephrocalcinosis is more pronounced in the renal medulla, with cellular damage and calcification occurring initially in the collecting ducts and long loops of Henle.

The typical radiologic appearance consists of clusters of stippled calcifications in both kidneys, most pronounced in the pyramids (Fig. 2–16), but also, in more severe cases, in the cortex. At first punctate and diffuse, the calcifications can later become conglomerate and dense. Among the causes of nephrocalcinosis are:

1. Hyperparathyroidism—most often the primary type.
2. Renal tubular acidosis (RTA) is the inability or diminished ability to excrete acid urine in response to systemic adidosis. If the defect is in the proximal tubule, there is loss of bicarbonate due to impaired tubular reabsorption of bicarbonate ions. With distal tubular defect, there is impairment of the secretion of hydrogen ions by the distal tubule, leading to cation wasting, including the loss in the urine of calcium ions. Thus, nephrocalcinosis occurs almost always with distal tubular defect, being rare in proximal renal tubular acidosis.[7]
3. Sarcoidosis—in most of the reported cases with nephrocalcinosis, there was also hypercalcemia. The mechanism for the occurrence of hypercalcemia in sarcoidosis has not been established; there may be an increased tissue sensitivity to normal vitamin D levels.
4. Bone dissolution, as with patient immobilization, bone metastases, and excess steroids (endogenous or exogenous).
5. Hypervitaminosis D.
6. Idiopathic hypercalciuria.
7. Milk-alkali syndrome.
8. Hypothyroidism (Fig. 2–17). In some of these patients there is apparently a hypersensitivity to vitamin D.[8]
9. Oxaluria. Increased amounts of oxalate in the urine can result from a primary metabolic defect. There is also an enteric hyperoxaluria, resulting from excess ingestion of oxalic-containing substances or from abnormalities in the intestinal tract, such as regional enteritis, distal small bowel resection (Fig. 2–18), and intestinal bypass operations for obesity, resulting in increased intestinal absorption of dietary oxalate.[9,10]
10. Wilson's disease (Fig. 2–19). Some of the patients with Wilson's disease have subnormal urinary acidifying capacity.[11]
11. Idiopathic hypercalcemia.

Prostatic Calcification

Prostatic calculi vary in size from a millimeter to several centimeters in diameter and occur in a patient from few to hundreds in number. Although found usually in men over 40 years old, they have been reported in young men and even children. The

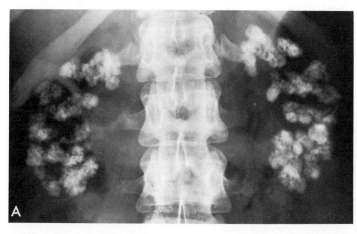
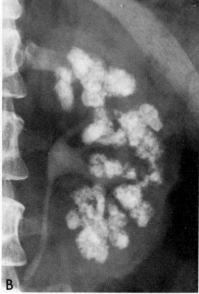

Figure 2–17. Nephrocalcinosis in 23-year-old woman with juvenile hypothyroidism. She has received thyroxine treatment for 14 years. *A,* Scout radiograph shows clusters of calculi in the renal parenchyma bilaterally. *B,* Urogram (left kidney) demonstrates that the calcifications are in the renal pyramids.

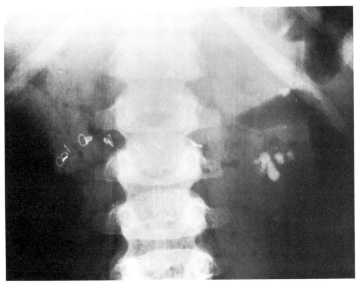

Figure 2–18. Nephrocalcinosis with hyperoxaluria. A two-year-old girl with hyperoxaluria following small bowel resection neonatally for midgut volvulus. Scout radiograph shows calculi in the parenchyma of the left kidney.

pathogenesis of these concretions is unknown; the most generally accepted theory is that they represent calcification of corpora amylacea, clumps of bacteria, blood clot, or pus. They may result from chronic prostatitis or, on the other hand, may act to cause an inflammatory process in the prostate. Prostatic calculi occur most commonly in the posterior and lateral lobes of the prostate, sometimes involving the gland diffusely and symmetrically, but at other times being asymmetrical and localized.

They usually have a characteristic radiologic appearance of many sharply defined homogeneous concretions clustered in the region of the symphysis pubis (Figs. 2–20 and 2–21), a midline location where pelvic phleboliths are uncommon. The location, size, and packing of the many concretions, sometimes faceted, are distinctive for prostatic calculi.

Tuberculosis can also produce calcification in the prostate gland, sometimes simulating the much more common nontuberculous calculous prostatitis. The calcifications of tuberculosis are apt to be less well defined and smudgy, without the sharp borders of prostatic calculi.

Foreign Material

Radiopaque medication in the rectum or vagina can produce radiographic densities which may

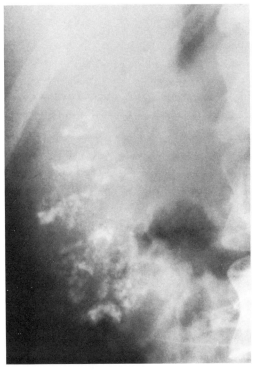

Figure 2–19. Nephrocalcinosis in a 23-year-old man with Wilson's disease. Scout radiograph of the right kidney shows clusters of small concretions in the renal parenchyma. There were similar calcifications in the left kidney.

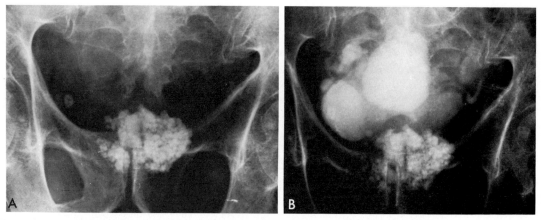

Figure 2-20. Prostatic calculi. *A,* Scout radiograph shows concretions of varying sizes involving an enlarged prostate, diffusely and symmetrically. The calcification near the right ischial spine is a phlebolith. *B,* Urography demonstrates the relation of the calcifications to the base of the bladder. Note the ureteral fish-hooking and the vesical pseudodiverticula, secondary to bladder outlet obstruction due to the enlarged prostate.

simulate bladder or prostatic calculi. Commercial preparations of rectal suppositories may contain calcium, bismuth, and zinc, in such compounds as calcium phosphate, bismuth subiodide, bismuth subgallate, bismuth resorcin, zinc oxide, and bismuth subcarbonate.[12] Also, some of the vaginal suppositories contain enough silver, mercury, or iodine compounds to produce opacities on the radiograph—compounds such as diiodohydroxyquin, phenyl mercuric acetate, silver picrate, and iodochlorohydroxyquin.[13] If the patient were to insert such a suppository just prior to the radiography, the resulting opacity could be misinterpreted as calcification associated with the bladder. Within 30 minutes or so the suppositories dissolve with a diffusion of the chemical substances, doing away with the possibility of confusing radiopacities.

Other foreign bodies in the rectum, vagina, uterus, bladder, or urethra are usually of distinctive enough configuration to preclude their being misinterpreted as calcific matter. Among such foreign bodies are catheters, thermometers, intrauterine contraceptive devices, and unusual substances inserted by disturbed patients. Radiopaque surgical devices or prostheses can also cause confusing densities (Fig. 2-22).

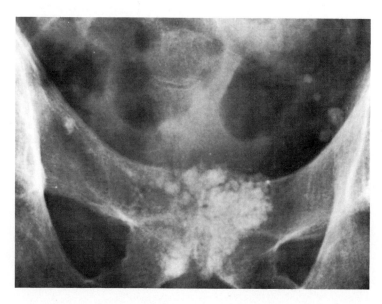

Figure 2-21. Prostatic calculi in asymmetrical distribution, being more pronounced in the left lobe. The concretions at the lateral aspect of the pelvis are phleboliths.

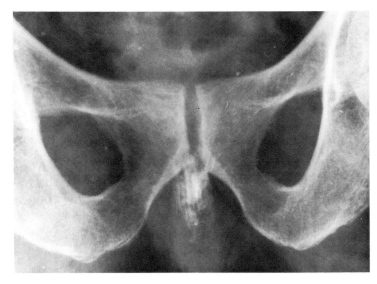

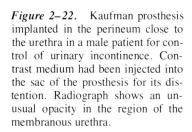

Figure 2–22. Kaufman prosthesis implanted in the perineum close to the urethra in a male patient for control of urinary incontinence. Contrast medium had been injected into the sac of the prosthesis for its distention. Radiograph shows an unusual opacity in the region of the membranous urethra.

Radiologic Characterization of Urinary Tract Concretions

In the evaluation of a radiopacity seen on an abdominal radiograph as to the possibility of its being a concretion of the urinary tract, the consideration of several factors can be of help:

1. Location
2. Density
3. Size
4. Shape
5. Axis
6. Mobility
7. Comparison with previous abdominal radiographs, if available.

Location. The location of the radiopacity is of utmost importance; it must be in the expected site of a component of the urinary tract (Figs. 2–23, 2–24, and 2–25). Yet it is important to remember that underlying abnormality of the urinary tract can place a component in an unusual location—e.g., marked dilatation of the renal pelvis, as in ureteropelvic junction obstruction; deviation of the ureter by an adjacent retroperitoneal mass; elevation and medial deviation of the terminal segment of the ureter by prostatic hypertrophy (Fig. 2–26); medial placement of inferior calyces in a horseshoe kidney.

Density. It is crucial to determine whether the radiopacity is of metallic, calcific, or other density, often judged by comparing its radiopacity with that of the spine for calcific or with that of the lead marker on the radiograph for metallic. If the radiopacity is of metallic density, consider things like: residual barium (e.g., in a colon diverticu-lum) from a previous GI series or barium enema; mercury in the intestinal tract from a ruptured balloon of an intestinal drainage tube; bullet fragment; etc. The radiopacity of a calcific structure depends not only on its content of calcium but also upon its

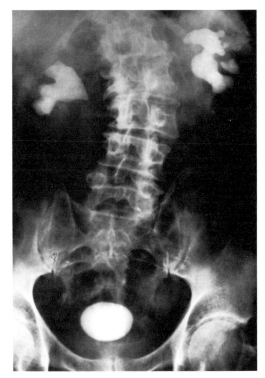

Figure 2–23. Scout radiograph shows bilateral staghorn calculi and a sharply defined, dense bladder calculus, all easily identified by their characteristic shape and location.

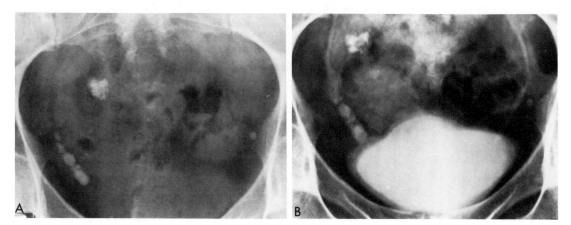

Figure 2–24. Ureteral calculi. *A,* Scout radiograph shows a line of homogeneously dense calculi, of different sizes and shapes, in the region and alignment of the lower segment of the right ureter. The triangular shape of some of the calculi would be most unusual for phlebolith. The concretion near the left ischial spine is round and has a central lucency, characteristic for phlebolith. The irregular, somewhat mottled calcification overlying the right border of the sacrum is in a uterine fibroid. *B,* Intravenous urogram demonstrates the relationship of the ureters to the various calcifications.

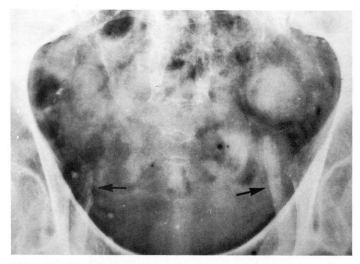

Figure 2–25. Ossification of the sacrotuberous ligaments (arrows). These could be misinterpreted as large ureteral calculi, but they extend too far caudally and at the wrong axes to be associated with the ureters.

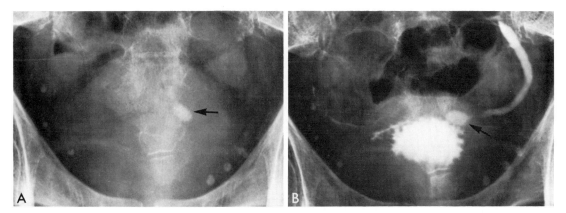

Figure 2–26. Ureteral calcification in unusual location and of unusual axis because of displacement of the ureter by prostatic enlargement. *A,* The ureteral calculus (arrow) is located much more medially and its axis is abnormal for the usual location of the ureter. The other rounded concretions are phleboliths. In addition, there are small linear flecks of calcification in pelvic arteries. *B,* Urogram demonstrates that the terminal segment of each ureter has been elevated by an enlarged prostate, the calculus (arrow) lying in the distal portion of the left ureter.

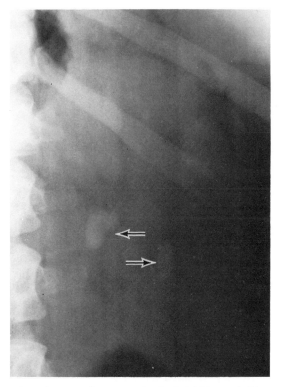

Figure 2–27. Faintly opacified cystine calculi (arrows) in the left kidney. A 22-year-old woman with cystinuria. Crystallographic analysis of the removed calculi showed 100 percent cystine.

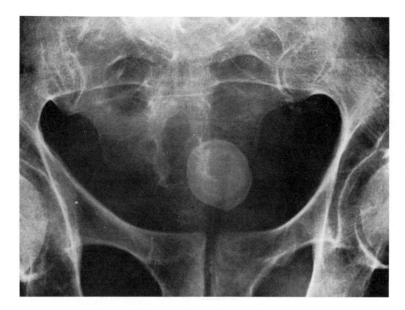

Figure 2–28. Poorly calcified vesical calculus with a sharply defined calcific rim.

size. For a given thickness, calcium oxalate concretions are more radiopaque than triple phosphate concretions. Cystine stones are less radiopaque than are calcium-containing stones (Fig. 2–27).

Urinary tract concretions are usually homogeneously dense but there are exceptions, such as: some faintly opaque bladder calculi with a peripheral ring of calcification (Fig. 2–28); extruded pa-

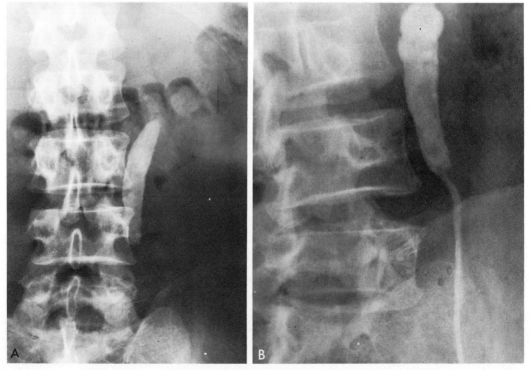

Figure 2–29. *A,* Scout radiograph shows a giant calculus in the left ureter. At urography there was no excretion of contrast medium by the left kidney. *B,* Left retrograde ureterography demonstrates the calcification to be in the ureter.

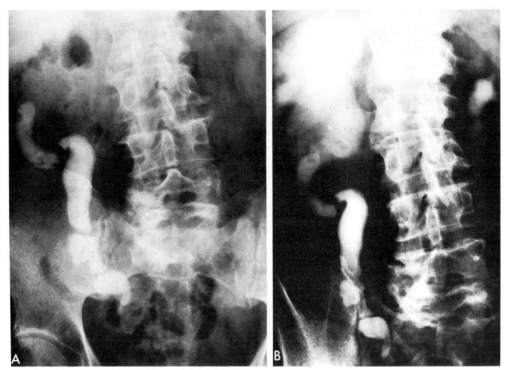

Figure 2–30. Giant calculi in the right ureter of a 63-year-old man with history of previous pyelolithotomy, ureterolithotomy, and partial nephrectomy for stones, all on the right side. *A,* Scout radiograph shows several large, dense calculi on the right, in a tortuous and dilated ureter. *B,* A 60-minute urogram demonstrates excretion by the right kidney, with obstructive uropathy.

pillae, triangular in shape, with a peripheral layer of calcification, as occurs in renal papillary necrosis.

Size. Concretions in the various components of the urinary tract are expected to be of generally specific sizes. However, there are exceptions, such as giant ureteral calculi (Fig. 2–29 and 2–30) or the giant calculus in the markedly dilated pelvis of ureteropelvic junction obstruction (Fig. 2–31).

Shape. With some urinary tract concretions, the shape is distinctive enough to be diagnostic, e.g., staghorn calculus of the renal pelvis, stellate bladder calculus, triangular calculus of renal papillary necrosis (Fig. 2–32), cup-shaped calculus which had formed in a calyx (Figs. 2–33 and 2–34).

Axis. If the calcification is linear or oval in shape, it is important to take account of its axis. Ureteral calculi often are not round, but have a long axis which should conform in direction with the expected course of the ureter (Figs. 2–35 and 2–36). Exceptions can occur; a calculus in a dilated ureter may present with its axis quite askew from the longitudinal course of the ureter.

Mobility. It is important to evaluate the mobility of the suspected concretion in relation to the urinary tract by making radiographs with change in patient position. A calculus in an undilated renal calyx will maintain a fixed position relative to the kidney as the position of the patient is changed. On the other hand, a calculus lying free in a sac of hydronephrosis will show movement within the soft-tissue density of the kidney. Similarly calculi within renal cystic structures usually move freely within the cyst, and multiple concretions (seed or milk of calcium) layer dependently when studied by a horizontal beam radiograph. Bladder calculi are usually freely mobile within the soft tissue outline of the bladder; the mobility is best demonstrated by supine vs. prone views or by decubitus views.

Previous Studies. Comparison of previous abdominal radiographs, if available, with the present radiograph can be most helpful. If a concretion seen now was also present, with little change in location or size, weeks or months or years ago, it is not likely to be a urinary tract calculus. The appearance of a concretion now in the location of the urinary tract but not present on a radiograph made days, weeks or even months ago is apt to be a urinary calculus (Fig. 2–37).

Also, the demonstration of movement on the

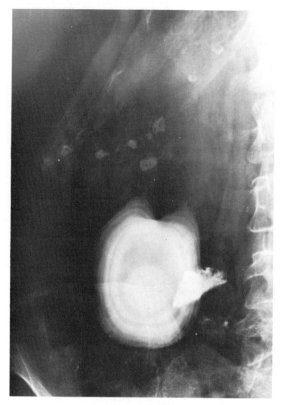

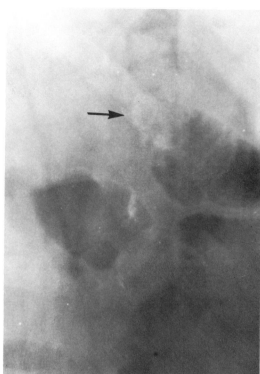

Figure 2–31   Figure 2–32

Figure 2–31.   Giant, laminated calculus in a dilated renal pelvis secondary to ureteropelvic junction obstruction. There is a triangular collection of barium in the bowel overlying the calculus. The circular calcifications cephalad to the calculus represent calcifications of costal cartilages.

Figure 2–32.   Calcification of extruded papillae in calyces in a patient with renal papillary necrosis. Scout radiograph shows faint rings of calcification. The arrow points to one such ring, triangular in shape.

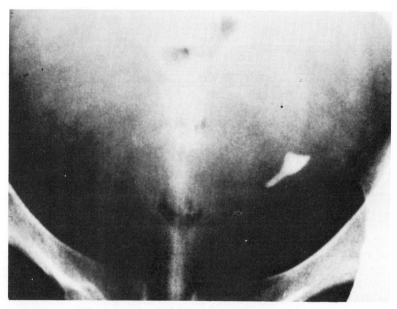

Figure 2–33.   Calculus in the lower segment of the left ureter, with the shape of the calculus reproducing the shape of a calyx in which it had formed and the axis of the calculus conforming to that of the ureter.

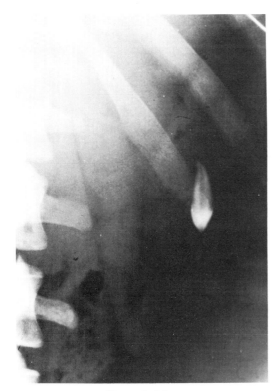

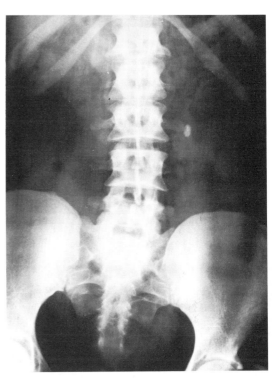

Figure 2–34   Figure 2–35

Figure 2–34.   A calcification of distinctive configuration in the region of the left kidney. The shape and structure are those of an adult tooth. This does not represent a tooth in a dermoid cyst. The patient had suffered facial trauma and a broken tooth had been swallowed. The tooth now is in the stomach, overlying the left kidney. (Courtesy of Dr. M. Rosenberg, Bridgeport, Connecticut.)

Figure 2–35.   Oval-shaped concretion just lateral to the transverse process of L3, at a position consistent with that of the left ureter and with its long axis conforming to the course of the abdominal ureter. This was a ureteral calculus.

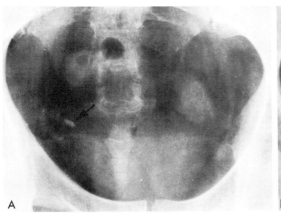

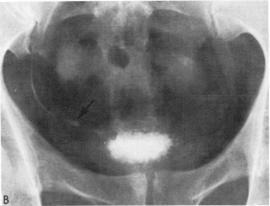

Figure 2–36.   Ureteral calculus. *A,* Oval-shaped concretion (arrow) with its long axis approaching the horizontal, consistent with the course of the terminal segment of the pelvic ureter. *B,* Urography proves that the calculus is in the ureter (arrow).

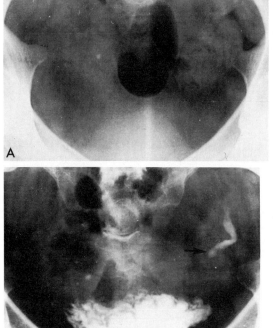

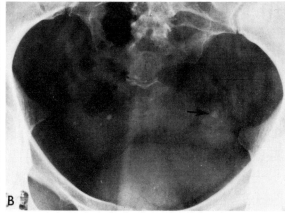

Figure 2–37. Ureteral calculus. *A,* Scout radiograph shows several small round concretions in the right side of the pelvis. These are phleboliths, most likely in a uterine vein. Note that there are no calcifications in the left side of the pelvis. *B,* Scout radiograph nine days later shows a triangular calcification in the left side of the pelvis (arrow). *C,* Urography proves that this new calcification is a ureteral calculus (arrow).

comparison radiographs is important. A concretion appearing now in the region of the lower segment of the ureter and shown to have been present in the region of the kidney on a previous radiograph can be confidently diagnosed as a urinary tract calculus (Fig. 2–38). In this regard, it is important to remember that calculi in the segment of ureter overlying the wing of the sacrum or overlying a transverse vertebral process can be hidden (obscured) by the bone density (Fig. 2–39). Hence, a calcification now present in the region of the lower segment of the ureter, not present on a radiograph made days or weeks ago, could have been in a segment of ureter obscured by bone; a careful comparative study may disclose the previously overlooked concretion.

Ureteral Calculus vs. Phlebolith

It is often difficult to differentiate on the abdominal radiograph a calculus in the lower segment of the ureter from a pelvic phlebolith. Several considerations can help in this differentiation. Urinary tract calculus is usually homogeneously dense; a phlebolith is apt to have a lucent center or several central lucencies. A phlebolith is usually round; a ureteral calculus may be angular (Fig. 2–40). Pelvic phleboliths are usually multiple; regard with suspicion what is thought to be a single pelvic phlebolith (Fig. 2–41). It has been said that ureteral calculi are not located caudally to a line drawn between the ischial spines; however, this is not a reliable sign, since angulation of the x-ray beam may project a calculus caudally. A change in the configuration or lie of a calcification speaks for ureteral calculus rather than phlebolith.

CONDUIT CALCIFICATION

Urinary tract conduits which may show calcification in their walls are the ureters, main renal arteries, and branches of the main renal arteries. Rarely, calcification occurs in the wall of a renal vein which has been "arterialized" secondary to a marked increase in its intraluminal pressure and blood flow, as with an arteriovenous fistula.

Calcification in the walls of the renal arteries has the same radiographic characteristics as calcifica-

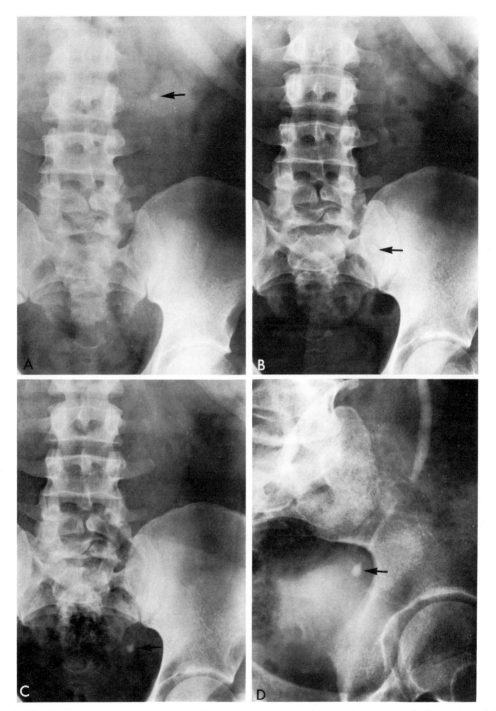

Figure 2–38. Ureteral calculus. *A*, Scout radiograph shows a round concretion (arrow) in the region of the-left kidney. *B*, Scout radiograph three days later shows no calcification in relation to the left kidney. However, note that the calcification (arrow) overlies the sacrum and is hidden by the bone density. *C*, Scout radiograph, seven days after *B*, demonstrates that the calcification (arrow) has moved caudally into the pelvis. *D*, Urography, in left posterior oblique position, proves the presence of a ureteral calculus (arrow).

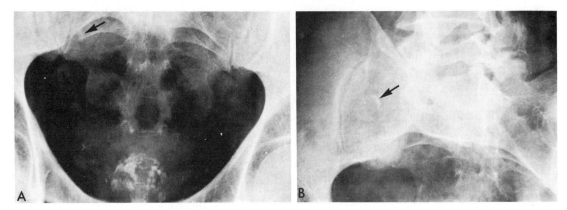

Figure 2–39. Ureteral calculus hidden by sacrum. *A,* Scout radiograph shows numerous prostatic calculi. There is a hardly visible calcification (arrow) overlying the right wing of the sacrum, the long axis of the calcification conforming to the expected course of the ureter. *B,* With the patient in the right posterior oblique position, the calculus (arrow) is seen more clearly. Subsequent urography proved the calcification to represent a ureteral calculus.

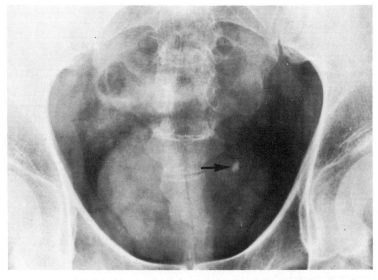

Figure 2–40. A single calcification (arrow), to the left of the sacrum, is angular rather than round. Subsequent urography proved it to be a ureteral calculus.

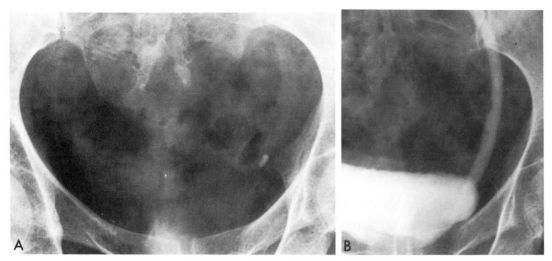

Figure 2–41. Ureteral calculus vs. phlebolith. *A,* Scout radiograph shows a single, oval concretion just medial to the left ischial spine. The long axis of the calcification conforms to the expected course of the ureter. These factors— single, oval, and course of axis—indicate calculus rather than phlebolith. *B,* Urogram proves that it is a ureteral calculus.

tion of other major branches of the aorta. The linear calcifications are typically of tramline configuration, with the longitudinal plaques of calcification being discontinuous due to separation

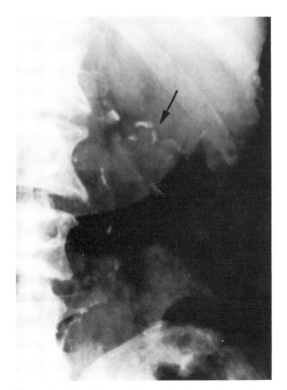

Figure 2–42. Scout radiograph shows discontinuous linear plaques of calcification, varying in width, in the aorta and left renal artery (arrow).

by uncalcified segments. The calcifications often vary in width, some being smooth and pencil thin, and others being chunky and irregular (Fig. 2–42). If the calcification extends to vessels peripheral to the main artery, the branching pattern of tramline calcification is distinctive (Fig. 2–43).

By far the most common cause of calcification of the ureteral wall is schistosomiasis (*Schistosoma haematobium*), usually with a continuous layer of wall calcification. The lower ureteral segments are involved most frequently, but the calcification can extend the entire length of the ureter to the renal pelvis. The calcification, stimulated by the dead ova, occurs primarily in the submucosa, but may also involve the muscle layers and the adventitia. The calcification appears on the radiograph as parallel thin, smooth lines defining the normal ureteral lumen, or, if the ureters are dilated and tortuous, as curvilinear calcifications (Fig. 2–44), or occasionally as mottled collections of calcification. Practically always there is also calcification of the bladder wall.

Tuberculosis of the ureter results usually in fibrotic narrowing of the lumen, with wall calcification occurring only infrequently and then usually in the lower ureteral segment.

CYST WALL CALCIFICATION

A number of types of renal cysts can have wall calcification, appearing on the radiograph as a smooth curvilinear calcific rim. The rim calcification need not be continuously complete; sometimes

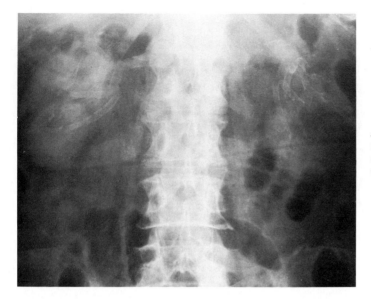

Figure 2–43. Both renal arteries and their branches are markedly calcified, showing the typical branching pattern of tramline calcification.

only a small segment of arcuate calcification can be seen. Characteristically, the smooth, sharp curvilinear calcification occurs at the very periphery of the mass. When the calcification is extensive and of irregular thickness, the radiographic appearance can be deceptive, presenting as a rim of calcification about a mass, with mottled calcification seemingly within the mass. However, the mottled calcification represents radiodensities on cyst surfaces not tangential to the x-ray beam but dense enough to be projected as radiopacities within the mass, simulating the appearance of solid mass calcification.

Simple renal cysts (Fig. 2–45) show radiographically demonstrable calcification in about 2 percent or less of cases as compared with an incidence of 10 percent or greater in various reports for renal cell carcinoma. Although calcification in renal neoplasms is of solid mass type, it can occasionally be of cyst wall type (Fig. 2–46). One or more cysts of the many which occur in an adult type polycystic kidney can rarely calcify; these are similar in appearance to the calcification of the simple renal cyst.[14,15] Rim-type calcification can also occur infrequently with parapelvic cyst, pararenal pseudocyst, and the rare multilocular cyst. However,

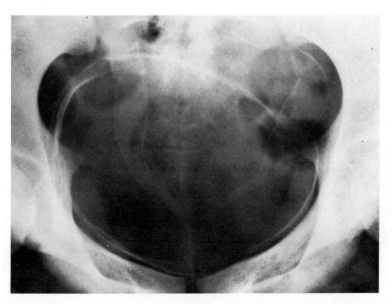

Figure 2–44. Schistosomiasis in a 16-year-old African female. Scout radiograph shows thin curvilinear calcification of the bladder wall. Thin lines of calcification define dilated and tortuous ureters. Because of fibrosis and distortion of the trigone, the ureteral orifices may be close to each other, as in this patient.

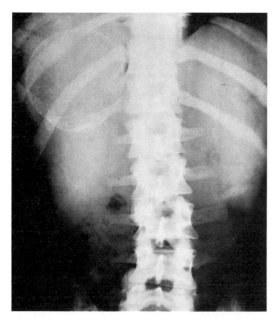

Figure 2–45. Renal cyst. Scout radiograph shows a large right upper quadrant mass with a continuous thin rim of calcification. At operation, this proved to be a renal cyst.

streaky and curvilinear calcification of diffuse solid mass type has been reported in a multilocular renal cyst, which had been irradiated three months previously.[16] Wall calcification or even ossification is occasionally seen in the walls of one or more of the cysts of the multicystic kidney in an adult patient (Fig. 2–47). Calcification is common in the walls of a renal echinococcus cyst, the simultaneous wall calcification of the main cyst and daughter cysts producing a distinctive radiographic appearance (Fig. 2–48); however, this characteristic appearance is often not present (Fig. 2–49).

Calcification occurs frequently in the wall of an aneurysm of the main renal artery or of an intrarenal aneurysm. Characteristically the neck of the aneurysm does not calcify; the radiograph might thus show a ring of calcification discontinuous at one small segment, representing the neck of the aneurysm (Fig. 2–50). Intrarenal aneurysms may be large and on the abdominal radiograph simulate a simple renal cyst with a calcified rim.

Infrequently, cyst type calcification about a part or all of the kidney represents calcification of the renal capsule resulting from a subcapsular hematoma (Fig. 2–51). It is likely that, similarly, he-

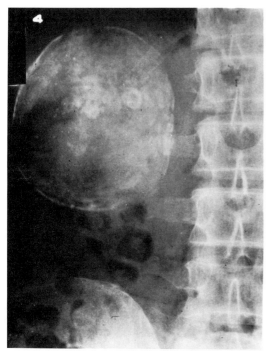

Figure 2–46. Renal adenocarcinoma with cyst wall type of calcification. Scout radiograph shows a large right upper quadrant mass with a thin, somewhat mottled rim of calcification. At operation, this proved to be a renal carcinoma.

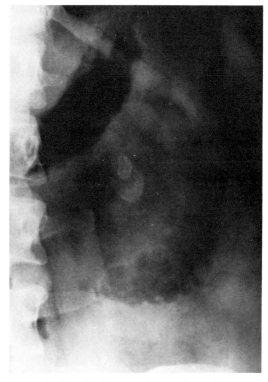

Figure 2–47. Multicystic kidney in a 39-year-old woman. Scout radiograph shows rims of calcification in two of the cysts.

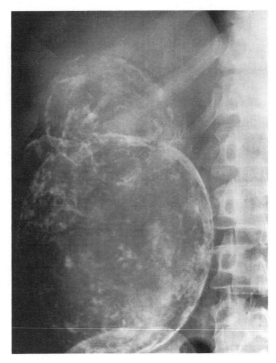

Figure 2-48. Echinococcosis in a 64-year-old man. Scout film shows rim type calcifications in the walls of the large main cyst as well as of the daughter cysts, located in the right kidney.

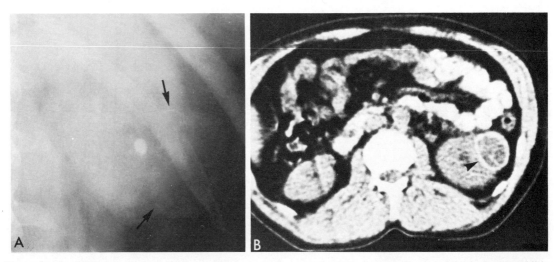

Figure 2-49. Echinococcosis in a 45-year-old man. *A,* Scout radiograph shows a dense renal calculus. In addition there is a protruding mass at the lateral lower pole of the kidney, with several thin curvilinear segments of faint calcification (arrows). *B,* CT scan shows a complete rim of calcification (arrowhead) at the periphery of the mass with several lines of calcification within the mass, representing calcification in the walls of daughter cysts.

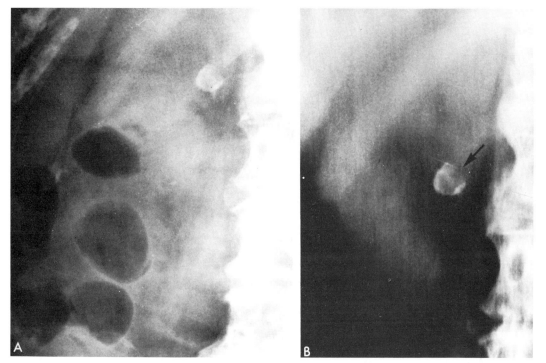

Figure 2–50. Renal artery aneurysm in a 70-year-old woman. *A*, Scout radiograph shows an irregularly thick incomplete ring of calcification in the region of the hilus of the right kidney. *B*, Tomography demonstrates more clearly the irregular thickness of the calcification in the wall of the aneurysm. The segment of discontinuous calcification (arrow) represents the location of the neck of the aneurysm.

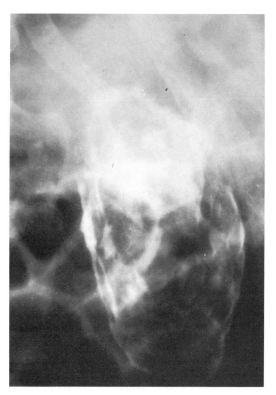

Figure 2–51. Calcification of renal capsule. Scout radiograph shows a peel of calcification surrounding the left kidney, probably the result of an old subcapsular hematoma.

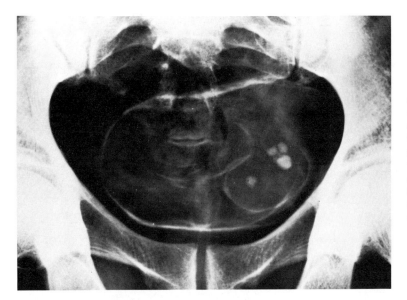

Figure 2–52. Schistosomiasis. Scout radiograph shows a thin continuous curvilinear calcification of the bladder wall. The incomplete rims of calcification within the bladder represent calcification in the walls of the terminal segments of dilated ureters, with several calculi in the left ureter.

matoma in the perirenal space could result in calcification of the renal capsule or of the renal fascia (Gerota's fascia).

Schistosomiasis of the bladder (*Schistosoma haematobium*) shows thin, continuous curvilinear calcification of cyst type (Fig. 2–52). However, since the bladder wall retains pliability, the smooth cyst type calcification of the full urinary bladder may appear irregular and corrugated when the bladder is empty (Fig. 2–53). With the development of carcinoma, a well-recognized complication of vesical schistosomiasis, the plain radiograph will show a discontinuity of the rim of calcification, this break resulting from invasion of

the bladder wall by the carcinoma. Uncommonly, the calcification is of flocculent type. The intensity of bladder calcification in schistosomiasis is related directly to the number of dead ova in the venules of the submucosa, muscularis, and adventitia. About one-half of the patients with vesical bilharziasis have radiologically demonstrable bladder-wall calcification.

SOLID MASS CALCIFICATION

Solid mass calcification is a term used for calcification in solid tissue, not necessarily a mass le-

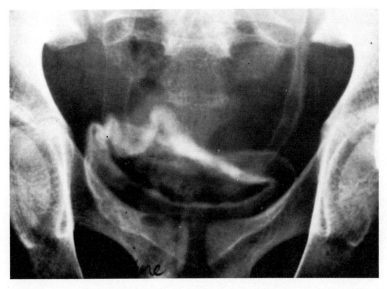

Figure 2–53. Schistosomiasis. Scout radiograph shows a continuous, partly wrinkled rim of calcification in the wall of the empty bladder of a 16-year-old male with schistosomiasis. Note the conduit type of calcification in the walls of the ureters.

sion. It is a type of dystrophic calcification, just as is cyst wall calcification, the calcification resulting very likely from tissue damage with localized electrolyte changes. With cyst wall type, the calcification does not occur in the fluid-containing part of the lesion but rather in the surrounding wall, yielding the characteristic appearance. With solid mass type, the zone of tissue damage is in a mass such as neoplasm, hamartoma, or granuloma, or in a nonmass zone of necrosis or inflammation.

The major feature is the varied internal calcific pattern, which may be speckled, mottled, streaky, amorphous, or a combination of these, interspersed with zones of no calcification or even radiolucency. The internal structure lacks geometric uniformity. If there is a mass, the marginal calcification is usually less pronounced than the internal calcification, the outer margin being discontinuous and irregular. Occasionally, the peripheral border is densely calcified and irregular, although smooth curvilinear borders do occur, mimicking the cyst wall type of calcification.

Neoplasms of the kidney, both benign and ma-

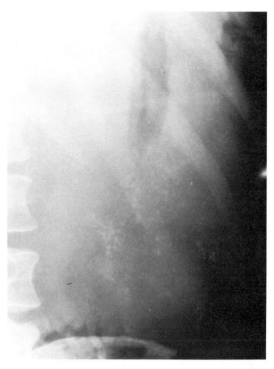

Figure 2–55. Adult Wilms tumor in a 62-year-old man. Scout radiograph shows speckled calcification, without marginal calcifications, in a large mass of the left kidney.

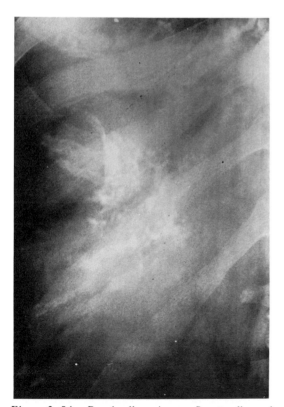

Figure 2–54. Renal cell carcinoma. Scout radiograph shows a large collection of streaky and amorphous calcification, without marginal calcification, in a large mass of the right kidney.

lignant, can show calcification (Figs. 2–54 and 2–55), the incidence in renal cell carcinoma usually reported as 10 to 15 percent. Phillips et al. stated that any renal mass containing calcification is probably tumor rather than cyst; their series of 225 cases of renal masses with pathologically proven diagnosis contained 72 simple cysts of which two (3 percent) were calcified and 66 renal cell carcinomas of which nine (14 percent) were calcified.[17] On occasion, renal cell carcinoma calcification can be smooth, thin, and curvilinear, simulating the calcification in the wall of a simple cyst (Fig. 2–56).[15,18,19] Cyst type calcification in solid neoplasms occurs usually in fibrous zones about areas of cystic degeneration, necrosis, or hemorrhage. Kikkawa and Lasser found radiographic calcification in only one of 51 renal cysts; in 60 renal cell carcinomas calcification could be demonstrated in 11 (18 percent), of which nine showed rimlike calcification.[19] With cancer the curvilinear calcification is most often present within the soft tissue mass of the neoplasm (Fig. 2–57), whereas with simple cyst the calcification is at the very periphery of the soft tissue mass. In a report of the analysis of 2709 renal masses, of which 111 contained radiograph-

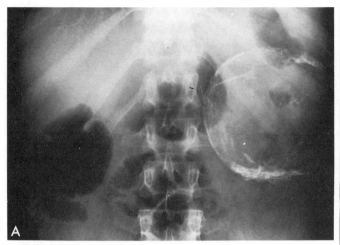
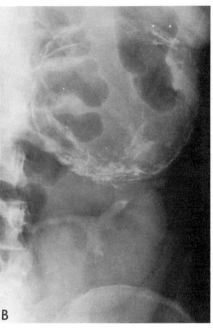

Figure 2–56. Renal cell carcinoma in a 47-year-old woman. *A,* Scout radiograph shows a large left upper quadrant mass with cyst type calcification. *B,* Urogram demonstrates the relationship of the mass to the left kidney. (Courtesy of Dr. Noel Nathanson, Brooklyn, N.Y.)

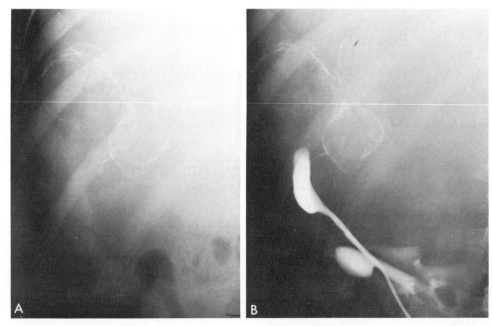

Figure 2–57. Renal cell carcinoma in a 32-year-old man. *A,* Scout radiograph shows linear and rimlike calcification in a right upper quadrant mass. *B,* Retrograde pyelogram demonstrates that the mass is in the right kidney and that the calcification is within the mass rather than at its periphery.

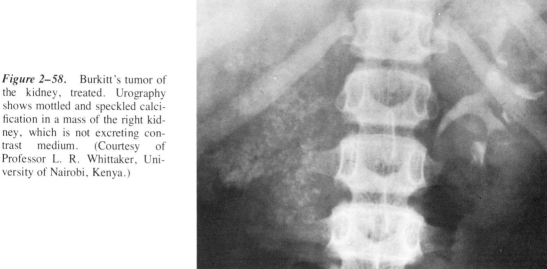

Figure 2–58. Burkitt's tumor of the kidney, treated. Urography shows mottled and speckled calcification in a mass of the right kidney, which is not excreting contrast medium. (Courtesy of Professor L. R. Whittaker, University of Nairobi, Kenya.)

ically visible calcium, Daniel et al. concluded that even though peripheral eggshell calcification without calcium within the mass was usually associated with benign simple cysts, the risk of malignancy was about 20 percent.[20]

Calcification is unusual in transitional cell carcinoma of the kidney (less than 1 percent). Primary osteogenic sarcoma, a very rare lesion which occurs in the elderly, shows heavy ossification. Osteogenic sarcoma metastatic to the kidney from a primary bone site is also rare, seen in the young, with ossification in the renal metastasis. Metastases to the kidney from other primary sites rarely calcify. However, lymphoma of the kidney, including Burkitt's tumor, can calcify after treatment by radiation or chemotherapy (Fig. 2–58). Adenomas of the kidney can show calcification, sometimes in the form of a smooth peripheral shell without internal calcification (Fig. 2–59) and thus simulating cyst wall calcification.[21]

Hamartoma of the kidney, angiomyolipoma or one without all three tissue elements (e.g., angiomyoma), sometimes shows solid mass type calcification (Fig. 2–60).

Among inflammatory diseases of the kidney, tuberculosis is most apt to show calcification. The calcification can be of any solid mass type: speckled, mottled, streaky, or amorphous (Figs. 2–61 and 2–62). Most distinctive and highly suggestive of tuberculosis is amorphous calcification in lobar distribution (Fig. 2–63), a reflection of the lobar type of parenchymal destruction around the calyces. Calcification in xanthogranulomatous pyelonephritis is most often calculi which predated and

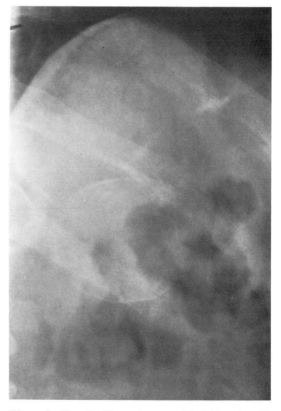

Figure 2–59. Papillary adenoma of the kidney in a 59-year-old man. Scout radiograph shows a thin rim of calcification in a mass in the left upper quadrant. Subsequent urography demonstrated the mass to be in the upper pole of the left kidney. Nephrectomy disclosed a cortical adenoma with cystic necrosis and hemorrhage.

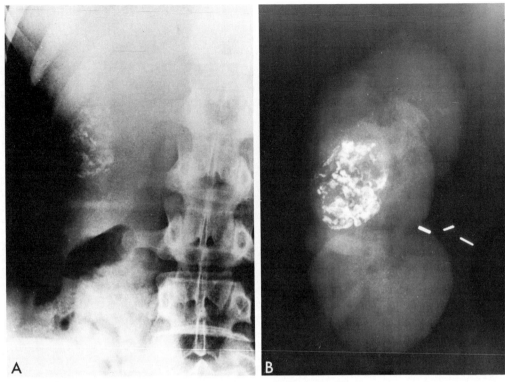

Figure 2-60. Renal hamartoma in a 27-year-old woman. *A,* Scout radiograph shows an oval collection of mottled calcification, without marginal calcification, in the right kidney. *B,* Nephrectomy was done because of the belief that the lesion was malignant. Radiograph of the specimen shows the nature of the calcification clearly. Pathologic diagnosis was angiomyoma, a hamartoma containing vascular and muscular elements.

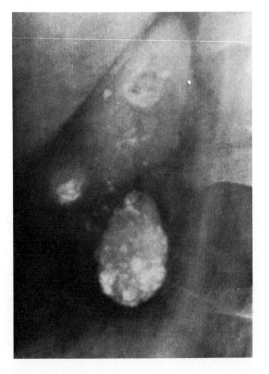

Figure 2-61. Renal tuberculosis. Scout radiograph shows a small right kidney with areas of amorphous and mottled calcification. Subsequent urography demonstrated no excretion of contrast medium by the right kidney.

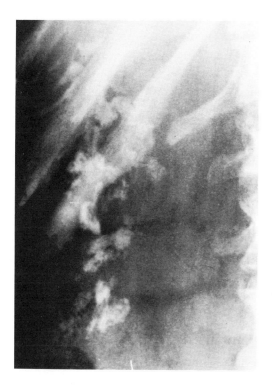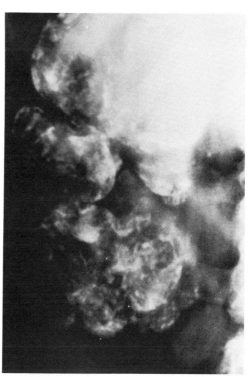

Figure 2–62. Renal tuberculosis. Scout radiograph shows scattered areas of amorphous calcification in the right kidney. Subsequent urography showed no excretion of contrast medium by this kidney.

Figure 2–63. Renal tuberculosis. Scout radiograph shows a large right kidney with amorphous and mottled calcification in lobar distribution. This kidney did not excrete contrast medium at urography.

Figure 2–64. Xanthogranulomatous pyelonephritis. Scout radiograph shows a zone of amorphous and streaky calcification, without marginal calcification, in an enlarged left kidney. This kidney did not excrete contrast medium at urography. (Courtesy of Dr. Robert Shapiro, New Haven, Connecticut.)

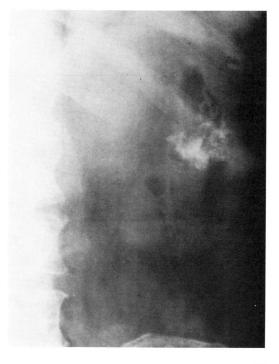

very likely produced the obstruction, which when secondarily infected led to the chronic infection and destruction of the renal parenchyma. However, dystrophic calcification of solid mass type can occur in the tissues damaged by the chronic infection (Fig. 2–64). Calcification occurs only infrequently in a chronic abscess of the kidney. It has been said that calcification occurs frequently in chronic pyelonephritis; that, however, has not been my experience.

Renal infarcts and intrarenal hematomas calcify only rarely. However, a specific type of renal ischemia, cortical necrosis, does calcify frequently if the patient can be kept alive beyond the acute episode, e.g., by dialysis. With ischemia of the cortex, possibly due to the thrombosis or severe spasm of the intrarenal arteries,[22] the cortex becomes necrotic except for a narrow zone of its periphery where perfusion is maintained by the capsular arteries and their perforation branches. Central to the necrotic layer is the still viable medulla. It is at the two interfaces of necrotic-viable tissue, one between the necrotic layer and the thin peripheral cortical rim and the other between the necrotic layer and the medulla, that calcification is deposited. The typical, but infrequently present, appearance is a tramline of calcification surrounding the kidney a few mm. below its capsule, an appearance first described in 1962.[23] After the acute ischemic episode, the kidneys initially enlarge, possibly owing to edema, and then gradually shrink with irregularity of the renal contour, the degree of irregularity and the extent of cortical calcification reflecting the distribution of the cortical necrosis.[24, 25] For the

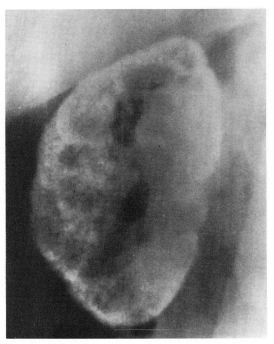

Figure 2–66. Chronic glomerulonephritis. Scout radiograph shows diffuse calcification in the cortex of the small right kidney. The left kidney had a similar appearance. The patient was a 46-year-old man with chronic renal failure.

appearance of radiologically demonstrable cortical calcification, the patient must survive the acute episode, the calcification usually appearing in four to eight weeks, with an occasional report of calcifi-

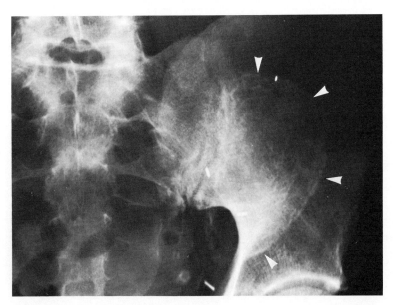

Figure 2–65. Calcification in a rejected renal transplant. Scout radiograph shows discontinuous linear calcifications of varying thickness in the cortex of the renal transplant (arrowheads). (Courtesy of Dr. Arthur Graham, Tampa, Florida.)

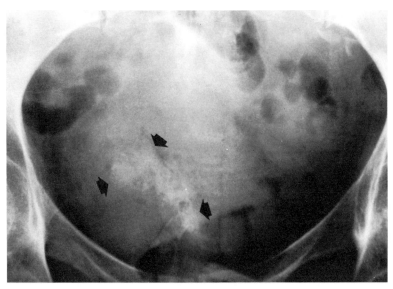

Figure 2–67. Squamous cell carcinoma of the bladder. Scout radiograph shows an ill-defined zone of hazy, amorphous calcification (arrows) in the region of the urinary bladder. (Courtesy of Dr. Stanford Goldman, Baltimore, Maryland.)

cation as early as three weeks. The calcification, which is scattered to extensive, may extend into the septa of Bertin (renal columns). Diffuse cortical calcification has also been reported in rejected renal transplants (Fig. 2–65).[26] Diffuse, mottled, or speckled calcification of the kidney, primarily in the cortex, occurs rarely in chronic glomerulonephritis (Fig. 2–66). Very few such instances have been described[27, 28] since the first report in 1947[29] of a young man, 28 years old at time of death. Autopsy showed both kidneys to be small (160 gm. and 180 gm.) with diffuse finely nodular calcification throughout the cortices, the calcifications measuring 1 to 2 mm. in diameter. Calcified casts were widely present in dilated, convoluted, and collecting tubules of the cortex.

As already mentioned in the discussion of renal concretions, the separated necrotic papillae in renal papillary necrosis may remain in the pelvicalyceal system, become encrusted by calcium salts, and take on the appearance of unusual, triangular-shaped calculi with a lucent center and completely calcific rim. However, it is also possible for the necrotic papilla to remain in place (necrosis in situ) and become calcified, the calcification being a solid mass type.

The incidence of calcification in bladder carcinomas, both transitional cell and squamous cell, is very low, about 0.5 percent.[30, 31] The roentgenologic appearance of the tumor calcification is finely granular, amorphous, or coarsely nodular, or a mixture of these types (Figs. 2–67 and 2–68). Also

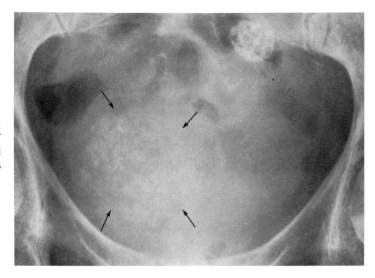

Figure 2–68. Undifferentiated carcinoma of the bladder. Scout radiograph shows a large collection of nodular, faint calcifications (arrows) in the region of the urinary bladder. The dense, mottled calcification at the brim of the pelvis is in a uterine fibroid.

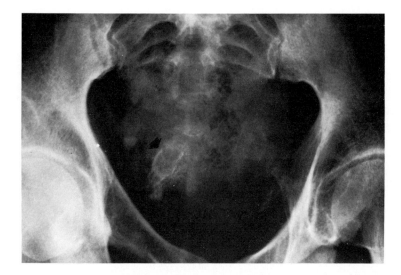

Figure 2–69. Keratinizing squamous cell carcinoma of the bladder. Scout radiograph shows several scattered zones of amorphous calcification, some with linear dense rims (arrow), in the region of the urinary bladder.

reported is hazy calcification with a dense rim (Fig. 2–69), simulating the appearance of a bladder calculus.[32] The calcification may be either within the tumor tissue, in zones of necrosis or hemorrhage, or on the surface of the tumor as encrustation of the tumor epithelium. Only a portion of the tumor mass is calcified, and the calcium may be distributed in a coarse, curvilinear pattern along the convex outer edge of the tumor. Calcification also occurs in the rare osteogenic sarcoma of the bladder, the tumor matrix producing calcium or osteoid. To be differentiated from calcification in a bladder neoplasm is postoperative ossification occurring in the scar of the muscles of the lower anterior abdominal wall (Fig. 2–70). Such heterotopic bone formation has been seen most often following sur-

gery on the stomach and urinary bladder, and when, on a radiograph, it projects over the location of the bladder, it can be confused with vesical calcification. The diagnosis can be made easily by physical examination, with the palpation of a stony hard mass or plaque in the surgical scar. Radiographically the opacity is usually much more dense and more sharply outlined than vesical neoplasm calcification. Also, obtaining a radiograph in the oblique projection demonstrates that the calcification is not related to the urinary bladder.

With urinary tract tuberculosis, renal calcification is relatively common, ureteral calcification infrequent, and bladder calcification rare. In the bladder the calcification can occur as dense clumps scattered diffusely in its wall, possibly represent-

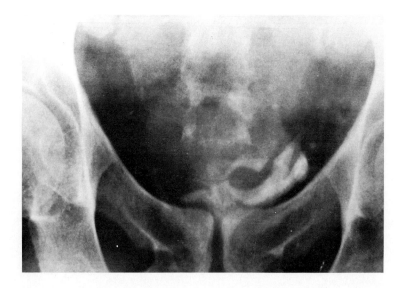

Figure 2–70. Ossification in abdominal surgical scars. Scout radiograph shows a zone of calcification (ossification), just above the symphysis and left pubic bone. The patient, a 58-year-old man, underwent cystostomy and two-stage urethroplasty for urethral stricture, about six months before.

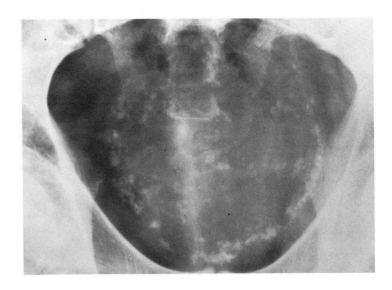

Figure 2–71. Tuberculosis of the urinary bladder. Scout radiograph shows scattered, poorly marginated calcific nodules of varying sizes in the wall of the bladder. (Courtesy of Dr. Joseph Toth, Montreal, Canada.)

ing calcification in zones of caseation in the mucosa (Fig. 2–71). Tuberculosis can also produce a faint and irregular rim of calcification in the bladder wall.[33] In addition to the conduit type of calcification that occurs in ureteral tuberculosis, already mentioned, there can, rarely, be intraluminal calcification of solid mass type.

Necrosis of the bladder mucosa from any cause in the presence of alkaline urine can result in calcium deposits on the bladder wall, the so-called alkaline encrusting cystitis.[33, 34] The initial cause for mucosal necrosis may be radiation therapy, cytoxan-induced cystitis, urinary infection, or chemical tissue toxins instilled into the bladder. The calcification consists of calcium phosphate or struvite. The highly alkaline urine can be due to infection by urea-splitting organisms or a high alkaline dietary load or renal acidification defect. The calcification is flocculent or nodular or curvilinear.

With amyloidosis, calcification infrequently occurs in the renal pelvis or ureter or bladder, being deposited submucosally and possibly related to tissue ischemia resulting from deposition of amyloid in blood vessels. The calcification is of nodular or coarsely granular type but may be linear in the ureter and renal pelvis.

REFERENCES

1. Healy T, Way BG, Grundy WR: Milk of calcium in calycine diverticula. Brit J Radiol 53:845–852, 1980.
2. Herman RD, Leoni JV, Matthews GR: Renal milk of calcium associated with hydronephrosis. Am J Roentgenol 130:572–574, 1978.
3. Benendo B, Litwak A: "Milk of calcium" in a renal cyst. Brit J Radiol 37:70–71, 1964.
4. MacMillan BG, Fritzhand MD, Spitz HB: Milk of calcium in the ureter. Radiology 127:376, 1978.
5. Friedman PS, Solis-Cohen L, Joffe SM: Urethral calculus: its roentgen evaluation. Radiology 62:248–250, 1954.
6. Paulk SC, Khan AU, Malek RS, Greene LF: Urethral calculi. J Urol 116:436–439, 1976.
7. Courey WR, Pfister RC: The radiographic findings in renal tubular acidosis: analysis of 21 cases. Radiology 105:497–503, 1972.
8. Bateson EM, Chander S: Nephrocalcinosis in cretinism. Brit J Radiol 38:581–584, 1965.
9. Chikos PM, McDonald GB: Regional enteritis complicated by nephrocalcinosis and nephrolithiasis: case report. Radiology 121:75–76, 1976.
10. Dowling RH, Rose GA, Sutor DJ: Hyperoxaluria and renal calculi in ileal disease. Lancet 1:1103–1106, 1971.
11. Fulop M, Sternlieb I, Scheinberg IH: Defective urinary acidification in Wilson's disease. Ann Intern Med 68:770–777, 1968.
12. Spitzer A, Caruthers SB, Stables DP: Radiopaque suppositories. Radiology 121:71–73, 1976.
13. Kaufman JJ: Medication simulating bladder stones. Radiology 78:227–228, 1962.
14. Kutcher R, Schneider M, Gordon DH: Calcification in polycystic disease. Radiology 122:77–80, 1977.
15. Shockman AT: The significance of ring-shaped renal calcification. J Urol 101:438–442, 1969.
16. Brown RC, Cornell SH, Culp DA: Multilocular renal cyst with diffuse calcification simulating renal-cell carcinoma. Radiology 95:411–412, 1970.
17. Phillips TL, Chin FG, Palubinskas AJ: Calcification in renal masses: an eleven-year survey. Radiology 80:786–794, 1963.
18. Cannon AH, Zanon B Jr, Karras BG: Cystic calcification in the kidney. Its occurrence in malignant renal tumors. Am J Roentgenol 84:837–848, 1960.
19. Kikkawa K, Lasser EC: "Ringlike" or "rimlike" calcification in renal cell carcinoma. Am J Roentgenol 107:737–742, 1969.
20. Daniel WW Jr, Hartman GW, Witten DM, et al: Calcified renal masses: a review of ten years experience at the Mayo Clinic. Radiology 103:503–508, 1972.
21. Jonutis AJ, Davidson AJ, Redman HC: Curvilinear calcifications in four uncommon benign renal lesions. Clin Radiol 24:468–474, 1973.

22. Hipona FA, Park WM: Calcific renal cortical necrosis. J Urol 97:961–964, 1967.
23. Lloyd-Thomas HG, Balme RH, Key JJ: Tram-line calcification in renal cortical necrosis. Brit Med J 1:909–911, 1962.
24. McAlister WH, Nedelman SH: The roentgenographic manifestations of bilateral renal cortical necrosis. Am J Roentgenol 86:129–135, 1961.
25. Whelan JG Jr, Ling JT, Davis LA: Antemortem roentgen manifestations of bilateral renal cortical necrosis. Radiology 89:682–689, 1967.
26. Harrison RB, Vaughan ED Jr: Diffuse cortical calcifications in rejected renal transplants. Radiology 126:635–636, 1978.
27. Arons WL, Christensen WR, Sosman MC: Nephrocalcinosis visible by x-ray associated with chronic glomerulonephritis. Ann Intern Med 42:260–282, 1955.
28. Palmer FJ: Renal cortical calcification. Clin Radiol 21:175–177, 1970.
29. Vaughan JH, Sosman MC, Kinney TD: Nephrocalcinosis. Am J Roentgenol 58:33–45, 1947.
30. Braband H: Incidence of urographic findings in tumours of urinary bladder. Brit J Radiol 34:625–629, 1961.
31. Miller SW, Pfister RC: Calcification in uroepithelial tumors of the bladder: report of 5 cases and survey of the literature. Am J Roentgenol 121:827–831, 1974.
32. Ferris EJ, O'Connor SJ: Calcification in urinary bladder tumors. Am J Roentgenol 95:447–449, 1965.
33. Pollack HM, Banner MP, Martinez LO, Hodson CJ: Diagnostic considerations in urinary bladder wall calcification. Am J Roentgenol 136:791–797, 1981.
34. Harrison RB, Stier FM, Cochrane JA: Alkaline encrusting cystitis. Am J Roentgenol 130:575–577, 1978.

Chapter 3

CALCIFICATIONS IN THE GALLBLADDER, LIVER, AND SPLEEN

Stephen R. Baker

CALCIFICATION IN THE BILIARY TRACT

An often observed finding on scout radiographs of the abdomen is one or more radiodensities in the right upper quadrant. Many of these are located in the biliary tract—frequently in the gallbladder lumen or wall, occasionally within the liver, and rarely in the extrahepatic biliary ducts. Calcified gallstones are, by far, the most common calcification but a number of other entities, some with a distinctive plain film appearance, will be seen from time to time. Localization of the calcification within the gallbladder or liver can usually be established with supine and oblique films. Upright and cross-table lateral projections will help determine motion and layering. Generally, with the exception of peripheral hepatic masses, it is not difficult to localize a calcified density of the liver or gallbladder. After position and mobility have been established, diagnostic possibilities will be further refined by consideration of the morphology of the calcification.

GALLBLADDER CALCIFICATION

Cholelithiasis

Gallstones may be caused by the precipitation of cholesterol salts or bilirubin pigments. A minority of calculi consists of combinations of these two constituents, and an occasional stone will be composed primarily of calcium carbonate. Roentgenographically visible calcification in gallstones almost always indicates the presence of bilirubin pigments within the calculi. Only 10 percent of gallstones are radiopaque but, considering the high

incidence of cholelithiasis in the general population, it is not surprising that calcified stones are often observed on plain films.[1] The radiographic appearance of calcified cholelithiasis is variable but in nearly every case it meets the criteria of concretion calcification. Multiple stones may be small, sometimes almost punctate in size (Fig. 1–2), while a single opaque calculus can become very large. When many stones are present they are often faceted and tend to be similar in size. However, occasionally large and small stones may be found together (Fig. 3–1). The margins of gallstones are usually smooth, and, if only an opaque rim is seen, its width is constant throughout the entirety of its

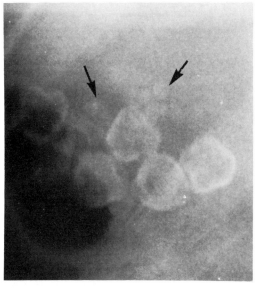

Figure 3–1. There are several faceted calcified gallstones as well as fainter, smaller calculi (arrows).

65

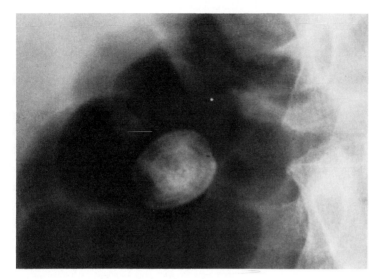

Figure 3–2. A single smooth gall-stone with concentric laminations.

perimeter. Occasionally, in obese patients or in those with faintly calcified stones, a complete rim of calcification may not be appreciated but tomographic cuts will usually reveal a continuous opaque

border. Stones will often be laminated with alternating bands of lucency and density, and nearly always the lamina will be concentric (Fig. 3–2). Infrequently, stones will have irregularly mixed dense and lucent centers (Fig. 3–3). Rarely, calcification will accumulate on only one surface of an otherwise lucent stone and will appear as an amorphous density with spicular contours. Irregularly calcified stones are most often situated in the cystic duct rather than free in the gallbladder lumen (Fig. 1–8). Gallstones should be readily distinguishable from other concretions of the right upper quadrant. Calculi in the renal pelvis and proximal ureter are often more dense and seldom have both a thin margin of calcification and a central lucency. Also, except for large stones in obstructed renal pelves, concretions in the genitourinary tract are less frequently laminated. Renal stones are more posterior and will stay near the spine on a right posterior oblique film, while the gallbladder will move far anteriorly in this projection. Rarely an appendicolith in a retrocecal appendix may simulate a gallstone both radiographically and clinically. Costal cartilage calcifications may also look like gallbladder concretions. They can usually be differentiated with oblique or inspiratory and expiratory films, which will demonstrate the fixation of cartilage calcification to ribs.

The Movement of Gallstones

The movement of gallstones during one examination or on serial films may provide diagnostic clues. A wide excursion of gallstones on recumbent and upright films or on sequential supine films suggests a large gallbladder.[2] When a stone be-

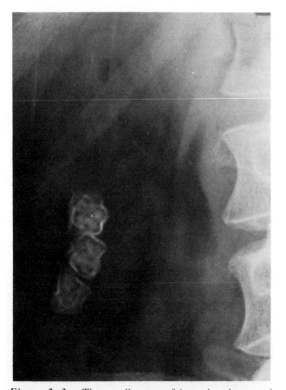

Figure 3–3. Three gallstones of irregular shape and mottled internal architecture. Note that in each stone the marginal calcification is uninterrupted.

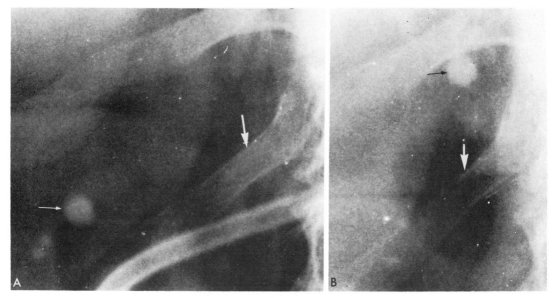

Figure 3–4. *A,* The horizontal arrow points to a gallbladder calculus and the vertical arrow indicates the 12th rib. *B,* One month later, the calculus has moved medially and superiorly and the patient has acute right upper quadrant pain. At operation an inflamed gallbladder and a single stone in the cystic duct were found. The impaction of the stone may have precipitated an attack of acute cholecystitis.

comes fixed in the cystic duct it can precipitate an attack of acute cholecystitis. Occasionally the lodging of a calculus in the cystic duct can be inferred on plain films from a lack of movement of previously mobile gallstones or from migration of a calculus superiorly and medially (Fig. 3–4, *A* and *B*).

Occasionally small stones will pass through the cystic duct into the common bile duct and then into the duodenum. While this phenomenon is infrequently observed radiologically, calculi up to 12 mm. in diameter have been known to traverse the ductal system without causing obstruction.[3,4] Stones may rarely perforate the gallbladder and be found in a number of unusual locations, including the peritoneum, anterior abdominal wall, pleura, and pericardial spaces.[5] However, the most common location of an ectopic gallstone is in the small or large intestine, where it may cause obstruction, the stone having passed into the bowel through a cholecystoenteric fistula (Fig. 4–12).

On rare occasions a gallstone will have both a calcific rim and an irregular lucent center, the interior of the stone being less dense than the surrounding soft tissues because it contains gas. The appearance of gas in a gallstone is labeled the "Mercedes-Benz" sign, so called because radiating lucencies from a central focus suggest the emblem of the motorcar (Fig. 3–5). Gallstones may have a crystalline structure which is subject to fissuring. As the stone ages, the crystalline lattice is

broken and gas present in solution in the small amount of fluid in the stone may then be liberated by shearing forces and enter the newly created internal crevices. The "Mercedes-Benz" sign is characteristically observed in noncalcific cholesterol stones, but occasionally a faint margin of calcification may occur.[6,7,8]

Cholelithiasis occurs typically in elderly and obese patients, with a distinct female preponderance. Pregnant and multiparous women have a higher incidence of gallstones than women with no children. There are also a few conditions in which the incidence of calcific stones is increased relative to gallstones of all types. In chronic hemolytic anemias red blood cell destruction leads to an elevated concentration of bilirubin in the bile and a greater risk for the development of bilirubin stones in the gallbladder. Phillips et al. found that 48 percent of patients with sickle cell anemia had cholelithiasis, and in 41 percent of this group the stones were opaque. Thus, in their series, 20 percent of all patients with sickle cell disease had calcified gallstones visible on plain films.[9]

Milk of Calcium

Milk of calcium or limy bile is an intraluminal opacity which will be seen within the gallbladder, but its appearance is different from that of a

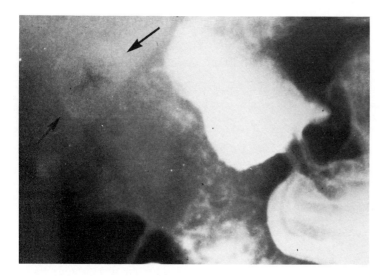

Figure 3–5. "Mercedes-Benz" sign. A faintly calcified gallstone (arrows) has central linear lucencies. The stone is lateral to the barium-filled duodenal bulb.

calculus. It may occupy the whole of the lumen and on supine films can conform to the shape of the gallbladder. There are no laminations in milk-of-calcium bile, but rounded densities representing lucent cholesterol stones may be contained within it (Fig. 3–6). Most cases of limy bile occur in patients with long-standing cystic duct obstruction,[10,11] but in rare instances the cystic duct may be patent. Chemical evaluation of the calcareous materials reveals calcium carbonate as the predominant constituent.

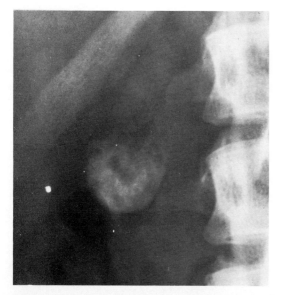

Figure 3–6. Limy bile with many filling defects caused by the coexistence of lucent cholesterol stones.

Milk of calcium consists of minute calculi of calcium carbonate held in suspension in bile. Cross-table lateral and upright films can frequently demonstrate a fluid level, as the heavier calcium carbonate calculi sink to a more dependent position in the gallbladder while clear bile layers superiorly (Fig. 3–7). Not all cases of limy bile show free mobility with change in position. Occasionally the calcification has a puttylike consistency. In this form, no fluid level will be noted. Limy bile generally should not be confused with other right upper quadrant opacities. However, if there is hepatomegaly and the gallbladder is then situated more inferiorly than normal, the semisolid limy bile could simulate a solitary calcified mesenteric lymph node. Several reports have documented the spontaneous passage of milk of calcium through the cystic and bile ducts but this is uncommon.[13,14]

Calcification in the Gallbladder Wall

Roentgenographically observed calcification in the gallbladder wall is not rare. We have collected 20 cases over a ten-year period at our institution. One retrospective review of cholecystectomy specimens revealed calcification in the gallbladder wall in 0.07 percent of patients.[15] Grossly, a calcified gallbladder is easily fractured and has a translucent bluish tint; hence the term "porcelain gallbladder." Other appellations for this condition are calcifying cholecystitis and cholecystopathia chronica calcarea. The precise mechanism for the deposition of calcium in the gallbladder wall is not known, but in all instances the gallbladder is chronically

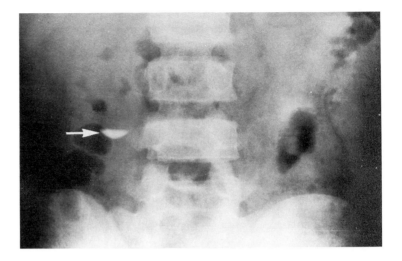

Figure 3–7. Upright view in a patient with limy bile demonstrates a clearly demarcated level caused by calcium carbonate calculi in the dependent position (arrow) and nonopaque bile above.

inflamed, the wall is thickened, the mucosa is irregularly denuded, and nearly always the cystic duct is obstructed.[16] Calcification occurs most often as strips or plaques in the muscular coat, but occasionally small concretions form in the Rokitansky-Aschoff sinuses.[17] Analysis of the dystrophic calcification in the porcelain gallbladder reveals predominantly calcium phosphate mixed with lesser amounts of calcium carbonate. Increased intraluminal pressure as a result of obstruction and the local trauma of coexistent gallstones lead to focal tissue necrosis with the laying down of calcium salts. Chronic inflammation and hemorrhage may also play a part in the calcifying process. Microscopically, calcium is deposited extracellularly in areas of hyaline degeneration (Fig. 3–8, *A* to *D*).

In a large series of patients with porcelain gallbladders, the mean age of the first appearance of calcification was 54 years, with a range of 38 to 70 years.[18] In our cases, the average age of onset was 68 and one 94-year-old patient was known to have had a calcified gallbladder for 20 years. The case of a 35-year-old female with thalassemia intermedia and a porcelain gallbladder has been reported.[19] Five times as many women as men are affected, a fact which may reflect the higher incidence of cholecystitis in females. For the most part, despite pathologic evidence of inflammation and obstruction, affected individuals are usually asymptomatic. Robb in 1928 stated:

> The calcified gallbladder is so quiescent, so unproductive of symptoms that the existence of many must never be known or even suspected and they are cast upon the rubbish heap of treasures whose only signpost is senile decay.[20]

However, another signpost of this entity has been recognized. While many calcified gallbladders are unsuspected clinically, awareness of their presence is important because they may be predisposed to gallbladder carcinoma. Etala reviewed 1,786 consecutive operations upon the biliary tract over a 23-year period. Seventy-eight patients had primary gallbladder carcinoma and 26 had calcified gallbladders. Sixteen of these, or 61 percent of patients with porcelain gallbladders, had concomitant gallbladder carcinoma. Thus, of the total of 78 malignancies of the gallbladder in this series, 16, or 20 percent, were associated with a calcified gallbladder. All tumors were invasive, and only two of 78 patients survived five years.[18] In another study, Cornell and Clark evaluated 4,271 cholecystectomies. There were 16 patients with porcelain gallbladders and two of the 16, or 12.5 percent, had primary carcinoma in the calcified gallbladder (Fig. 3–9).[21]

Because of the association between cancer of the gallbladder and calcification in the gallbladder wall, it has been suggested that patients with porcelain gallbladders should undergo prophylactic cholecystectomy. While this appears to be good advice in general, two caveats must be heeded. First, there is little known about the temporal relationship of calcifications to cancer. It is not clear how long after the gallbladder calcifies the cancer will appear or if some calcified gallbladders are destined never to harbor a malignant neoplasm. The fact that some individuals live with a calcified gallbladder for a long time suggests that there may be a differential susceptibility to carcinoma. Second, many patients with a calcified gallbladder are elderly and may not be candidates for an elective operation whose value has not been conclusively proved.

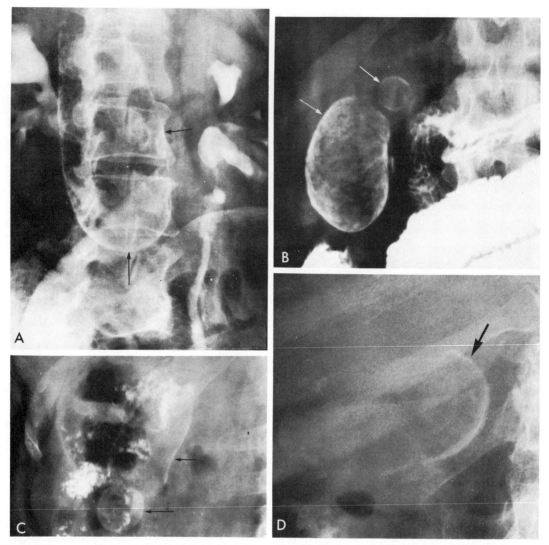

Figure 3–8. A spectrum of calcified gallbladders: *A*, An oblique film shows an enlarged porcelain gallbladder (arrows) projected over the lumbar vertebrae. *B*, Calcification in a gallbladder (lower arrow), and the cystic duct (upper arrow). *C*, Calcification in a gallbladder (upper arrow) with a Phrygian cap (lower arrow). Note the narrowing of the lumen near the fundus. The density overlying the gallbladder is unconjugated Telepaque in the large bowel. *D*, Curvilinear calcifications occupying only a part of the gallbladder wall (arrow).

The plain film appearance of a calcified gallbladder is usually distinctive, consisting of an ovoid or pear-shaped conglomeration of flakes or plaques of calcium in the right upper quadrant or right mid-abdomen. The cystic duct may sometimes be seen also as a rounded or tubular opacity, medial and superior to the gallbladder. Unlike the appearance of cysts, both the inner and outer borders of the flakes of calcification in a porcelain gallbladder can be irregular. A well-defined double track of calcium may be noted, representing opacification in both the mucosa and the muscularis. Some calcified gallbladders appear rounded, while others have a more complex shape, especially if the gallbladder contains a Phrygian cap or is otherwise folded upon itself.

Sometimes the differentiation between a porcelain gallbladder and cysts in other organs is difficult to make on a single supine film. The gallbladder will move far anteriorly on a right posterior oblique film. Calcified cysts in the liver may also be ventrally positioned. However, cystic calcifica-

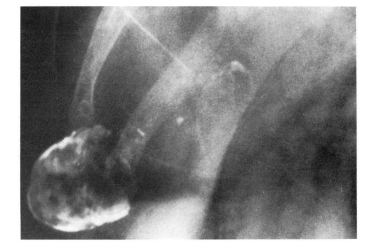

Figure 3–9. A porcelain gallbladder which at operation contained carcinoma in its proximal portion. The tumor was invasive, extending into the second portion of the duodenum. (Courtesy of Dr. Harry Miller, Bronx, New York.)

tions are almost always smooth at their outer contour, while the margins of gallbladder walls may be irregular. It is important to distinguish also a single large calculus in the gallbladder from a calcified gallbladder wall because of the association of porcelain gallbladders with carcinoma. Almost always gallstones are calcified continuously throughout the entirety of their circumference, while gallbladder wall calcification is discontinuous. However, if the gallbladder is densely calcified, the differentiation between these two entities on plain films may be difficult or even impossible.

That is not to say that patients with calcified gallbladders do not have coincident cholelithiasis. In fact, almost all of them do have at least one calculus.[22] Surprisingly, it is very uncommon to observe a stone in a calcified gallbladder. Usually, gallbladder calculi are either radiolucent or much less dense than the gallbladder wall and are therefore not seen on plain films. It is conceivable that a carcinoma growing in a porcelain gallbladder may be recognized by the resorption of calcification at the site of the enlarging tumor. However, this phenomenon has not yet been recognized radiographically. Occasionally, only a part of the gallbladder wall will become radiopaque.[23,24]

Calcification in Gallbladder Carcinoma

Carcinoma of the gallbladder is not rare; several thousand cases are reported each year. In women it is the fifth most common malignancy of the gastrointestinal tract, following cancer of the colon, pancreas, stomach, and esophagus. The tumor is rarely resectable because it has almost always spread beyond the gallbladder before it is detected. Plain film studies hardly ever give an inkling of the presence of the tumor. There have only been a few reports of calcification in a primary gallbladder carcinoma observable on plain films of the abdomen. In most cases there was fine punctate calcification in the region of the gallbladder fossa.[25,26] Scattered calcification overlying the liver shadow is not specific for a gallbladder carcinoma because it may also be found in primary hepatic tumors and metastatic disease to the liver.

CALCIFICATIONS WITHIN THE LIVER

Compared with adjacent organs, calcification in the liver is unusual. In fact, unless the opacity is highly specific for an intrahepatic entity, densities seen on supine films of the abdomen should be presumed to be outside the liver. Single concretions in this area are more likely to be in the gallbladder or kidney. Multiple concretions that cross the midline are almost always pancreatic in origin. Cystic lesions, with the exception of the cysts of *Echinococcus granulosus,* are very rare, as are calcifications in intrahepatic vessels. The vast majority of ill-defined opacities overlying the liver are calcifications in costal cartilage. Solid calcifications overlying the liver may also be in the skin, abdominal wall, lower lung fields, peritoneum, spleen, stomach, or adrenal glands. Intrahepatic solid calcification is quite uncommon and often very faint, and therefore may be missed if not searched for carefully.

Nonetheless, there is a wide spectrum of hepatic disorders that can present with radiodense lesions on plain films. Many times their appearance is suf-

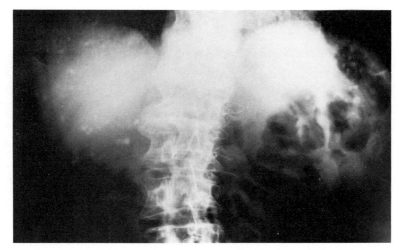

Figure 3–10. Histoplasmosis. Multiple punctate calcifications in the liver and spleen.

ficiently characteristic to suggest the diagnosis before additional procedures are undertaken. Mostly, the calcifications will be a manifestation of a quiescent condition of long standing. But on occasion plain film recognition will be of diagnostic and prognostic importance because it will reveal a rapidly progressive disease. The following discussion will proceed along the lines of the morphologic analysis offered in Chapter 1. Also included will be examples of noncalcific opacities in the liver. Pediatric diseases that may be associated with hepatic calcification will be discussed separately in Chapter 10.

MULTIPLE CALCIFICATIONS IN THE LIVER

Infectious Disease

Many conditions may produce multiple calcifications in the liver but calcified granuloma is by far the commonest worldwide. Most inflammatory granulomas represent tuberculosis or histoplasmosis infection. In endemic regions, multiple well-defined match-head-sized densities in the liver, seen along with similar calcifications in the lung and the spleen, suggest histoplasmosis (Fig. 3–10). In other locales, small rounded calcifications in the liver, even in the absence of radiographic changes in the lung or spleen, point to tuberculosis. These calcifications are mostly uniformly dense but may have a laminated or even a mottled appearance. Most of the time hepatic tuberculomas are associated with granulomas in the spleen. While there may be only a few calcified tubercles in the spleen, in the liver

they may often be too numerous to count (Fig. 3–11).

Not all multiple tuberculous granulomas are very small. Some may be greater than one cm. in diameter and have shaggy borders and dense granular interiors. For example, occasionally tuberculous nodes in the porta hepatis will calcify and may be seen in the absence of other intrahepatic densities (Fig. 8–15).[27,28]

Brucellosis is another chronic inflammatory disease that may calcify in the liver. All three species

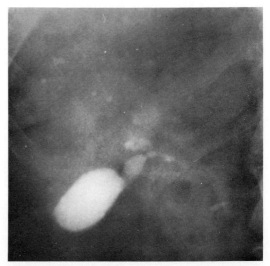

Figure 3–11. Tuberculous granulomas in the liver. A film from an oral cholecystography shows a visualized gallbladder and multiple calcified granulomas in the liver.

of brucellosis—*B. abortus, B. melitensis,* and *B. suis*—can cause infection, but only with *B. suis* are there also calcific lesions. Typically the intra-hepatic abscesses in brucellosis infection are multiple rounded densities 1 to 2 cm. in diameter which are almost always associated with calcifications of similar size and configuration in the spleen.[29]

Armillifer armillatus is a parasite found in the rain forests of West Africa and the Philippines. The adult parasite lives in the respiratory tract of pythons and other snakes. Eggs are released in snake saliva and may be inadvertently ingested by man. The larvae migrate to the peritoneum and liver where they become encysted and calcified. This infestation causes no symptoms and its only interest is its pathognomonic appearance on plain films of the abdomen. The parasites appear as C-shaped or incomplete ring shadows, 4 by 6 mm. in length by 1.5 mm. in width. Seen on end, the calcified worms look like dash marks, but almost always enough C-shaped forms are observed to make a diagnosis (Fig. 3–12).[30, 31]

Metastatic Tumor Calcification

An ever-lengthening list of metastatic tumors have been reported with multiple calcifications in the liver. The radiographic appearance ranges from dense, well-defined masses to faint multifocal collections of calcifications that may be missed on cursory examination. Calcification in metastatic disease usually occurs in large livers and in patients in whom the presence of a primary tumor is already known. However, on occasion, the recognition of hepatic calcifications may be the first sign of malignancy.

Colonic Carcinoma Metastases

The most common primary tumors with multiple calcified metastatic deposits in the liver are adenocarcinoma of the colon and serous cystadenocarcinoma of the ovary. Metastatic colonic tumors appear as faint amorphous masses of closely arrayed punctate or stippled calcifications. Sometimes the calcifications are so close together that they impart a granular appearance to areas of the liver. Calcium deposition may be a consequence of tissue necrosis but histologic specimens have shown calcification in colonic metastases in the absence of cell death. Another explanation for calcification in colonic tumors is that mucin-producing masses have an avidity for calcium. Yet this proposed mechanism does not account for all cases of radiopaque colonic metastases. In a series of 21 patients, the

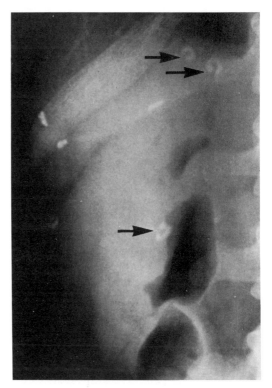

Figure 3–12. *Armillifer armillatus:* the arrows point to C-shaped encysted larvae within the liver—a pathognomonic finding. (Courtesy of Dr. Esmond Mapp, Philadelphia, Pa.)

presence of calcium in the hepatic metastases from colon malignancy was found to be unrelated to the duration of the tumor or the maturity of the malignant cells.[32] Calcified metastasis may appear along with calcification in the primary mass, but in many cases only the hepatic metastases are radiodense. The finding of finely speckled or punctate calcifications in the liver and the absence of calcifications elsewhere should suggest colonic malignancy more than any other condition.[33–35] Care must be taken in the observation of faint calcifications, for they can be simulated by such conditions as feces coated with opaque material in the adjacent hepatic flexure or transverse colon. Sequential films taken a day apart may show a change in the pattern of intraluminal densities in the large intestine, but calcific metastases in the liver will be unchanged on multiple films taken within an interval of a few days.

Metastatic Ovarian Carcinoma

Metastatic serous cystadenocarcinoma will calcify in 20 to 30 percent of cases, and infrequently

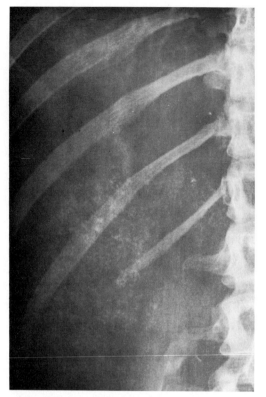

Figure 3–13. Psammomatous calcification in the liver from an ovarian cystadenocarcinoma. Multiple faint speckled opacities in the right lobe of an enlarged liver. The primary tumor in the pelvis was also calcified.

calcification will be seen over the liver on plain films.[36] Metastatic deposits can be found in the substance of the liver, on the liver capsule, or in the peritoneal cavity adjacent to the liver. Ovarian carcinoma calcification occurs in intracellular psammoma bodies and is not related to tissue necrosis. However, the radiographic appearance of individual metastasis is similar or even identical to that of colon carcinoma. Calcific densities in this tumor may be speckled, smudgy, and sometimes barely perceptible (Fig. 3–13). Calcification of the liver from serous cystadenocarcinoma of the ovary almost never occurs without coincident calcification elsewhere, usually in the peritoneum or in the primary tumor (Fig. 3–14). This is an important diagnostic consideration because few other conditions will produce simultaneous calcified peritoneal and liver metastasis. Occasionally, ovarian metastases in the liver will become more opaque after radiotherapy.

Other Metastatic Tumors to the Liver

Usually calcification in metastatic tumor to the liver is an insidious process with gradual intensification of radiopacity and visualization of an increasing number of foci on sequential films. However, calcifications may occur rapidly, with the liver becoming diffusely dense within a few weeks (Fig. 3–15). There are a number of tumors which, while rarely associated with calcific hepatic densities, can produce a characteristic picture of nodules scattered throughout the hepatic mass. Some of the nodules may be well-defined and markedly opaque, but often they have indistinct margins and may have central lucencies. Generally both lobes of the liver are involved. Included in this group of neoplasms are metastatic islet cell tumors of the pancreas,[37,38] carcinoma of the breast,[39,40] malignant melanoma,[41,42] and mesothelioma.[37,43]

Calcification in Primary Tumors

Much more rarely, primary liver tumors will calcify. Hepatocellular carcinoma and cholangiocarcinoma may be unifocal or can present as sev-

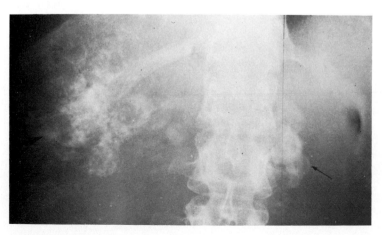

Figure 3–14. Dense psammomatous calcification in the peritoneum (small arrow) and the liver (large arrow) from an ovarian cystadenocarcinoma. Calcified peritoneal deposits, in addition to liver densities, are characteristic of this tumor.

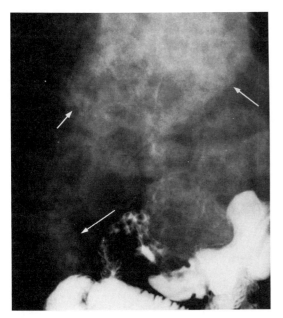

Figure 3–15. Multifocal, cloudlike calcified metastases in the liver (arrows) from a retroperitoneal mesenchymoma. One month before, there were no opacities in the liver.

eral separate masses in the hepatic parenchyma. When calcification is multiple, it is usually coarser and denser than that seen in ovarian or colonic metastases.[44,45] A rare tumor with a propensity to calcification is mixed malignant tumor of the liver. This neoplasm contains both hepatocellular and mesenchymal elements. Often patients also have pulmonary osteoarthropathy.[46] Mixed malignant tumors are slow-growing masses, appearing on plain films as calcified globular densities up to 2 cm. in diameter scattered throughout the liver.[46] If a calcified primary hepatic cancer is identified, there should be a strong suspicion of mixed malignant tumor. For example, in a series of 23 cases of calcified primary carcinomas, 13 were mixed malignant tumors.[48]

SOLITARY SOLID CALCIFICATION IN THE LIVER

Inflammatory Lesions

Several inflammatory processes may calcify in the liver as a single solid mass. While many of these entities may be common clinically, roentgenographically visible calcification in the liver is very rare. Intrahepatic tuberculous granuloma may cal-

cify, with the focus of opacity usually found in an area of caseation.[49] There have been several widely scattered reports of calcified hepatic gummas. The liver may be the organ that most often harbors a luetic mass, but calcification is exceedingly rare, and, when present, a well-defined mottled density several centimeters in diameter will be noted.[50,51] Calcified healed pyogenic and amebic abscesses have also been mentioned in case reports. Improvements in diagnosis and therapy will undoubtedly make these inflammatory masses rarer still in the years to come.[52] A parasitic disease that may cause a single focus of hepatic calcification is fascioliasis, caused by *Fasciola gigantica,* a liver fluke found in equatorial Africa and Southeast Asia. Calcification of the liver may be the result of a tissue response to migrating larvae passing into the parenchyma of the liver. Usually a single lobulated mass with irregular lucencies is seen on plain films.[53]

Metastatic Disease

Most single solid hepatic calcifications are calcified metastases. Again, the most common primary sites are the colon and the ovary (Fig. 3–16). A single focus of calcification, in fact, may be more common than multiple calcifications in the liver from these tumors. Primary hepatic tumors can also be seen as single lesions. Included in this group

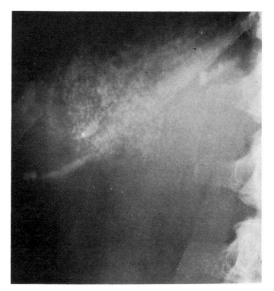

Figure 3–16. Localized granular calcification in the liver from carcinoma of the colon. The primary tumor was not calcified. (Courtesy of Dr. Larry Oliver, Reading, Pa.)

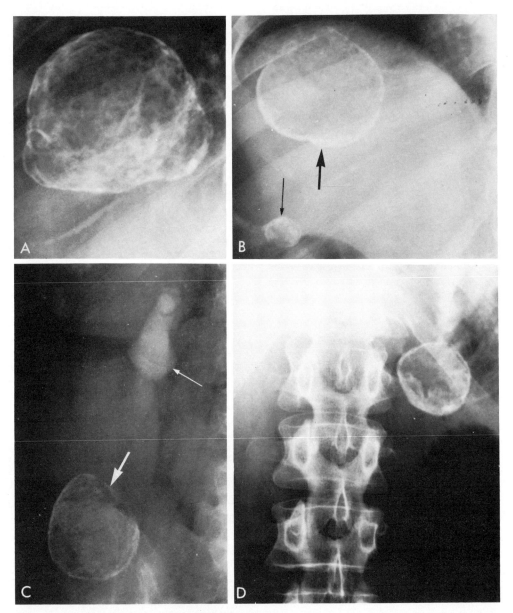

Figure 3–17. A spectrum of *Echinococcus granulosus* calcification: *A,* Dense calcification of a cyst in the liver, with slight irregularity of its inferior border. *B,* Two hepatic echinococcal cysts. The larger one (upper arrow) is not calcified circumferentially. *C,* A single echinococcal cyst attached to the capsule of the liver (lower arrow). The gallbladder is opacified with contrast material (upper arrow). Sometimes an echinococcal cyst resembles a calcified gallbladder. *D,* A cyst in the left lobe of the liver. There is dense calcification throughout the wall of the cyst.

are bile duct and hepatocellular carcinomas,[45] but, once more, the rare mixed malignant tumor of the liver is the most common primary liver carcinoma presenting as a single focus of calcification.[48]

Benign Tumors

Pathologically, the most frequent benign hepatic tumor is cavernous hemangioma. For the most part, hemangiomas are clinically silent and radiographically inconspicuous. However, they may occasionally calcify. First reported by Aspray in 1945,[54] only a few additional cases have been recorded. Most calcified hemangiomas are dense masses with irregular projections extending from the main calcific conglomeration.[55,56] Several cases have shown more than one focus of calcification. Usually, the radiographic features are not sufficiently characteristic of hemangioma to differentiate it from other solid lesions. While hemangioma calcification in other organs such as the spleen, stomach, and colon is manifested by discrete opacification in the form of phleboliths, this pattern has not yet been observed in the liver.

CYSTIC CALCIFICATION

Echinococcus Granulosus

When a calcified cystic lesion is shown to be intrahepatic, the first diagnosis must be hydatid disease. The most common type of hydatid disease is caused by the larva of *Echinococcus granulosus,* a parasite with a world-wide distribution but found most often in the Mediterranean Basin and the Middle East. Man is an accidental and intermediate host and acquires the infestation by ingestion of the echinococcal ova. The parasites enter the portal circulation after passing through the small intestinal wall. They may settle in the hepatic parenchyma or pass through the liver into the heart and other organs. In the liver, they form a cyst composed of two walls; the endocyst or inner wall contains the germinal layers, scoleces, and daughter cysts, and the encircling pericyst is composed of compressed hepatic tissue. The rimlike calcifications seen in plain films in approximately 15 percent of cases are due to calcium deposition in the pericyst.[57]

The liver is by far the most common site for infestation by *E. granulosus.* Calcification usually develops from 5 to 10 years after initial infestation and is often associated with hepatomegaly. The presence of calcium does not necessarily indicate an inactive cyst, but the heavier the calcific rim, the more likely the cyst is quiescent. While multiple calcified cysts may be observed, solitary calcification is more common. If calcified cysts are present in other organs, they are usually also present in the liver.

Radiographic Appearance

Like cystic calcification elsewhere, marginal opacities are arclike but need not be continuous. Usually the outer wall of a cyst of *Echinococcus granulosus* is smooth, but at times a portion of the wall may be irregularly calcified. Often the cyst may not be perfectly round but can be deformed by adjacent structures. Occasionally, focal intracystic densities are seen within the cyst, and at times the presence of both pericystic and smaller daughter cyst calcifications produces a polyhedral appearance (Fig. 3–17).[58]

The radiographic configuration of *Echinococcus granulosus* must be distinguished from that of the rarer but more malignant form of hydatid disease, *Echinococcus multilocularis.* This parasitic infestation is found in Northern Canada, Alaska, and Central Europe, and a definitive host is the fox. *Echinococcus multilocularis* usually does not present as cystic lesions. Rather, the pattern of calcium deposition may resemble that seen in metastatic disease with multiple solid densities that are dense and amorphous. In a few cases confluent calcifications with arcuate and solid components are observed. Calcification occurs in 68 percent of cases and in approximately 16 percent both the right and left lobes are involved simultaneously. Multiple ill-defined solid densities scattered throughout the liver in an ill patient from an endemic area with known exposure should suggest the diagnosis.[59,60]

Other Cysts

Benign noninflammatory cysts occur in the liver frequently, but these hardly ever calcify.[61] Metastases from ovarian mucinous cystadenocarcinoma calcify with both cystic and solid components (Fig. 3–18). Usually calcification is also present in the peritoneal cavity. There have been a few reports of calcification in polycystic disease and in amebic abscesses.[62] However, the finding of cystic calcification in the liver should strongly suggest hydatid disease as the cause.

CONDUIT CALCIFICATION

Vessels in the region of the liver uncommonly calcify. On rare occasions calcifications may occur

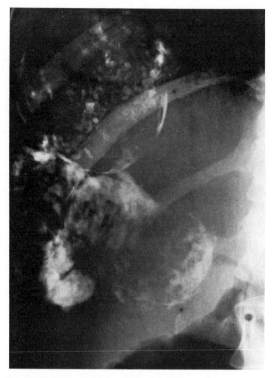

Figure 3–18. Mixed solid and cystic calcification in liver metastases from mucinous cystadenocarcinoma of the ovary. Often these tumors are associated with cystic calcification in the peritoneum. (Courtesy of Dr. Paul Cohen, Amsterdam, The Netherlands.)

in the hepatic or gastroduodenal arteries, and in both arteries aneurysms also calcify. The portal vein, the intrahepatic portion of the inferior vena cava, and the hepatic veins may also have roentgenographically visible calcium in their walls or in intraluminal clots. The topic of conduit calcification in both arteries and veins will be discussed in Chapter 7.

CALCULI IN THE LIVER AND DUCTAL SYSTEM

Stones in both the intrahepatic and extrahepatic portions of the biliary tree, exclusive of the gallbladder, are rarely seen on plain films of the abdomen. The incidence of calculi in the biliary ducts varies from less than 1 percent to 6 percent in patients with coincident cholelithiasis. However, most calculi in the biliary ducts are not radiopaque. Occasionally stones in the common hepatic or common bile duct will be seen. Usually these concretions are similar in size and shape to the coincident calculi present in the gallbladder (Fig. 3–19). At times, after cholecystectomy a calcified stone is retained in the common bile duct and can be observed on plain films of the abdomen (Fig. 3–20).

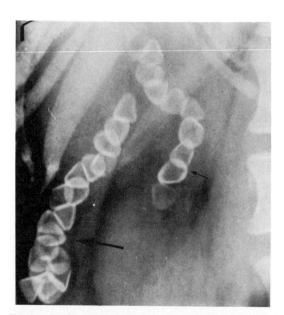

Figure 3–19. Stones in the common bile duct and gallbladder. The large arrow points to numerous gallbladder stones. The small arrow points to multiple similar calculi in the common bile duct.

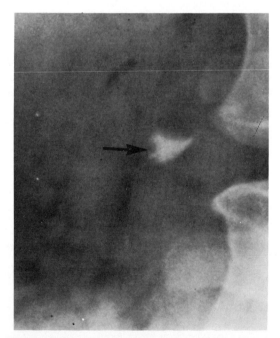

Figure 3–20. An irregularly shaped calcific stone in the common bile duct. This patient had his gallbladder removed five years before. (Courtesy of Dr. Murray Rosenberg, Bridgeport, Connecticut.)

Rarely, there can be calcified stones in the intra-hepatic radicles without cholelithiasis. In Caroli's disease, which is a congenital dilatation of the bile ducts, calculi may be seen within the dilated ductal system.[63] There have also been isolated reports of calcified stones in biliary radicles in the absence of structural abnormalities in the ducts.[64] Also, several cases of milk of calcium in the common bile duct have been noted.[65]

DIFFUSE OPACIFICATION OF THE LIVER

There are several conditions that may give an opaque cast to the liver. Most are caused by a deposition of elements other than calcium; viz., thorium, iron, and thallium sulfate.

Thorotrast

Thorotrast is a colloidal suspension of thorium dioxide which has been employed as a contrast agent. It was first available for diagnostic radiology in 1928,[66] but was banned in the early 1950's except for experimental studies which continued to at least 1964.[67] Its predominant use was as an intravascular contrast material for cerebral angiography. Almost from the outset it was a controversial agent because thorium 232 is radioactive with a half-life of 400 years and with 90 percent of its emitted radiation as alpha particles.[68] Moreover, several of the daughter products of thorium are also radioactive. Between 50,000 and 100,000 individuals have received Thorotrast and many are still alive today.

The untoward effects of thorium have been well documented. After an intra-arterial injection, thorium will deposit in the liver, spleen, and nearby lymph nodes. In the liver, Thorotrast causes hepatic fibrosis and cirrhosis and predisposes to hepatic malignancies. Half the tumors resulting from Thorotrast injection are cholangiocarcinomas and hepatic cell carcinomas. The other half are the otherwise rare angiosarcomas.[69] Soon after administration thorium will concentrate in the liver and spleen, rendering both organs diffusely dense. Over the course of several years, there is a gradual drainage of thorium from the liver to adjacent lymph nodes. The liver decreases in opacity and a feathery or lacy pattern is seen in association with dense, well-defined peripancreatic lymph nodes and a very dense small mottled spleen (Fig. 3–22).[70] The association of densities in the spleen, peripancreatic

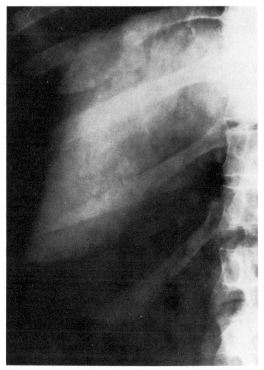

Figure 3–21. Early appearance of Thorotrast in the liver. Soon after intra-arterial administration, colloidal thorium is deposited diffusely in the liver. The liver appears homogeneously dense. This appearance is of historical interest only because the use of thorium has been discontinued.

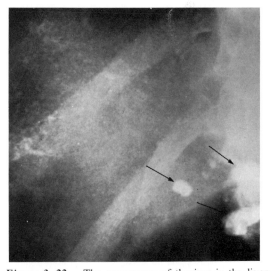

Figure 3–22. The appearance of thorium in the liver long after the administration of Thorotrast. This 45-year-old man had received Thorotrast 29 years previously. The findings of a fine linear pattern of radiodensity in the liver and dense opacification of peripancreatic lymph nodes (arrows) are characteristic.

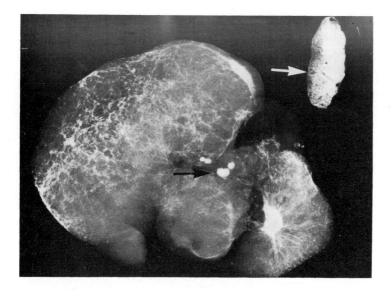

Figure 3–23. Radiograph of a section of the liver and spleen and peripancreatic nodes removed at autopsy from a patient who received Thorotrast. Observe the feathery linearity of densities in the liver, the dense nodes (black arrow), and the mottled opacity of the spleen (white arrow).

lymph nodes, and liver is pathognomonic for Thorotrast retention (Fig. 3–23).

Iron Overload

A homogeneously dense liver and spleen can be seen with iron overload owing to excessive ingestion, repeated transfusions, or idiopathic hemochromatosis.[71,72] Hepatic and splenic densities are the result of excessive deposition of hemosiderin. In primary hemochromatosis both the liver and spleen can be homogeneously opaque. Occasionally faint opacification of retroperitoneal nodes may also be seen, as these too are sites for iron deposition (Fig. 8–14). A single case of increased density simulating iron overload has been seen after the ingestion of an excessive amount of thallium sulfate.[73]

CALCIFICATION AND OTHER DENSITIES IN THE SPLEEN

Radiodensities in the spleen occupy a narrower spectrum than those in the liver (Table 3–1). While various entities may produce similar patterns of opacity in the hepatic parenchyma, the diagnostic choices are limited and usually clear-cut when one is confronted with a splenic density. Except for splenic cysts, where many different histologic types can produce identical images, radiographic appearances are frequently characteristic or even pathognomonic. Thus, plain film recognition is usually informative, and careful evaluation may obviate the necessity of further studies to reach a diagnosis.

Multiple Discrete Calcifications

Tuberculosis

Worldwide, calcified tuberculous granuloma is the most common cause of splenic densities. In one series of patients with splenic calcifications, the underlying cause was tuberculosis in over 90 percent.[74] Sweany's observation in 1940 that "The spleen is affected more with tuberculosis calcification and perhaps less with non-tubercular calcification than any other abdominal organ"[75] applies today in spite of the declining prevalence of this disease. Most often, calcified tubercles occur

Table 3–1. Radiodensities in the Spleen

I. Multiple Discrete Densities
  A. Common
    Tuberculosis
    Histoplasmosis
  B. Uncommon
    Brucellosis (*B. suis*)
  C. Rare
    Hemangioma
    Hamartoma
II. Cystic Calcification
  A. Congenital
    Epidermoid Cyst
    Cystic Hemangioma
  B. Acquired
    Echinococcus
    Hemorrhagic Cysts
    Serous Cysts
  C. Splenic Artery Aneurysms
  D. Metastatic Mucinous Adenocarcinoma of the Ovary
  E. Calcification of the Splenic Capsule
III. Solid Calcification or Opacification
    Sickle Cell Disease
    Thorotrast
    Hemosiderosis

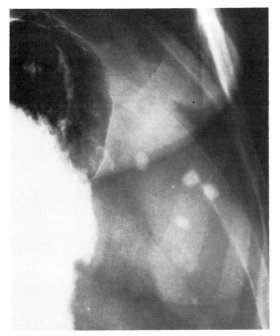

Figure 3–24. A few calcified granulomas in the spleen.

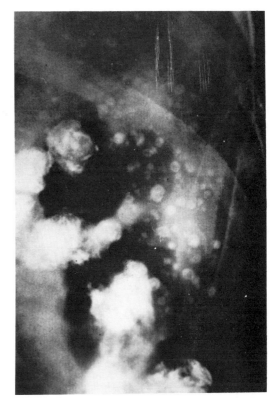

Figure 3–25. Multiple tuberculous granulomas in the spleen. Many have central lucencies and resemble phleboliths.

in a normal-sized spleen and in an asymptomatic patient. Infrequently, calcified granulomas may also be present in the liver. It takes several years for the calcification of splenic granulomas to be detected radiographically. Calcium is first laid down in the caseous center of the granuloma and then in the surrounding capsule. Consequently, younger granulomas may have irregular contours, but the more mature foci of inflammation have smoother outlines. Most calcifications in tuberculous infections of the spleen are approximately 5 mm. in diameter (Fig. 3–24), but the size of multiple opacities is not uniform. Generally, only a few calcifications are found in the spleen but this is not an inviolate rule; in some cases, granulomas may be numerous (Fig. 3–25).[76]

Histoplasmosis

In endemic areas, such as the Ohio Valley, the predominant cause of multiple discrete opacities in the spleen is histoplasmosis. In 44 percent of spleens observed at postmortem examinations in Cincinnati, Ohio, calcified granulomas were present, compared with 30 percent in splenic specimens removed at autopsy in New York City and 2 percent in specimens obtained in Rotterdam, The Netherlands.[77] Microscopic examination revealed evidence of histoplasmosis in most of the Cincin-

nati cases. The occurrence of well-defined multiple calcifications in the spleen correlates well with positive skin tests for histoplasmosis in regions where the disease is common.[78]

As in tuberculosis, the granulomas in the spleen may caseate at their centers and calcium may be laid down within the central mass of necrotic and infected tissue. Calcium may also deposit at the fibrous margins of the granuloma. Often there is a noncalcified band separating these two foci of calcification. Occasionally the granuloma may appear as a laminated concretion, which is a distinctive feature in histoplasmosis. However, not all calcified granulomas have this characteristic appearance. In contrast to tuberculosis, there are almost always many calcifications in the spleen (Fig. 3–26). Typically, they are round, smooth, and less than 5 mm. in diameter and often associated with similar calcifications in the liver and chest.[79]

Brucellosis

Brucellosis is a third infectious disease with a predilection for splenic calcifications. Untreated

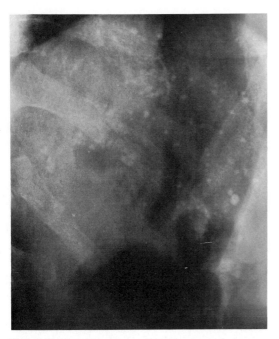

Figure 3–26. Histoplasmosis. Many calcified granulomas are scattered throughout the spleen.

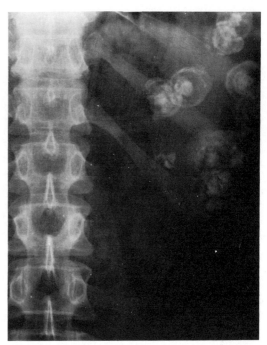

Figure 3–27. Calcified *Brucella suis* abscesses in the spleen. There are multiple "target" lesions with marginal calcifications and dense centers. (Courtesy of K. C. Demetropoulos, Detroit, Michigan. Reprinted with the permission of the Journal of the Canadian Association of Radiologists.)[82]

patients may have repeated episodes of fever and malaise, alternating with asymptomatic intervals. The disease may be caused by three species of Brucella, but as in the liver, only *Brucella suis* will cause calcification. Interestingly, the calcifications are often so distinctive in brucellosis that a plain film diagnosis can be made with assurance. Granulomas contain a flocculent central nidus averaging 5 to 10 mm. in diameter. Emanating from the central focus are irregular linear densities, and a separate encircling margin of calcification can be seen. In some cases the calcification represents a snowflake or a target (Fig. 3–27). Calcified granulomas are multiple, never confluent, and usually associated with splenomegaly.[80-83]

Tumors of the Spleen

In the older literature, frequent mention was made of the presence of phleboliths in the spleen. Both tuberculosis and histoplasmosis may simulate the appearance of phleboliths closely. Histologic examination almost always reveals that what resemble phleboliths roentgenographically are really granulomas. Thus, the presence of phleboliths in the spleen in the absence of a mass lesion should be considered very rare. Even in hemangioma, which is the most common benign tumor of the spleen, the observation of radiographically visible phleboliths is very uncommon. Most hemangiomas of the spleen are small and undetectable on plain films.[84] When phlebolithic calcification does occur, the multiple densities usually have central lucencies and are greater than 5 mm. in diameter (Fig. 1–10). In these patients, the tumors are large and there is splenomegaly.

Hamartomas are very rare tumors of the spleen which are occasionally included with hemangiomas in a classification of splenic neoplasms, but they should really be considered as a separate entity. Since the number of hamartomas are so few, it is not clear if they have a characteristic pattern of calcification.[85]

CYSTIC LESIONS IN THE SPLEEN

There are many kinds of splenic cysts. A few, such as epidermoid cysts and cystic hemangiomas, are congenital.[86,87] Many are acquired either as a result of parasitic infestation or as a consequence of trauma. Several categorizations have been proposed, based on such factors as cytology, histology, or etiology. The classification offered in Table 3–1 considers only those entities that have been

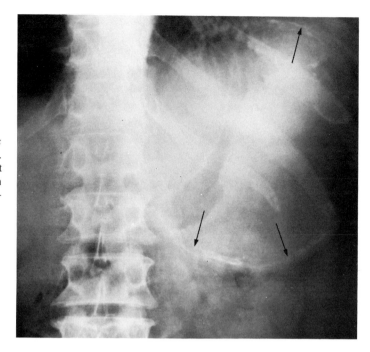

Figure 3–28. Large *Echinococcus granulosus* cyst (arrows) in the spleen. The etiology of a calcified splenic cyst usually cannot be determined by plain films alone in the absence of other lesions.

reported with calcification observable on plain films.

Two-thirds of all reported splenic cysts are caused by *Echinococcus granulosus* (Fig. 3–28).[88] Cystic lesions may occur in the spleen in the absence of cysts elsewhere, but most often the liver is also involved. The spleen is the second most common site of calcification with *Echinococcus granulosus.* Usually the walls of the cysts are heavily calcified and the spleen is enlarged. Pathologically, multiple cysts are more common but usually only one will calcify.[89]

Of the remainder of calcified acquired cysts, 80 percent are hemorrhagic cysts[90] usually secondary to trauma.[91] The mechanism of formation is unclear, but it may be the result of liquefaction of a hematoma. It is not known why some traumatized spleens will rupture and others form cysts. Cystic degeneration is a rare event, considering the large number of cases of splenic trauma.[92] Serous cysts, which make up approximately 20 percent of all non-echinococcal acquired cysts of the spleen, also have a traumatic etiology (Fig. 1–18). Like hemorrhagic cysts they have a fibrous lining.[93] Perhaps serous cysts are hemorrhagic cysts in which the blood has been totally resorbed and only a fibrous wall and clear fluid remain. Hemorrhagic and serous cysts are found most often in women of childbearing age for reasons which remain obscure.

A small percentage of cystic lesions are true cysts with epithelial or endothelial linings and these may

calcify infrequently. Calcified epidermoid cysts and cystic hemangiomas have been observed on occasion but are much less common than acquired cysts. For the most part, all splenic cysts either are asymptomatic or cause vague sensations of discomfort or fullness in the left upper quadrant. They can grow to large size before detection. Sometimes plain films of the abdomen obtained for other reasons may reveal calcified cysts that were completely unexpected.

Radiographically, calcifications in the various types of splenic cysts have no reliable distinguishing characteristics. Hydatid cysts look remarkably similar to hemorrhagic or epidermoid cysts. When small, splenic cysts tend to calcify circumferentially with a continuous smooth outer wall and a less distinct and more irregular inner wall. Large cysts may demonstrate only interrupted arcs of opacity, but heavily calcified margins can also be seen in cysts of massive dimensions (Fig. 3–29).[94]

The differential diagnosis of calcified splenic cysts includes many other conditions. Echinococcal cyst of the left lobe of the liver can simulate a splenic mass. Enlargement of the liver tends to displace the stomach laterally, while tumors of the spleen deviate the stomach toward the midline. Calcified renal tumors are usually smaller than splenic cysts. Mesenteric cysts can elevate the transverse colon and splenic flexure. Splenic cysts usually enlarge the spleen and displace adjacent organs from it. For example, calcified splenic masses

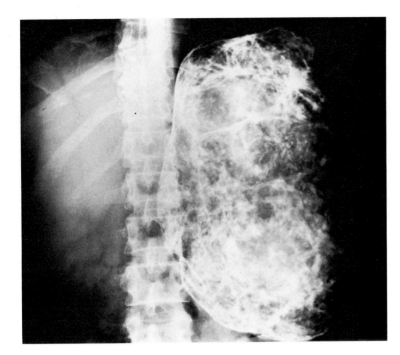

Figure 3–29. Enormous, heavily calcified splenic cyst of unknown etiology.

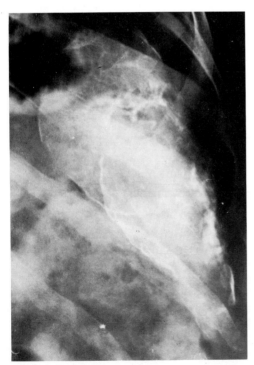

Figure 3–30. Extensive calcification involving the splenic capsule.

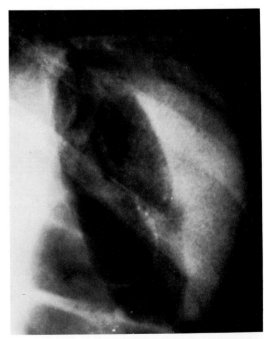

Figure 3–31. Dense mottled calcification of the spleen in a patient with sickle cell anemia. Subsequent films revealed that the spleen had decreased in size and had become denser.

are apt to displace the kidney medially and inferiorly and depress the splenic flexure. Understanding the principle of displacement by enlarging organs can help determine if a calcified mass in the left upper quadrant is indeed in the spleen. Calcified pancreatic cysts are extremely rare but may not be differentiable from splenic cysts. On plain film examination calcified aneurysms of the distal splenic artery can be misinterpreted as splenic cysts. It is very rare for splenic cysts to be multiple[95] but more common for splenic artery aneurysms to have several contiguous annular calcifications.[96] The absence of splenomegaly and the presence of calcification in other parts of the artery also suggest splenic artery aneurysms.

There is one other type of arcuate calcification that is always multiple in the spleen, i.e., metastatic mucinous adenocarcinoma of the ovary. This tumor may involve the spleen with cystic deposits either on the surface or within the organ. Usually calcification is also present in metastases in the peritoneal cavity and in the liver.[97]

Calcification in the margin of the spleen is rare. It usually occurs as a result of subcapsular hematoma formation. The radiographic appearance can simulate that of calcified cysts if only a small portion of the capsule is radiopaque. However, if most of the spleen is enveloped by hematoma, smooth rimlike calcification will assume the appearance of the spleen itself (Fig. 3–30).

DIFFUSE OPACIFICATION OF THE SPLEEN

Diffuse opacification of the spleen can be seen in only a few conditions. In each of these the appearance of the spleen is characteristic, and ancillary radiologic findings in other organs will usually permit a definitive diagnosis on plain films.

Sickle Cell Disease

Opacification of the spleen has been observed in 2 to 10 percent of adolescent and young adult patients with homozygous sickle cell anemia.[98,99] Increased radiodensity in the spleen is probably due to a combination of hemosiderin deposition, which gives a generalized increased density to the spleen, and focal deposition of calcium in areas of hemorrhage, infarct, and fibrosis.

The exact relationship between the laying down of calcium and the presence of hemorrhage and scarring is unclear. The spleen may appear diffusely opaque, but most often multiple 1 to 2 mm. punctate densities give the spleen a coarsely granular appearance (Fig. 3–31).[100–102] Opacification can occur initially in both large and small spleens, and as the spleen decreases in size, it usually becomes more dense.[103] Rarely, in adults with a mixed hemoglobinopathy such as thalassemia S, the spleen will become opaque but remain enlarged.[104] Almost always splenic densities and sickle cell anemia are associated with other changes characteristic of the disease, such as aseptic necrosis of the humeral heads, cardiomegaly, and gallstones.

Increased Density Due to Iron

In patients overloaded with iron because of idiopathic hemochromatosis, excessive ingestion, or repeated transfusions, hemosiderin will be laid down in the spleen. As in sickle cell disease, the

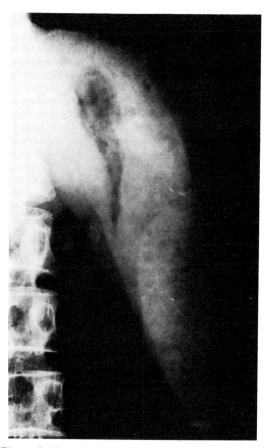

Figure 3–32. A patient who recently received Thorotrast. The spleen is enlarged and diffusely radiopaque.

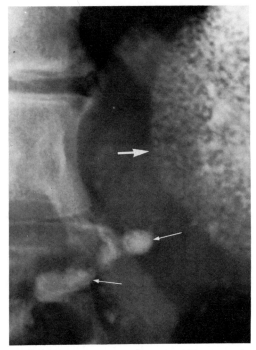

Figure 3–33. A patient who received Thorotrast long ago. The spleen is very dense and mottled (large arrow) and there is opacification of peripancreatic lymph nodes (small arrows).

opacification involves the entire spleen. The roentgenographic appearance is a generalized homogeneous density without the punctate granularity seen in sickle cell disease. Usually the spleen is enlarged at initial presentation and remains big. There may be a similar increase in density of the liver and retroperitoneal lymph nodes.

Thorotrast

After intravascular administration, Thorotrast will be retained by the spleen (Fig. 3–32). The roentgenographic appearance is pathognomonic. Initially the spleen is homogeneously dense. After several years, the density becomes mottled and there are associated opacifications of peripancreatic lymph nodes as well as very fine feathery density throughout the liver (Fig. 3–33).[105]

REFERENCES

1. McNulty JG: Radiology of the Liver. Philadelphia, WB Saunders Company, 1977.
2. Young BR: Roentgen examination of the acute abdomen—the Carman Lecture. Radiology 64:481–497, 1955.
3. Richards P: Spontaneous migration of gallstones. N Engl J Med 266:299–300, 1962.
4. Hansson K, Lundh G, Ranberg L: Spontaneous and total disappearance of stones from the gallbladder. Acta Chir Scand 127:176–180, 1964.
5. Scanlan RL, Young BR: The roentgen diagnosis of gallbladder and biliary tract disease without cholecystography. Am J Roentgenol 72:639–643, 1954.
6. Cancelmo JJ: Stellate fissuring in gallstones. Radiology 64:420–423, 1955.
7. Meyers MA, O'Donohue N: The Mercedes-Benz sign—Insight into the dynamics of formation and disappearance of gallstones. Am J Roentgenol 119:63–70, 1973.
8. Wright FW: The 'Jack Stone' or 'Mercedes-Benz' Sign—A new theory to explain the presence of gas within fissures in gallstones. Clin Radiol 28:469–473, 1977.
9. Phillips JC, Gerald BE: The incidence of cholelithiasis in sickle cell disease. Am J Roentgenol 113:27–28, 1971.
10. Phemister DB, Rewbridge AG, Rudisill H Jr: Calcium carbonate gallstones and calcification of the gallbladder following cystic duct obstruction. Ann Surg 94:493–516, 1931.
11. Knutsson F: On limy bile. Acta Radiol 14:453–462, 1933.
12. Ochsner SF, Orgeron EA: Opaque gallstones showing pliability during cholecystographic visualization. Am J Roentgenol 82:1024–1026, 1959.
13. Marquis JR, Densler J: The disappearing limy bile syndrome. Radiology 94:311–312, 1970.
14. Schwartz A, Feuchtwanger M: Radiographic demonstration of spontaneous disappearance of limy bile. Gastroenterology 40:809–812, 1961.
15. Ochsner SF, Carrera GM: Calcification of the gallbladder ("Porcelain Gallbladder"). Am J Roentgenol 89:847–853, 1963.
16. Ochsner SF: Intramural lesions of the gallbladder. Am J Roentgenol 113:1–10, 1971.
17. Berk RM, Armbruster TG, Saltzstein S: Carcinoma in the porcelain gallbladder. Radiology 106:29–31, 1973.
18. Etala E: Cancer de la vesicula biliar. Prensa Med Argent 49:2283–2299, 1962.
19. Aksoy M, Camli N, Dirvana S et al: "Porcelain Gallbladder" in a case of thalassemia intermedia. Radiology 95:265–266, 1970.
20. Robb JJ: Observations on calcification of the gallbladder—with the presentation of a case. Brit J Surg 16:114–119, 1928.
21. Cornell CM, Clarke R: Vicarious calcification involving the gallbladder. Ann Surg 149:267–272, 1959.
22. Polk H C Jr: Carcinoma of the calcified gallbladder. Gastroenterology 50:582–585, 1966.
23. Gunn A: Calcified cyst attached to the gallbladder. Brit J Radiol 39:68–69, 1966.
24. Lambert Leder G, Lombard R: Diverticule calcifié du bas fond vésiculaire. Acta Gastroint Belg 31:175–181, 1968.
25. Rogers LF, Lastra MP, Lin KJ et al: Calcifying mucinous adenocarcinoma of the gallbladder. Am J Gastroenterol 59:441–445, 1973.
26. Parker GW, Joffe M: Calcifying primary mucus-producing adenocarcinoma of the gallbladder. Brit J Radiol 45:468–469, 1972.
27. Astley R, Harrison N: Miliary calcification of the liver. Report of a case. Brit J Radiol 22:723–724, 1949.
28. McCullough JAL, Sutherland CG: Intra-abdominal calcification: interpretation of its roentgenologic manifestations. Radiology 36:450–451, 1941.
29. Spink WW: Suppuration and calcification of the liver and spleen due to long-standing infection with *Brucella suis*. N Engl J Med 257:209–210, 1957.

30. Bretland PM: *Armillifer armilatus* infestation—Radiologic diagnosis in two Ghanaian soldiers. Brit J Radiol 35:603–608, 1962.

31. Steinbach HL, Johnstone HG: The roentgen diagnosis of armillifer infection (porocephalus) in man. Radiology 68:234–237, 1957.

32. Green PA: Hepatic calcification in cancer of the large bowel. Am J Gastroenterol 55:466–470, 1971.

33. Miele AJ, Edmonds HW: Calcified liver metastases; A specific roentgen diagnostic sign. Radiology 80:779–785, 1963.

34. Appleby A, Hackins DM: Calcification in hepatic metastases. Brit J Radiol 31:449–450, 1958.

35. Wells J: Calcified liver metastases. N Engl J Med 253:639–640, 1956.

36. Fred AL, Eiband JM, Collins LC: Calcifications in intra-abdominal and retroperitoneal metastases. Am J Roentgenol 91:138–148, 1964

37. Darlak JT, Moskowitz M, Kattan KE: Calcifications in the liver. Radiol Clin North Am 18:209–219, 1981.

38. Zimmer FF: Islet-cell carcinoma treated with alloxan: Associated with calcified hepatic metastases and thyrotoxic myopathy. Ann Intern Med 61:543–549, 1964.

39. Shonfeld ED, Guarino AV, Bessolo RJ: Calcified hepatic metastases from carcinoma of the breast. Case report and review of the literature. Radiology 106:303–304, 1973.

40. Saghatoeslami M, Khodarghmi K, Epstein BS: Calcified intra-hepatic metastases from carcinoma of the breast. JAMA 181:1139–1140, 1962.

41. Maddock WG, Lien RM: Calcified liver nodules from metastatic primary melanoma: Ocular primary 15 years previously. Quart Bull Northwestern Univ Med School 29:374–378, 1955.

42. Karras BG, Cannon AA, Zanon B Jr: Hepatic calcification. Acta Radiol 57:458–468, 1962.

43. Persaud V, Bateson EM, Bankay CD: Pleural mesothelioma associated with massive hepatic calcification and unusual metastases. Cancer 26:920–928, 1970.

44. Allen RW, Holt AH: Calcification in primary liver carcinoma. Am J Roentgenol 99:50–52, 1967.

45. Meyers MA: Calcifications in cholangio-carcinoma. Brit J Radiol 41:65–66, 1968.

46. Ludwig J, Grier MW, Hoffman HM et al: Calcified mixed malignant tumors of the liver. Arch Pathol 99:162–166, 1975.

47. Morgan AG, Walker WC, Mason MK et al: A new syndrome associated with hepato-cellular carcinoma. Gastroenterology 63:340–354, 1972.

48. Hall PM, Winkelman EI, Hauk WA et al: Calcification in the liver, an unusual feature of ductal cell hepatic carcinoma. Cleveland Clin Quart 37:93–105, 1970.

49. Zipser RD, Rau JE, Ricketts RR et al: Tuberculous pseudotumor of the liver. Am J Med 61:946–951, 1976.

50. Alergant CD. Gumma of the liver with calcification. AMA Arch Intern Med 98:340–343, 1956.

51. Haddow RA, Kemp-Harper RA: Calcification in the liver and portal system. Clin Radiol 18:225–236, 1967.

52. D'Alessandro A, Leja J, Vera MA: Cystic calcifications of the liver in Colombia; echinococcus or calcified abscesses. Am J Trop Med 15:908–913, 1966.

53. Grange D, Dhumeaux D, Couzineau P, et al: Hepatic calcification due to *Fasciola gigantica*. Arch Surg 108:113–115, 1974.

54. Aspray M: Calcified hemangioma of the liver. Am J Roentgenol 53:446–453, 1945.

55. Muehlbauer MA, Farber MG: Hemangioma of the liver: Some interesting clinical and radiological observations. Am J Gastroenterol 45:355–365, 1966.

56. Plachta A: Calcified cavernous hemangioma of the liver: Review of the literature and report of 13 cases. Radiology 79:783–788, 1962.

57. Gonzalez LR, Marcos J, Illanos M et al: Radiologic aspects of hepatic echinococcosis. Radiology 130:21–27, 1979.

58. Bonakdarpour A: Echinococcus disease: Report of 112 cases from Iran and a review of 611 cases from the United States. Am J Roentgenol 99:660–667, 1967.

59. Thompson WM, Chisholm OP, Tank R: Plain film roentgenographic findings in alveolar hydatid disease—*Echinococcus multilocularis*. Am J Roentgenol 116:345–358, 1972.

60. Heilbrun M, Klein AJ: Massive calcification of the liver: Case report with a discussion of its etiology on the basis of alveolar hydatid disease. Am J Roentgenol 55:189–192, 1946.

61. Caplan LN, Simon M: Non-parasitic cysts of the liver. Am J Roentgenol 96:421–428, 1966.

62. Kutcher R, Schneider M, Gordon DH: Calcification in polycystic disease. Radiology 122:77–80, 1977.

63. Mathias K, Waldman D, Daikler G: Intrahepatic cystic bile duct dilatation and stone formation. A new case of Caroli's disease. Acta Hepato Gastro 25:30, 1978.

64. Bassler A, Peters AG: Hepatic calculi. Am J Med Sci 214:427–430, 1947.

65. Simmonds HT Jr: Milk of calcium bile in the common duct. Am J Roentgenol 78:1020–1023, 1957.

66. Mackenzie KGF, Preston CD, Stewart W et al: Thorotrast retention following angiography. A case report with postmortem studies. Clin Radiol 13:157–162, 1962.

67. Talley RW, Poznanski AK, Heslin JH et al: Laminagrams of Thorotrast-opacified liver in evaluation of chemotherapy for metastatic cancer. Cancer 17:1214–1219, 1964.

68. Janower ML, Miettimen OS, Flynn MJ: Effects of long term thorotrast exposure. Radiology 103:13–20, 1972.

69. Curry JL, Johnson WG, Feinberg DH et al: Thorium induced hepatic hemangioendothelioma. Am J Roentgenol 125:671–677, 1975.

70. Kuisk H, Sanchez JS, Mizuno N: Colloidal thorium dioxide (Thorotrast) in radiology with emphasis on hepatic cancerogenesis. Am J Roentgenol 99:463–475, 1967.

71. Joffe N: Siderosis in the South African Bantu. Brit J Radiol 37:200–209, 1964.

72. Shambron E, Zheutlin M: Radiologic signs in hemosiderosis. JAMA 168:33–35, 1958.

73. Grunfeld O, Aldana L, Himostroza G: Radiologic aspects of thallium poisoning. Radiology 80:847–849, 1963.

74. Gray EF: Calcifications of the spleen. Am J Roentgenol 51:336–351, 1944.

75. Sweany HC: On the nature of calcified lesions with special reference to those in the spleen. Am J Roentgenol 44:209–229, 1940.

76. Massoud MG, Shafei AZ: Calcified miliary tuberculosis of the spleen. Brit J Radiol 30:101–102, 1957.

77. Schwarz J, Silverman FM, Adriano SM, et al: The relationship of splenic calcifications to histoplasmosis. N Engl J Med 252:887–889, 1955.

78. Okudaira M, Straub M, Schwarz J: The etiology of discrete splenic and hepatic calcification in an endemic area of histoplasmosis. Am J Pathol 39:599–611, 1961.

79. Serviansky B, Schwarz J: The incidence of splenic calcification in positive reactors to histoplasmosis and tuberculin. Am J Roentgenol 76:53–59, 1956.

80. Yow EM, Brennan J, Nathan MH et al: Calcified granulomata of the spleen in longstanding brucellar infection. Ann Intern Med 55:307–313, 1961.

81. Arcomano JP, Pizzolato MF, Singer R et al: A unique type

of calcification in chronic brucellosis. Am J Roentgenol 128:135–137, 1977.

82. Demetropoulos KC, Lindenauer SM, Rapp R et al: Target
calcification of the spleen in chronic brucellosis
(*Brucella suis*). J Canad Assn Radiol 25:161–163,
1974.

83. Case Records of the Massachusetts General Hospital. Case
(42461) N Engl J Med 255:950–962, 1956.

84. Benjamin BI, Mohler DH, Sandusky WR: Hemangioma of
the spleen. Arch Intern Med 115:280–284, 1965.

85. Komaki S, Gombas OF: Angiographic demonstration of a
calcified splenic hamartoma. Radiology 121:77–78,
1976.

86. Greene WW, Foroughi E: Calcified epidermoid cyst of the
spleen. Amer Surgeon 29:613–616, 1963.

87. Coleman WO: Epidermoid cyst of the spleen: Report of
two cases. Am J Surg 100:475–479, 1960.

88. Witter JA, Brekke VG: Solitary calcified cyst of the spleen.
Am J Surg 76:315–318, 1948.

89. Soler-Bechara J, Soscia JL: Calcified echinococcus (hydatid) cyst of the spleen. JAMA 187:62–63, 1964.

90. Fowler RH: Collective review—non-parasitic benign cystic tumors of the spleen. Surg Gynecol Obstet 96:209–
215 1953.

91. Forde WJ, Finby N: Splenic cysts. Clin Radiol 12:49–54,
1961.

92. Asbury GF: Calcified pseudocyst of the spleen. AMA Arch
Surg 76:148–150, 1958.

93. McClure RD, Altemeier WA: Cysts of the spleen. Ann
Surg 116:98–102, 1942.

94. Culver G, Becker C, Koenig EC: Calcified cystic tumor of
the spleen. Radiology 39:62–68, 1942.

95. Kierulf E: A calcified cyst of the spleen, demonstrated
roentgenographically. Acta Radiol Scand 27:43–46,
1946.

96. Riemenschneider PA: Multiple large aneurysms of the
splenic artery. Am J Roentgenol 74:872–873, 1955.

97. Papavasiliou CG: Calcification in secondary tumors of the
spleen. Acta Radiol 51:278–281, 1959.

98. Macht SH, Roman PW: Radiologic changes in sickle cell
anemia. Radiology 51:697–707, 1948.

99. Ehrenpreis B, Schwinger HH: Sickle cell anemia. Am J
Roentgenol 68:28–36, 1952.

100. Jacobson G, Zucherman SD: Roentgenographically demonstrable splenic deposits in sickle cell anemia. Am
J Roentgenol 76:47–52, 1956.

101. Hemley SD, Mellins HZ, Finby N: Punctate calcifications
in the spleen in sickle cell anemia. Am J Med 34:483–
485, 1963.

102. Seligman BR, Rosner F, Smulewicz JJ: Splenic calcification in sickle cell anemia. Am J Med Sci 265:495–
499, 1973.

103. Smith EH, Balthazar E, Moskowitz H: Roentgenographic
signs of splenic atrophy in sickle cell disease. J Canad
Assn Radiol 23:133–135, 1972.

104. Whitley JE, Cooper HW, Hayes DM et al: Radiodensities
of the spleen associated with thalassemia-S disease.
Am J Roentgenol 91:900–902, 1964.

105. Samuel E: Thorotrast spleen. Brit J Radiol 28:204–205,
1955.

Chapter 4

CALCIFICATIONS AND OTHER DENSITIES IN THE STOMACH AND INTESTINES

Stephen R. Baker, M.D.

Many widely varying conditions in the gastrointestinal tract may be recognized on plain films by the presence of single or multiple opacities. The lumina of the stomach, small intestine, appendix, and large intestine should, in a sense, be considered extracorporeal, and these organs may contain pills, bones, and other ingested foreign bodies. Calculi may form in the intestines and appendix or enter the gastrointestinal tract through a fistula. An awareness of the appearance of the various types of gastrointestinal concretions and other radiodensities may be crucial for the diagnosis and management of serious abdominal disorders. Also, the walls of these hollow organs can be the site of calcification in both benign and malignant masses, some of which have a characteristic radiographic appearance on plain films.

In the discussion that follows, for both the stomach and the intestines, a distinction will be made

Table 4–1. Calcifications and Other Densities in the Stomach

Mural Calcification
Carcinoma of the stomach
Gastric leiomyoma
Hemangioma
Calcified duplication cyst
Intraluminal Densities
Foreign bodies
Pills
Gallstones
Opaque liquid medication coating bezoars

between intraluminal and extraluminal densities. Little attention will be given to readily recognizable foreign bodies. Rather, the focus will be on densities that are not so clearly discerned. Emphasis will be placed on pattern recognition and clinical implications of the various densities both endogenously produced and introduced from outside.

CALCIFICATIONS AND OTHER OPACITIES IN THE STOMACH

Mural Lesions

Calcification in the wall of the stomach is rarely encountered. The most common cause of such calcification is adenocarcinoma of the stomach. In recent years, there has been a growing list of small series and single case reports of calcified gastric malignancy. It is striking how similar all the cases appear. On plain films the gastric air shadow is often narrowed and a large infiltrating mass is suggested by numerous homogeneously punctate or granular calcifications which are most often faintly opaque (Fig. 4–1). Occasionally the calcifications may be so closely spaced that they give a hazy, poorly defined pattern of opacity, but usually individual densities can be recognized.[1] Calcification in adenocarcinoma of the stomach is rarely flocculent or streaky, a diagnostic point which serves to differentiate it from the less commonly observed calcified gastric leiomyoma.

Calcified gastric carcinoma, also known as pet-

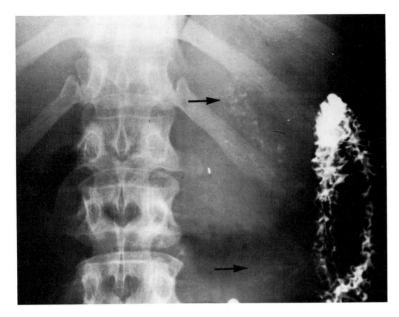

Figure 4–1. Calcified adenocarcinoma of the stomach. The arrows point to two areas with mottled calcification within the tumor. Almost the whole stomach is infiltrated with carcinoma. (Courtesy of Dr. D. Randall Radin, Bronx, New York.)

rified stomach, almost always is a large lesion when discovered.[2,3] It generally behaves no differently from other bulky stomach carcinomas. It can metastasize to the liver but calcification in hepatic deposits is extremely rare. While initial reports suggested that calcified tumors appear in younger individuals, later series indicated that the age of onset is roughly the same as that of gastric adenocarcinomas in general.[4–7] The cause of calcification is still a matter of conjecture. On microscopic section, calcium salts are extracellular and are usually found in necrotic sections of the tumor. According to Gemmell, areas of ischemia are associated with a diminution of cellular respiration and an increase in carbon dioxide concentration and alkalinity.[8] Dystrophic calcification occurs in the petrified stomach, supposedly because the tumor has outgrown its blood supply.[9] Hence, in the well-vascularized stomach, calcification does not occur until the tumor becomes large. However, this theory fails to account for the fact that most large gastric carcinomas may grow rapidly and contain areas of necrosis and yet fail to calcify.

Batlan and others, noting that calcification occurs only in mucin-producing tumors, offer a different explanation.[10,11] They claim that mucin is a glycoprotein with a special avidity for calcium. It has a chemical composition similar to the cartilage in the provisional zone of calcification at the epiphysis of a growing bone. This is an intriguing but still unsubstantiated suggestion that fails to explain why only some tumors concentrate calcium in sufficient amount to be seen on a plain film of the abdomen.

Leiomyoma of the Stomach

Leiomyoma of the stomach is a common neoplasm that can range from an insignificant wall lesion to a huge, mostly exophytic mass, larger than the stomach itself. While microscopic calcification may often be found in gastric leiomyomas, roentgenographically visible opacities are exceedingly uncommon. In fact, only a few cases have been reported. Perhaps more sensitive imaging techniques such as computed tomography will reveal a closer correlation between pathologic and radiologic findings, but usually there is insufficient calcium in these tumors for plain film detection. Unlike carcinoma of the stomach, leiomyoma calcification tends to be mottled, coarse, and dense, with irregular streaks and clumps. The calcifications project away from the gastric lumen rather than encircling it (Fig. 4–2).

It is not always possible to distinguish carcinoma from leiomyoma by the pattern of calcification. Calcifications in leiomyomas can be simulated by radiodense solid lesions in the left adrenal or left kidney or spleen. At times, the calcification may extend a distance from the stomach.[12–15] For example, a gastric leiomyoma presenting as a calcified mediastinal mass has been reported.[16]

Other Gastric Masses

Other calcifying gastric tumors arising from the stomach are rare. Milk of calcium in a duplication

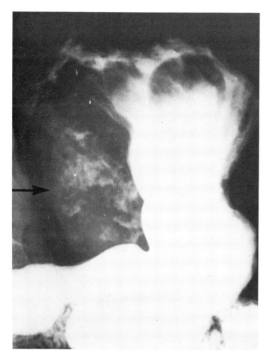

Figure 4–2. Calcified leiomyoma of the stomach. A film from an upper gastrointestinal series shows a large exophytic mass with dense clumps of calcification (arrow).

cyst arising from the upper lesser curvature of the stomach has been observed (Fig. 4–3). Phlebolithic calcification has been noted in hemangiomas of the stomach, although the presence of radio-paque phleboliths in this tumor is very infrequent.[17] In a series of 26 cases of hemangioma of the stomach, only one example of a mass with calcified phleboliths was recognized on plain films.[18]

Intraluminal Opacities

Calcified concretions are formed and remain opaque in an alkaline environment. Hence, the acid contents of the lumen of the stomach do not favor calcium deposition. Thus, opaque gastric calculi forming de novo do not occur here. Bezoars are radiolucent and will be seen on plain films only if they are coated by an opaque material such as liquid bismuth compounds.[19]

While calcified gallstones may rarely pass in a retrograde fashion through the pyloric sphincter, almost all discrete intraluminal opacities in the stomach represent ingested substances.[20] Pills are the most frequently observed radiopaque objects in the stomach. To be seen in the stomach a pill must be both radiodense and remain undissolved. Most medications opaque enough to be seen on plain films will either pass through the stomach quickly or break apart and enter into solution in the gastric lumen. In general, to visualize an intragastric density, an abdominal film must be taken soon after the ingestion of the substance. Occasionally, however, some pills will resist dissolution and remain intact in the stomach. In particular, iron-containing medications may be seen as well-defined densities

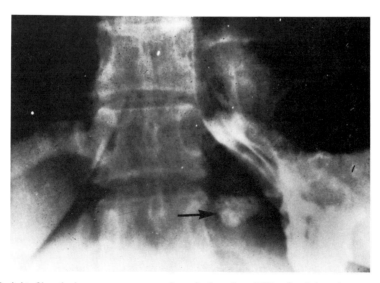

Figure 4–3. Upright film during an upper gastrointestinal series. Milk of calcium in a gastric duplication cyst (arrow). A level demarcating the boundary between the calcified contents in the cyst and the radiolucent fluid above is seen.

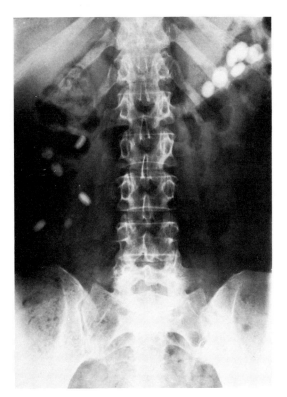

Figure 4–4. Dense pills in the stomach and colon. This patient was known to be a frequent consumer of iron-containing vitamin tablets.

Table 4–2. Calcifications and Other Densities in the Small Bowel

Intramural lesions
Carcinoid tumors
Hemangiomas
Intraluminal opacities
Ingested materials
Solid opaque medication
Metallic objects
Bones
Calcareous clay
Mercury globules
Enteroliths
Intraluminal stones
Meckel's stones
Stones entering through a fistula
Gallstones

tery.[23–25] The calcifications are fixed and do not change position on successive films.

Approximately 5 percent of small bowel hemangiomas contain radiographically demonstrable phleboliths.[26] Hemangiomas are soft, often bulky tumors that do not restrict movement of the small bowel during peristalsis. These masses and their calcific phleboliths may change position in sequential films. Occasionally, hemangiomas cause intussusception, forcing the tumor to traverse a long distance. Hemangiomas may occur anywhere in the small bowel but are most frequent in the distal jejunum and ileum.[26]

Leiomyomas of the small bowel are relatively common tumors, but calcification within them is exceedingly rare. No example of calcification in primary small bowel carcinoma has been reported, but there has been one case in which pelvic and retroperitoneal metastases calcified while the primary site remained unopacified.[27]

within the stomach lumen.[21] Often other iron pills that have passed beyond the stomach into the small intestine will also be observed on the same radiograph (Fig. 4–4).

OPACITIES IN THE SMALL INTESTINE

Intramural Lesions

Calcifications in small bowel tumors are very uncommon. Carcinoid tumors calcify occasionally and they represent the majority of lesions in the small bowel with detectable calcification on plain films. Most of the reported cases have revealed small, scattered, well-defined spherical calcifications, similar to but somewhat larger than phleboliths.[22] Less often, combinations of flecks and arcuate lines of radiodensity may be seen with this tumor. All reported examples of calcified carcinoid tumors arise from the ileum, and the opacities are usually located away from the lumen in the midst of an area of sclerosis in the adjacent mesen-

Intraluminal Opacities

Ingested Substances

The ingested substances most often visible in the small bowel are medications. Liquid preparations containing calcium or other high-atomic-number elements such as bismuth are infrequently recognized because they are diluted by gastric juices and rapidly disperse through the intestines with peristalsis. On the other hand, solid medications are often seen in the small bowel. Pills will be observed if they are sufficient in radiopacity and if they have resisted disintegration in the stomach and small intestine.[8]

Medications containing iron are the most commonly observed foreign bodies in the small bowel. These pills often resist dissolution and may appear intact anywhere in the small or large intestine. The sizes and shapes of iron-containing medications vary because ferrous sulfate and ferrous gluconate may be incorporated into a number of pharmaceuticals, including vitamin complexes.[21]

Enteric coating is often applied to iron medications to render the active ingredient of a pharmaceutical resistant to decomposition. The purpose of enteric coating is to protect the integrity of the pill from breakdown in the stomach and thereby allow greater small bowel absorption. However, sometimes the coating may be so impregnable that the drug will not be released. Most often this occurs in elderly patients and in pills with a long shelf life. Some enteric coated medications such as potassium chloride can be faintly radiopaque, owing to the chemical composition of the coating material.[29] Unfortunately, information about the constituents of the protective coating are generally unavailable to consumers and physicians because the ingredients are often trade secrets.

Iodine-containing pills are radiodense but are usually not seen because they dissolve rapidly in the stomach or proximal small bowel. Occasionally nonabsorbed Telepaque, an iodine compound, will appear as clumps of density in the distal small bowel and colon (Fig. 4–5). This is to be distinguished from the amorphous appearance of conjugated Telepaque which has been absorbed in the small bowel, transported to the liver and biliary ductal system, and then reentered the gut through the enterohepatic circulation. Conjugated Telepaque will occasionally be seen in the small bowel, often as a diffuse increase in density, confined to small bowel loops.[30]

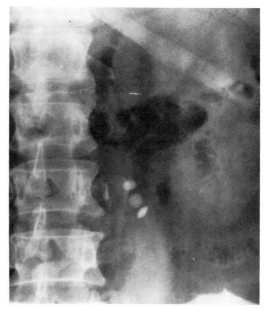

Figure 4–6. Three disc-shaped opaque pills in the small bowel. The radiographic beam passes through the long axis of the upper and lower pills. Hence, they appear more dense than the middle pill, which is aligned with its narrow axis to the beam.

Radiographic Appearance. Most pills can be easily recognized on a scout radiograph, but if they are small they can be confused with concretions. Pills are sometimes disc-shaped, a conformation seldom seen with stones. Also, they are homogeneous, with their radiodensity varying directly with their thickness (Fig. 4–6). Consequently, ovoid or round pills are less dense at the periphery. On the

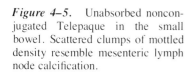

Figure 4–5. Unabsorbed nonconjugated Telepaque in the small bowel. Scattered clumps of mottled density resemble mesenteric lymph node calcification.

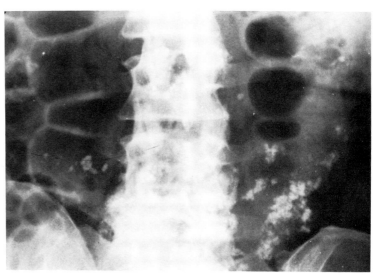

other hand, concretions may be laminated or at least have a band of increased density at their margins.

The recognition of pills in the gut can be significant in modifying patient management. If a medication is intact in the colon, then it is most probable that it is of no benefit to the patient because it will not be absorbed.[29] A switch to another agent may be necessary. Also, the presence of many pills, such as ferrous sulfate, in the intestine when none are prescribed may be an indication of overdose.[21]

Any radiopaque material passing through the stomach intact can be seen in the small bowel. Large objects like pins and coins will rarely cause diagnostic difficulty, for their appearance is readily discerned. However, small objects ingested in large quantities may look like contrast material and without historical information may be misinterpreted on plain films (Fig. 4–7).

In West Africa primarily, but also in parts of the southern United States, geophagy is practiced. After

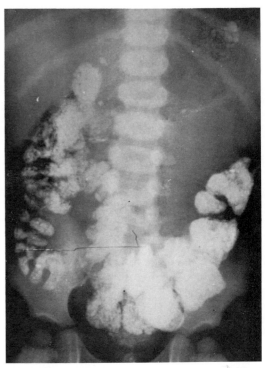

Figure 4–8. Undigested radiopaque material fills the colon and a smaller amount is present in the fundus of the stomach. The patient is a child who regularly ingested clay.

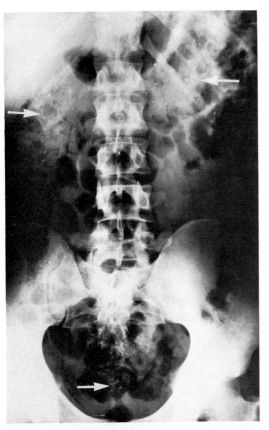

Figure 4–7. Numerous small fragments of metal are scattered throughout the colon (arrows). They represent fragments of razor blades ingested by a disturbed patient to induce gastrointestinal bleeding.

the ingestion of calcareous clay, undissolved opacities can be seen throughout the gastrointestinal tract, from stomach to rectum. If much clay is consumed, the calcific densities may simulate the appearance of barium (Fig. 4–8). After the inadvertent rupture of a mercury bag attached to a long intestinal tube, elemental mercury may move freely through the small intestine. Since mercury is very dense and is a liquid at body temperature, it will assume the shape of small radiopaque globules in the small and large bowel (Fig. 4–9).

Enteroliths

Occasionally, concretions may form in the small bowel lumen. Sometimes undigested vegetable matter, such as plum or prune pits, serves as a nidus (Fig. 4–10).[31] However, in most instances there is no nucleus of insoluble material.[32] The formation of enteroliths requires retardation in flow of intestinal contents. Hence they will be found proximal to a stenosis or in a diverticulum with a narrowed neck.[33] Calcified intestinal stones will occur only if there is both stasis and a favorable pH for

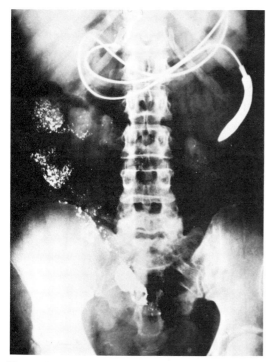

Figure 4-9. Globules of mercury in the colon after the rupture of a mercury bag attached to a long intestinal tube.

calcium deposition.[14] In the upper small bowel the intestinal contents are too acidic for the precipitation of calcium. Here nonopaque choleic acid stones may be present, occurring almost always in women and often located in duodenal diverticula.[31] Calcified enteroliths are encountered only in the distal small intestine where the bowel contents are more alkaline. In the ileum the pH of intestinal secretions may reach 9.0.[34] Analysis of distal small bowel enteroliths usually reveals calcium oxalate or calcium carbonate as the main chemical constituent.[33] They have been reported in patients with Crohn's disease, intestinal tuberculosis, and other abnormalities causing bowel constriction, even carcinoma of the cecum.[35-37] Usually multiple calculi are present, and, while the shape of the stones may vary, they are often of a similar size. Enteroliths are rarely laminated and usually have a thin complete rim of calcification and a lucent or faintly opaque center (Fig. 4-11).[34]

Most small bowel diverticula have wide mouths which permit easy inflow and egress of intestinal contents. Therefore, they are not likely sites for stone formation. However, if there is diverticulitis, the neck may be narrowed and the contents of the diverticulum can be trapped. A prime example is

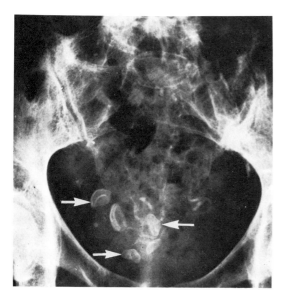

Figure 4-10. Enteroliths in the distal small bowel with prune pits as the nidi of the stones. The patient has intermittent obstruction owing to the descent of ileum into a femoral hernia. (Courtesy of Dr. Harry Miller, Bronx, New York.)

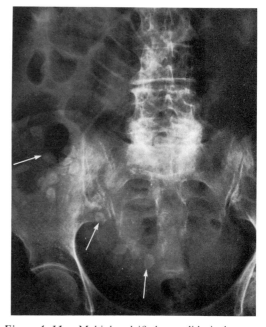

Figure 4-11. Multiple calcified enteroliths in the cecum and distal ileum (arrows). This patient has a constricting carcinoma in the proximal ascending colon. Note also marked small bowel dilatation. (Courtesy of Dr. Daniele Salvioni, New York.)

an inflamed Meckel's diverticulum, where both stasis and an alkaline environment promote calcium precipitation. Only a few cases of opaque calculi in Meckel's diverticulum have been reported and most of these were in men, even though the incidence of Meckel's diverticulum is equal in both sexes.[38] Most of the stones in small bowel diverticula are single and round, but multiple, faceted concretions have also been noted.[39,40] When a diverticulum is large, movement of the stone on successive films can be observed. In one report, a stone moved from the lower abdomen to the right upper quadrant within a single giant diverticulum.[41]

Differential Diagnosis of Enteroliths. Enteroliths, either in a diverticulum or proximal to an obstruction, can usually be distinguished from other calculi. Appendiceal stones are more densely calcified and fixed in position. Multiple gallstones are almost always confined to the gallbladder while enteroliths may move within loops of bowel.[42] Ureteral calculi and phleboliths are usually smaller than intestinal stones. Generally, enteroliths cause no symptoms in themselves but their presence on plain films should alert one to the possibility of significant intestinal narrowing or diverticular inflammation.

Stones Entering the Bowel Lumen through an Abnormal Opening

Stones and other calcifications formed outside the intestinal tract can pass into the lumen of the bowel and cause obstruction. In almost all cases, these concretions are gallstones that have passed through a cholecystoenteric fistula. Common sites for obstruction by gallstones are the second portion of the duodenum, the duodenal-jejunal junction, distal ileum, ileocecal valve, and sigmoid colon.[43]

The classic radiologic triad of gallstone impaction in the intestines (more commonly known as gallstone ileus) consists of air in the biliary tree caused by fistulous communication with the gastrointestinal tract, intestinal obstruction, and calculus in the lumen of the bowel. When all three features are present, the diagnosis is secure and no further preoperative studies need be done (Fig. 4–12).[44] However, at times air in the biliary tract may be inapparent. Gallstones calcify approximately 10 percent of the time, but between 40 and 50 percent of obstructing stones are calcified and can be seen on plain films.[45] Usually only one large nonfaceted stone will be observed, and often the obstructing calculus will be greater than 2.5 cm. in diameter. In questionable cases, it is helpful to examine previous films of the abdomen. If the stone

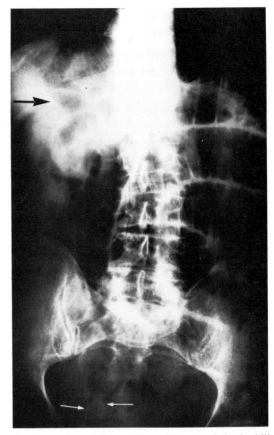

Figure 4–12. Gallstone ileus. There is air in the biliary tree (black arrow), small bowel obstruction, and a faintly calcified gallstone in the distal ileum (white arrows).

was formerly in the right upper quadrant and is now in the lower abdomen, the diagnosis is further corroborated.

The overwhelming majority of patients with gallstone ileus are middle-aged and elderly females. More than half will have a history of gallbladder disease.[46] Since between 1 and 5 percent of all small bowel obstructions are due to gallstone ileus, this condition will be seen occasionally in any busy radiology department. It is important to recognize the distinctive plain film findings of gallstone ileus so that surgery can be performed promptly after radiographic recognition.

Calcifications in the Appendix

Appendicoliths

Stones in the appendix are not rare. Among the many names that have been given to them, the most popular are coproliths, fecoliths, stercoliths, and

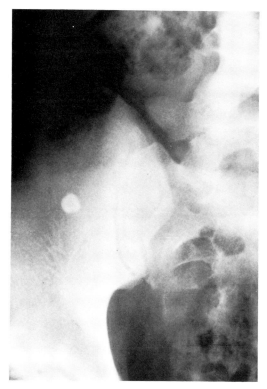

Figure 4–13. Typical appearance of an appendicolith. There is a dense, sharply outlined concretion in the right lower quadrant.

appendicoliths.[47] The best term is appendicolith because it signifies the origin of the stone and serves to distinguish it from other intraluminal calculi in the gastrointestinal tract. Stones in the appendix were first noted in 1813, and Weisflog in 1906 provided the initial description of the radiologic ap-

pearance of calcified appendicoliths.[48,49] Since the turn of the century, appendiceal stones have been observed with increasing frequency. Initial reports stated that they were very rare, but now they are not considered unusual.

Not all stones are calcified. In a study of 100 surgically removed noninflamed appendices, four stones were found but only one was calcified. However, in 100 patients with acute appendicitis, 17 calculi were present and 12 were seen preoperatively on plain films (Fig. 4–13).[50] Another study claimed that up to 60 percent of resected and diseased appendices contained stones but that calcification occurred in no more than 30 percent of them (Fig. 14 *A* and *B*).[51] Opaque calculi are of clinical importance because they are frequently associated with perforation, especially in children with abdominal complaints. Brady found that 32 of 34 children with calcified appendicoliths had perforation at the time of operation.[52] Hence, it is generally agreed that in a symptomatic patient with a demonstrated appendiceal calculus an appendectomy should not be delayed.

The formation of appendicoliths requires the inspissation of fecal material, which serves as a nidus for calcium deposition. Stasis associated with bacterial infection promotes calcification. If the developing stone is fixed in the lumen, it grows gradually with concentric laying down of calcium salts, often giving a laminated appearance (Fig. 1–4).[53] The nidus is usually nonabsorbable vegetable material, but any particulate substance trapped in the appendix may serve as a nucleus for a stone. Occasionally, after barium enema or upper GI series, barium may remain in the appendix. As water is reabsorbed, the barium remains and a stone may form around it. Indians in northern

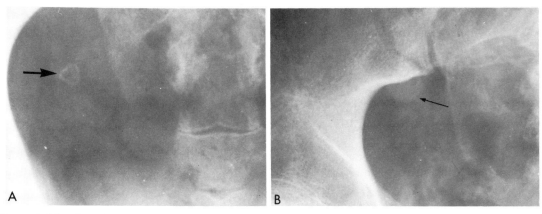

Figure 4–14. Sometimes appendicoliths may be faintly calcified. In *A* only a marginal rim of calcification is seen (arrow). The appendicolith in *B* (arrow) is diffusely but minimally calcified, and if all of it were to overlie the iliac bone, it might be missed.

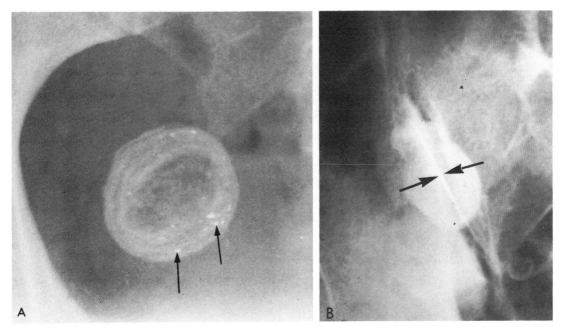

Figure 4–15. *A,* Laminated appendicolith containing flecks of barium (arrow). *B,* The nidus of this large appendicolith is a straight pin (converging arrows). (Courtesy of Dr. Harry Miller, Bronx, New York.)

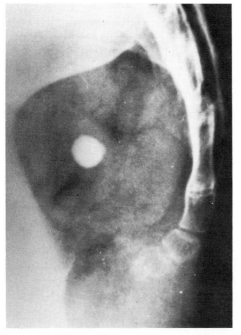

Figure 4–16. Lateral film of the rectum. A dense appendicolith in a retrocecal appendix occupies a low position in the pelvis.

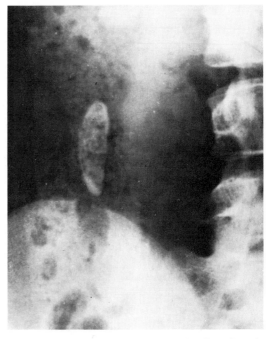

Figure 4–17. Large oblong appendicolith. Occasionally an appendicolith has an elongated configuration.

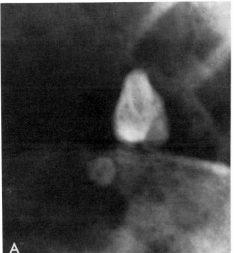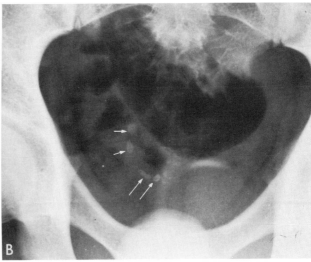

Figure 4–18. Multiple appendicoliths. *A,* Two appendicoliths of dissimilar size and appearance. The upper stone is triangular and the rounded lower stone resembles a phlebolith. *B,* Four appendicoliths occupying the lumen of a low-lying appendix. They should not be confused with phleboliths, which are usually positioned more laterally.

Quebec derive much of their protein from the ingestion of game killed with shotguns. Appendicitis is surprisingly high in this population and shot is often found within the appendiceal stone.[54] Elongated foreign material such as a straight pin or flecks of contrast material may serve just as well as the focus upon which stones form (Fig. 4–15, *A* and *B*).

Appendicoliths can occur wherever the appendix is located. Usually they are seen in the right lower quadrant. If the appendix is low-lying they will be found in the pelvis (Fig. 4–16), and if the appendix is retrocecal and posterior, they can be seen in the right upper quadrant (Fig. 1–36). In one case of a patient with malrotation of the colon, an appendiceal calculus was observed in the left upper quadrant.[52] Rarely, stones may be free in the peritoneal cavity. Like other concretions, appendiceal stones are sharply marginated with curvilinear or faceted borders. Occasionally small irregularities may appear on one surface, but generally they assume a regular geometric shape. Appendicoliths are frequently densely calcified and approximately three-fourths are clearly laminated. Stones up to four cm. in diameter have been noted.

Most of the time appendicoliths can be easily distinguished from mesenteric lymph nodes in the right lower quadrant because the latter have irregular margins and mottled interiors. Ureteral calculi are usually smaller and less prominently laminated, but occasionally differentiation between the two is difficult without oblique films or intravenous urography. Phleboliths are also smaller and have a central lucency, which is an uncommon finding in appendiceal stones. Moreover, phleboliths are generally restricted to pelvic locations while most appendiceal calculii are located more superiorly. Appendicoliths occur at any age but are most frequent in older children and young adults. In a patient with a right lower quadrant concretion the diagnosis of appendicolith should be suggested and if the patient has the appropriate symptoms, immediate operative intervention must be considered.

Mucocele Calcification

Sometimes obstructed appendices do not form stones, even if the luminal blockage is persistent. Especially when infection is absent and there is continuous production of mucus by appendiceal epithelial cells, accumulation of fluid may distend the appendix. If the obstruction persists and mucus formation continues, a mucocele can develop. These are rare lesions found in less than 0.3 percent of all appendices removed at operation.[56,57] Occurring primarily in middle age, they are slightly more common in males. Some may be clinically silent, but often there is a history of multiple episodes of right lower quadrant pain.[58,59] Generally, mucoceles are detected as filling defects on gastrointestinal contrast studies, but in a small percentage of patients, calcification in the wall of the cyst can be seen on plain films (Fig. 4–19).

Mucocele calcification resembles that seen in cysts elsewhere. A thin, often continuous rim of calcification is present in the wall of the cyst. There

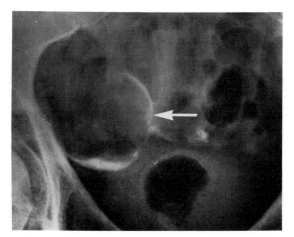

Figure 4–19. Calcified mucocele. A large cystic mass with an incomplete rim of calcification (arrow).

Table 4–3. Calcifications and Other Densities in the Large Intestine

Intraluminal Densities
    Concentration of liquid substances
        Bismuth
        Conjugated Telepaque
    Ingested objects
        Pills
        Metallic objects
        Bones
    Concretions
        Enteroliths
        Gallstones
        Coating of feces in the distal colon
    Foreign bodies introduced per rectum
Intramural Calcifications
    Adenocarcinoma
    Hemangioma

are no laminations or angulations in the annular opacity. Often, mucocele calcification is faint and, since the appendix usually overlies the iliac bone, oblique films may be helpful in revealing the lesion. A cystic lesion in the right lower quadrant is not specific for mucocele. Rarely, mesenteric cysts may also be found here. Occasionally an echinococcal cyst may project from the inferior margin of the liver in the region of the right colon. Since appendiceal mucoceles accompany the right colon, they may be present in the pelvis. In women, leiomyoma of the uterus may occasionally have a cystic appearance and can be confused with mucoceles. Also benign cystadenomas and dermoid cysts of the ovary may have annular calcification. One case of a hydrocele of a right spermatic cord in a middle-aged man presented as a rimlike calcification in the right pelvis and looked exactly like a mucocele.[60]

Myxoglobulosis

Approximately 5 percent of cystic lesions of the appendix contain free-floating intracystic solid bodies. Since the solid material contains mucin and assumes a globular shape, the term myxoglobulosis has been given to this uncommon variant of mucocele. The particulate densities within the cyst are termed globoid bodies. One explanation for their formation is that the lining cells of mucoceles may slough and become nidi for the development of concretions containing mucin and cellular debris. Infrequently, globoid bodies may calcify and appear as multiple concretions within the mucocele. Usually the wall of the cyst is not calcified. Because globoid bodies may move freely in the cyst, they can change their location with respect to each other; this is a point of differentiation from multi-

ple appendicoliths, which are usually fixed in a narrow lumen.[61-64]

RADIOPACITIES IN THE LARGE INTESTINE

Liquid Substances

The large bowel resorbs water and forms, stores, and expels feces. Nonabsorbable radiopaque substances suspended in luminal fluid may first be-

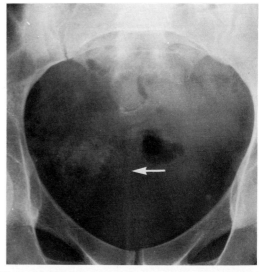

Figure 4–20. Concentration of bismuth in the right colon. Two days before, this patient took four ounces of bismuth subsalicylate by mouth. With resorption of water in the cecum, bismuth concentrates and becomes radiopaque as it coats feces (arrow).

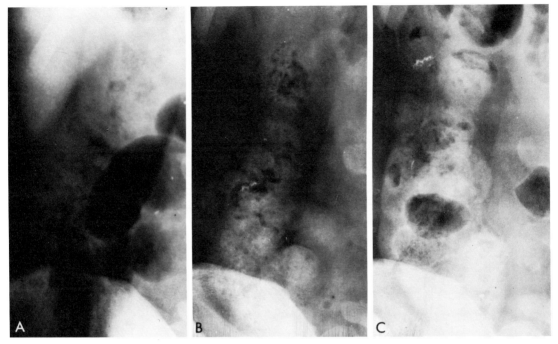

Figure 4–21. Coating of feces with conjugated Telepaque. Films of the right colon on three successive days. *A,* Day one of an oral cholecystogram. There is no opacity in the colon. A single dose of Telepaque was just given by mouth. *B,* Day two—faint coating of feces in the right colon. A second dose of Telepaque was then given. *C,* Day three—bright coating of feces in the colon caused by the accumulation of conjugated Telepaque.

come concentrated in the cecum as water is resorbed. Opaque liquid medications taken orally can concentrate in the right colon, and may be observed in the large intestine on plain films (Fig. 4–20).

Conjugated Telepaque is another substance that may become visible in the large bowel. Orally administered Telepaque can enter the enterohepatic circulation and pass through liver cells into the ductal system and then enter the duodenum through the common bile duct. While usually not seen in the small bowel, it becomes visible in the right colon where it coats feces (Fig. 4–21, *A, B, C*).

Bones

Solid radiopacities may appear in the colon for a variety of reasons. Ingested foreign bodies can pass through the large bowel and become fixed at some point. Most small and smooth objects will usually cause no problem, but larger angulated items can obstruct the colonic lumen or perforate the wall of the large bowel. The swallowing of radiopaque foreign bodies is more apt to occur in demented, inebriated, or neurologically impaired individuals.[65] It has also been observed in elderly denture wearers. In the aged, tactile sensation in the oral cavity is generally depressed, and the wearing of a dental prosthesis further decreases awareness of unchewed material. The calcified foreign body most often recognized in the colon is a chicken breastbone. Frequently, it is inadvertently swallowed in soups, sandwiches, and salads, or other food where the patient does not expect to encounter a bone.[66] Chicken bones may be long and pointed and can penetrate the intestinal wall at any point.

Common sites for obstruction and penetration of chicken bones are the second portion of the duodenum, the duodenal-jejunal junction, Meckel's diverticulum, the ileocecal region, and the colonic flexures.[67,68] Moreover, in the aged, where there is a high incidence of diverticulosis, the sigmoid becomes a frequent site for obstruction, perforation, and abscess formation (Fig. 4–22). Even if a chicken bone is calcified, it may not be seen on plain films because it can overlie the pelvic bones. In a patient predisposed to inadvertent ingestion of foreign bodies and who also presents with symptoms of obstruction and diverticulitis, careful search of plain films should be made for the presence of a foreign body. After contrast material is introduced into the colon, it may become more difficult to ascertain the presence of a bone or other opacity.

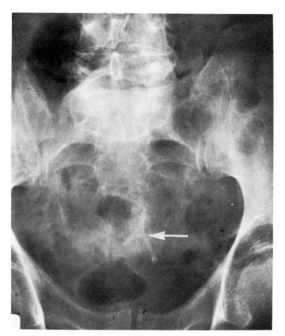

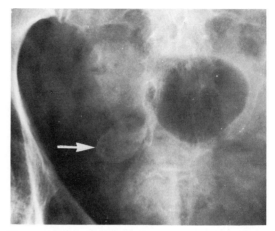

Figure 4-23. Single calculus in a sigmoid diverticulum. A large faintly calcified stone (arrow). On films following barium enema, its position within a diverticulum was noted.

Figure 4-22. Chicken bone in the sigmoid colon. An ingested chicken bone perforated a sigmoid diverticulum causing a diverticular abscess. While diverticulitis may be diagnosed with a barium enema, a chicken bone or other density that precipitates acute inflammation may be missed if no preliminary film is obtained.

Concretions

Just as in the small intestine, concretions may be noted in the large bowel. The colon is a frequent site of obstruction in gallstone ileus. Cecal and ascending colon obstruction promotes the formation of calculi in the same way that enteroliths may form in the small bowel lumen and in Meckel's diverticulum. Diverticula are common in the left colon, but calcific stones are unusual (Fig. 1–43). This is surprising because of the prolonged transit time in patients with diverticulosis, the narrowed necks of colonic diverticula, and the alkaline pH of intraluminal contents. All these favor the formation of large bowel stones (Fig. 4–23).[69-71]

Little has been written about the incidence of concretions in the distal colon. Some state that opaque calculi are uncommon in this area as compared to small bowel enteroliths. We have observed a number of patients who had transient opacifications of feces in the absence of obstruction. In several patients, arcuate calcification coated fecal material on one day, and after a bowel movement both feces and their marginal opacities had been evacuated. In some instances transient opac-

ification was extensive (Fig. 4–24, *A* and *B*). Most of the patients in whom this finding was observed were elderly but some were young and had no chronic colonic abnormalities. It is conceivable that transient elevations in pH could provide a favorable environment for calcium deposition. Undoubtedly, in other patients, accumulations of radiopaque material such as bismuth at the margin of feces may be detectable on plain films.

Solid substances can enter the intestine per rectum. Usually the recognition of opaque objects in the rectum or distal colon poses no difficulty. Occasionally, dissolving suppositories may simulate masses or concretions. Most rectally administered medications are radiolucent, but hemorrhoid preparations containing bismuth and zinc can be seen on plain films.[72] Within minutes after insertion, opaque suppositories are rapidly fractured and dissolve. If a radiograph is taken soon after administration of such a suppository, the demonstrated radiodensities may resemble phleboliths (Fig. 4–25, *A* and *B*), prostatic calculi, or calcification in solid masses.

Mural Lesions

Carcinoma of the Large Intestine

The most common cause of calcification in the wall of the large intestine is mucin-producing adenocarcinoma. The cecum and rectum are the most frequent sites, but calcified malignancies have also been noted in other sections of the large bowel.[73] Typically, these tumors present with a mottled,

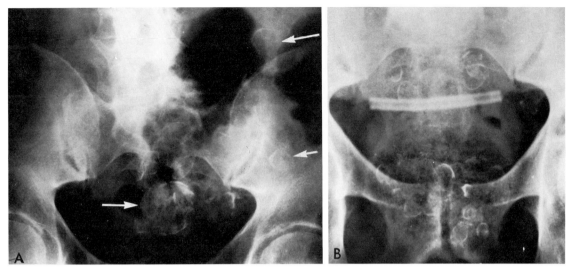

Figure 4–24. Two examples of transient intraluminal opacities in the colon. *A,* Multiple curvilinear densities in the rectum, sigmoid, and descending colon (arrows). They were not present on subsequent films obtained the next day. *B,* Many rounded opacities which appear to coat feces. After an enema, they were evacuated from the colon.

speckled, or granular pattern of calcification, which may extend away from the intestinal lumen (Fig. 4–26). Occasionally, instead of numerous punctate opacities, only a few densities will be seen. At times only the metastatic deposits from the primary colonic tumor will be radiopaque. By far the most common location of calcified metastases is the liver. Occasionally, calcified metastases appear in retroperitoneal lymph nodes. However, peritoneal calcific deposits are extremely unusual in colonic cancer. This is an important point of differentiation

from ovarian serous cystadenocarcinoma, in which psammomatous calcification may simulate exactly the appearance of primary colonic tumors. However, with ovarian malignancies, calcified peritoneal metastases are common. Sometimes ossification may occur in rectal carcinomas. Generally, bone-forming carcinomas are small and slow-growing, but they can also extend rapidly into adjacent pelvic muscles (Fig. 4–27).[74–76]

Many patients with calcified carcinoma are below age 40 at the time of initial recognition of the

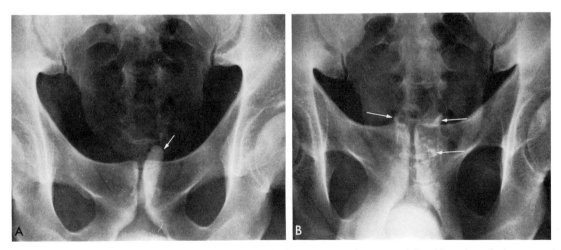

Figure 4–25. The appearance of radiopaque suppositories. A suppository containing bismuth and zinc was administered rectally. *A,* Immediately after placement, the opaque suppository is intact (arrow). *B,* Fifteen minutes later, the suppository had fragmented into multiple densities (arrows).

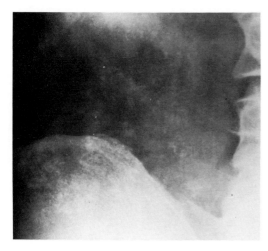

Figure 4–26. A large ascending colon adenocarcinoma. It contains innumerable speckled calcifications.

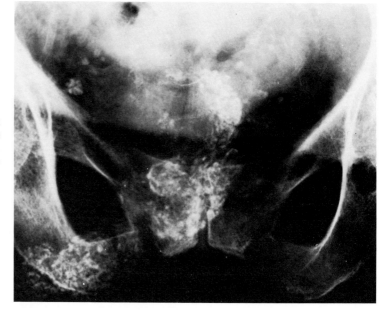

Figure 4–27. Calcified carcinoma of the rectum growing directly into the soft tissues of the right buttock. (Courtesy of Dr. Paul Cohen, Amsterdam, The Netherlands.)

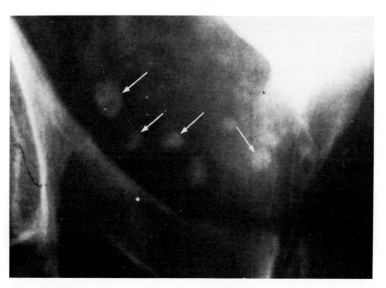

Figure 4–28. Hemangioma of the rectum. There are several discrete calcifications (arrows) in this large tumor that simulate phleboliths. (Courtesy of Dr. Thomas Beneventano, Bronx, New York.)

disease. Yet, while there appears to be a predilection for younger age groups, only rarely has a calcified adenocarcinoma been reported in a patient with pre-existing ulcerative colitis.

Hemangioma

Another colonic tumor that presents with calcification on plain films is hemangioma. Colonic and rectal hemangiomas are uncommon lesions and may occasionally have radiopaque phleboliths within them. In the rectum, hemangiomas may be suggested by any abnormal position of phleboliths (Fig. 4–28). In the more proximal colon, phleboliths and hemangiomas may move considerable distances with peristalsis.[78–80]

REFERENCES

1. Bloch C, Peck HM: Calcification in gastrointestinal malignancy: An important clue in radiologic diagnosis. Mt Sinai J Med 38:405–416, 1971.
2. Myo Lwin TO, Soodeen TH: A case report on calcified mucinous adenocarcinoma of the stomach. J Canad Assn Radiol 24:370–373, 1973.
3. Ghahramani GG et al: Calcified primary tumors of the gastrointestinal tract. Gastrointest Radiol 2:331–339, 1978.
4. Kendig TA, Gaspar MD, Secrest PG: Calcification in gastric carcinoma: Case report. Radiology 68:80–82, 1957.
5. Hermann G, Rozin R: Calcification in gastro-intestinal carcinomata. Clin Radiol 15:139–141, 1964.
6. Balthazar E, Rosenthal M: Calcifying mucin producing adenocarcinoma of the stomach. NY State J Med 73:2704–2706, 1973.
7. Thomas RL, Rice RP: Calcifying mucinous adenocarcinoma of the stomach. Radiology 88:1002–1003, 1967.
8. Gemmell NI: Calcification within a gastric carcinoma. Am J Roentgenol 91:779–783, 1964.
9. Robertson JW, Osterhout S: Calcification in scirrhous carcinoma of the stomach. Am J Surg 83:830–832, 1952.
10. Batlan LE: Calcifications within the stomach wall in gastric malignancy. Am J Roentgenol 72:788–794, 1954.
11. Khilnani MT: Calcifying mucous-cell carcinoma of the stomach. Am J Dig Dis 5:479–483, 1960.
12. Leigh TF: Calcified gastric leiomyoma: Report of case. Radiology 55:419–422, 1950.
13. Garbarini J, Price HP: Calcified leiomyoma of the stomach. N Engl J Med 243:406–407, 1950.
14. Crummy AB Jr, Juhl JH: Calcified gastric leiomyoma. Am J Roentgenol 87:727–728, 1962.
15. Koloski EL, Shallenberger PL, Hawk AW: Large partially calcified gastric leiomyoma. Am J Surg 80:245–248, 1950.
16. Graham JC Jr, Blanchard IT, Scatliff JH: Calcified gastric leiomyoma presenting as a mediastinal mass. Am J Roentgenol 114:529–531, 1972.
17. Kerekes ES: Gastric hemangioma: A case report. Radiology 82:468–469, 1964.
18. Flannery MG, Caster MP: Hemangioma of the stomach with a roentgenologic diagnostic point. Am J Roentgenol 77:38–40, 1957.
19. Canlas EM, Fildes CE: Radiopaque phytobezoar: A case report. Radiology 60:261–264, 1953.
20. Afflerbaugh JK, Cole HA: Intragastric gallstone. Radiology 64:581–583, 1955.
21. Staple TW, McAlister WH: Roentgenographic visualization of iron preparations in the gastrointestinal tract. Radiology 83:1051–1056, 1964.
22. Boijsen E, Kaude J, Tylén U: Radiologic diagnosis of ileal carcinoid tumor. Acta Radiol (Diagnosis) 15:65–83, 1974.
23. Case records of the Massachusetts General Hospital. Case 34–1973. N Engl J Med 289:419–424, 1973.
24. Kaude JV: Calcification in carcinoid tumors. N Engl J Med 289:921, 1973.
25. Noonan CD: Calcified carcinoid of the small bowel: A case report. Radiol Clin Biol 41:115–120, 1972.
26. Marine R, Lattomus, WW: Cavernous hemangioma of the gastrointestinal tract: Report of case and review. Radiology 70:860–863, 1958.
27. Rosenfield AJ: Widespread calcified metastases from adenocarcinoma of the jejunum. Am J Dig Dis 20:990–993, 1975.
28. Handy CA. Radiopacity of oral non-liquid medications. Radiology 98:525–533, 1971.
29. Hinkel CL: The significance of opaque medications in the gastro-intestinal tract with special reference to enteric coated pills. Am J Roentgenol 65:575–581, 1951.
30. Nathan MH, Newman A: Conjugated iopanoic acid (Telepaque) in the small bowel: An aid in the diagnosis of gallbladder disease. Radiology 109:545–548, 1973.
31. Shapiro JH, Rubinstein B, Jacobson HG et al: Enteroliths in the small intestine. Am J Roentgenol 75:343–348, 1956.
32. Grettve S: A contribution to the knowledge of primary true concrements in the small bowel. Acta Chir Scand 95:387–410, 1947.
33. Blix G: Contribution to chemistry of primary calculi of the small intestine. Acta Chir Scand 76:24–34, 1935.
34. Katz I, Fischer RM: Enteroliths complicating regional enteritis; A report of two cases. Am J Roentgenol 78:653–660, 1957.
35. Brettner A, Euphrat E: Radiological significance of primary enterolithiasis. Radiology 94:283–288, 1970.
36. Bery K, Virmani P, Chawla S: Enterolithiasis with tubercular intestinal strictures. Brit J Radiol 37:73–75, 1964.
37. Gundersen AL, Kreiter RL: Cecal lithiasis. Secondary to cecal stenosis. JAMA 205:462–463, 1968.
38. Enge I, Frimann-Dahl J: Radiology in acute abdominal disorder due to Meckel's diverticulum. Brit J Radiol 37:775–780, 1964.
39. Dovey P: Calculus in a Meckel's diverticulum—a preoperative radiological diagnosis. Brit J Radiol 44:888–890, 1971.
40. Feldman MI: Calculi in Meckel's diverticulum. Radiology 86:541–543, 1966.
41. Bischoff ME, Stampfli WP: Meckel's diverticulum with emphasis on the roentgen diagnosis. Radiology 65:572–577, 1955.
42. Altaras J: Calculi of the small intestine. Brit J Radiol 29:684–686, 1956.
43. McLaughlin CW Jr, Craimer M: Obstruction of the alimentary tract from gallstone. Am J Surg 81:424–430, 1951.
44. Donner MW, Weiner S: Diagnostic evaluation of abdominal calcifications in acute abdominal disorders. Radiol Clin North Am 2:145–159, 1964.
45. Eisenmann JI, Finck EJ, O'Laughlin BJ: Gallstone ileus: A review of the roentgenographic findings and report

of a new roentgen sign. Am J Roentgenol 101:361–366, 1967.

46. Bridenbaugh RB, Bridenbaugh JH, Berg HM: Gallstone ileus: report of four cases. Am J Roentgenol 77:684–689, 1957.
47. Felson B, Bernhard CM: The roentgenologic diagnosis of appendiceal calculi. Radiology 49:178–191, 1947.
48. Ducharme JC, Hurtubise M, Anouty J: Calcified appendiceal fecolith in children: Incidence and significance. J Canad Assn Radiol 17:155–157, 1966.
49. Weisflog: X-ray diagnosis of enteroliths in the appendix. Fortschr Geb Röentgenstr 10:217–219, 1906.
50. Faegenburg D: Fecaliths of the appendix: Incidence and significance. Am J Roentgenol 89:752–759, 1963.
51. Thomas SF: Appendiceal coproliths: Their surgical importance. Radiology 49:39–49, 1947.
52. Brady BM, Carroll DS: The significance of the calcified appendiceal enterolith. Radiology 68:648–653, 1957.
53. Berg RM, Berg HM: Coproliths. Radiology 68:839–844, 1957.
54. Carey LS: Lead shot appendicitis in northern native people. J Canad Assn Radiol 28:171–174, 1977.
55. Bunch GH, Adcock DF: Giant faceted calculus. Ann Surg 109:143–146, 1939.
56. Norman A, Leider LS, del Carman J: Mucocele of the appendix, Am J Roentgenol 77:647–651, 1957.
57. Euphrat EJ: Roentgen features of mucocele of the appendix. Radiology 48:113–117, 1947.
58. Peyton Barnes J: Calcified mucocele of the appendix. Am J Surg 76:323–327, 1948.
59. Bonann LJ, Davis JG: Retroperitoneal mucocele of the appendix: A case report with characteristic roentgen features. Radiology 51:375–382, 1948.
60. Ferris EJ, Shauffer IA: Hydrocele of the spermatic cord: With roentgenographic findings simulating a mucocele of the appendix. Am J Roentgenol 94:395–398, 1965.
61. Milliken G, Poindexter CA: Mucocele of appendix with globoid body formation. Am J Pathol I:397–402, 1925.
62. Probstein JG, Lassar GM: Mucocele of the appendix with myxoglobulosis. Ann Surg 127:171–176, 1948.
63. Miller D: Mucocele and myxoglobulosis of the appendix. Surg Clin North Am 27:337–343, 1947.
64. Felson B, Wiot JF: Some interesting right lower quadrant entities. Radiol Clin North Am 7:83–95, 1969.
65. Maglinte DDT, Taylor SD, Ng AC: Gastrointestinal perforation by chicken bones. Radiology 130:597–599, 1979.
66. Bunker PG: The role of dentistry in problems of foreign bodies in the air and food passages. J Am Dent Assoc 64:782–787, 1962.
67. Katz I, Arcomano J: Roentgen findings in a case of perforation of the cecum by a bone. Radiology 63:411–414, 1954.
68. Berk RN, Reit RJ: Intra-abdominal chicken bone abscess. Radiology 101:311–313, 1971.
69. Zbornik RC: Large fecal stones—the sigmoid. Am J Roentgenol 113:355–359, 1971.
70. Harland D: A case of multiple calculi in the large intestine with a review of the subject of intestinal calculi. Brit J Surg 41:209–211, 1953.
71. Thompson R, Barry WF Jr: Rectal calculus. Radiology 96:411–412, 1970.
72. Spitzer A, Caruthers SB, Stables DP: Radiopaque suppositories. Radiology 121:71–73, 1976.
73. Fletcher BD, Morreels CL, Christian WH III, et al: Calcified adenocarcinoma of the colon. Am J Roentgenol 101:301–305, 1967.
74. Van Patten HT, Whittirk JW: Heterotopic ossification in intestinal neoplasia. Am J Pathol 31:73–91, 1955.
75. Hall CW: Calcification and osseous metaplasia in carcinoma of the colon. J Canad Assoc Radiol 13:135–139, 1962.
76. Engel S, Dockerty MD: Calcification and ossification in rectal malignant processes. JAMA 179:345–350, 1962.
77. Shockman AT: Calcified carcinoma of the colon superimposed on chronic ulcerative colitis. Am J Dig Dis 14:683–687, 1969.
78. Bell GA, McKenzie AD, Emmons H: Diffuse cavernous hemangioma of the rectum: Report of a case and review of the literature. Dis Colon Rectum 15:377–382, 1972.
79. Bailey JJ, Barrick CW, Jenkinson EL: Hemangioma of the colon, JAMA 160:658–659, 1956.
80. Hollingsworth G: Haemangiomatous lesions of the colon. Brit J Radiol 24:220–222, 1951.

Chapter 5

CALCIFICATION IN THE PANCREAS, ADRENAL GLANDS, AND RETRO-PERITONEUM

Stephen R. Baker, M.D.

The pancreas, adrenal glands, and adjacent retroperitoneal connective tissues are infrequent sites for calcification. Yet, often the spectrum of diagnostic possibilities suggested by the pattern of calcification may be narrow and, especially in the pancreas, the plain film findings can point to the identity of a radiopacity so strongly that further radiologic studies may not be needed. In other instances, plain film findings are not definitive and more sophisticated modalities must be employed to best characterize a lesion. However, in all cases, evaluation of the position and pattern of calcification on plain films can supply important diagnostic information.

PANCREAS

Concretions

By far, the most common cause of pancreatic calcification is chronic calcifying pancreatitis. Long-standing ductal obstruction and inflammation promote the precipitation of protein and the denudation of mucosal cells which serve as a nidus for the deposition of calcium. Small stones consist mainly of protein, but larger concretions contain increasing percentages of calcific compounds. Cut sections of pancreatic calculi usually demonstrate multiple opaque laminae composed of calcium carbonate in the form of calcite.[1-4]

Common findings in pancreatitis are ductal nar-

rowing and obstruction. Proximal to the point of stenosis, both the duct of Wirsung and tributary ducts may dilate and, after a period of time, more and more calculi will be accommodated within their larger lumens. On occasion, multiple calculi may plug both large and small ducts, furthering the process of proximal dilatation. Atrophy of glandular tissue accompanies the increase in duct size. Frequently, calcifications progress to such an extent that the entire organ appears calcified. In the past, this was called diffuse calcification of the pancreas and thought to represent opacification in acinar cells. Careful microscopic analysis has revealed that even in the most heavily calcified pancreases the small intralobular ducts contain stones, but parenchymal cells are free of calcium.[5-7] Fat necrosis,

Table 5–1. Pancreatic Calcification

Concretions
Pancreatitis
Chronic calcifying pancreatitis from alcohol abuse
Nutritional pancreatitis
Hyperparathyroidism
Cystic fibrosis
Hereditary pancreatitis
Idiopathic Pancreatic Calculi
Solid Calcification
Cystadenoma
Cystadenocarcinoma
Lymphangioma
Islet Cell Tumors
Adenocarcinoma
Cystic Calcification
Calcification in Pseudocysts

107

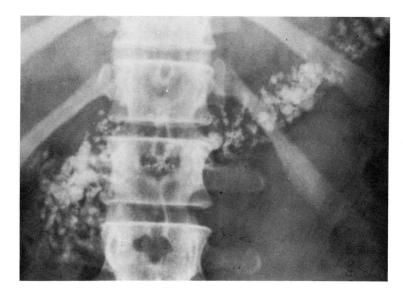

Figure 5–1. Innumerable dense calculi in the pancreas extending from head to tail.

another feature of pancreatitis, has been implicated as a cause of calcification, but calcium deposition in this process is not extensive enough to be seen on plain x-ray. Hence, the multiple pancreatic calcifications seen in chronic pancreatitis are exclusively concretions within ducts.

Radiographic Appearance

The typical appearance of chronic calcifying pancreatitis on abdominal films is that of multiple dense, discrete opacities that cross the midline at the level of L1–L2 and conform to the shape of the pancreas. On the right the densities are close to the midline, but on the left the limit of calcification may extend far peripherally, sometimes pointing upwards toward the left hemidiaphragm and in other instances traversing a horizontal course toward the lateral abdominal wall (Fig. 5–1). While the individual calcifications are distinct and separable, the chain of calcification is usually continuous. In approximately 25 percent of cases, opaque concretions are present in the head of the pancreas alone [7] (Fig. 5–2). Calcification confined to the tail or body only is very uncommon (Fig. 5–3). Occasionally, it is difficult to discern concretions in the section of the pancreas that overlies the spine, but films taken in varying degrees of obliquity will move the

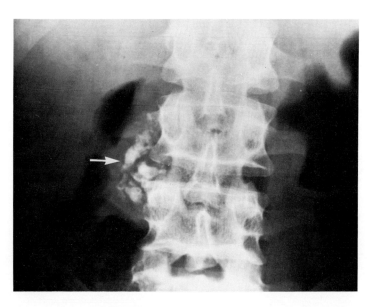

Figure 5–2. Calcification confined to the pancreatic head (arrow). Note that some of the concretions are elongated.

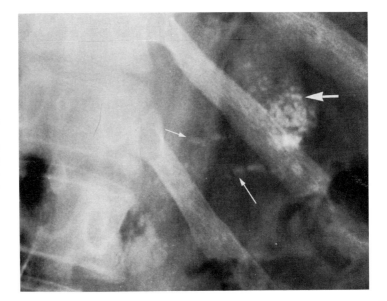

Figure 5–3. Most of the pancreatic calcifications in this 37-year-old alcoholic male are in the tail (large arrow). Scattered calculi are also present in the body (small arrows). However, the head is free of stones. This is an unusual pattern of pancreatic calcification.

vertebrae away from the pancreas and show the uninterrupted course of calcification. When only the pancreatic head contains calcification, the conglomeration of closely packed stones may simulate the appearance of a calcified solid mass. Here, again, oblique or lateral films can show that the pattern of calcification consists of multiple unconnected, sharply outlined densities (Fig. 1–33).

Individual concretions will often vary in shape. In fact, it is unusual for pancreatic stones to have a monotonous appearance. Predominantly, they have rounded or irregularly angulated contours, but elongated and even branched stones may be seen. Almost without exception, stones are completely marginated and often they are very opaque. They may be laminated or contain small central or eccentric lucencies (Fig. 5–4). Multiple stones characteristically differ in size. It is common to see calculi of widely varying dimensions in the same gland, and occasionally individual stones may reach a diameter of 2 to 3 centimeters (Fig. 5–5).

The diagnosis of multiple pancreatic calculi is easy when stones extend from the head to the tail. There is no other entity consisting of numerous stones that cross the midline in the general location of the pancreas. Rarely, lymphangioma of the pancreas can occur with phlebolithic calcifications. These concretions are generally few compared to

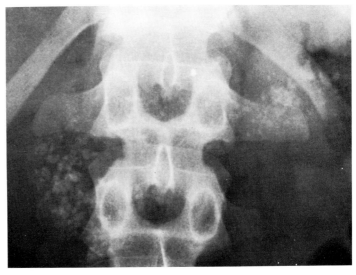

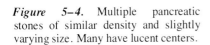

Figure 5–4. Multiple pancreatic stones of similar density and slightly varying size. Many have lucent centers.

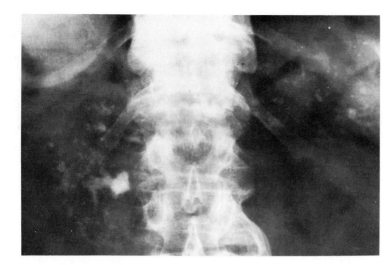

Figure 5–5. Pancreatic lithiasis of widely varying size. In the head, there is a very large stone with branching extensions.

the multiplicity of stones seen in chronic pancreatitis.[8] After a single intravascular injection of Thorotrast, colloidal thorium will gradually be taken up in peripancreatic lymph nodes and remain there indefinitely. They will be observed on x-ray as multiple, large, very dense opacities along the course of the pancreas. However, Thorotrast deposition in peripancreatic nodes is always accompanied by Thorotrast in the liver and in the spleen and should never cause confusion with the appearance of chronic calcifying pancreatitis[9] (Fig. 5–6).

Rarely, only a few large stones will be present. If the calculi are confined to a portion of the pancreas and are of similar size and shape, they can be confused with gallbladder or urinary calculi[10,11] (Fig. 5–7). The disappearance of pancreatic stones has been noted in pancreatic carcinoma and in pancreatic pseudocysts.[12–14] The mechanism for the dissolution of stones is unclear. A pseudocyst can also displace stones as it stretches and deforms the pancreas (Fig. 5–8).

Etiology

In North America, Europe, and the temperate regions of Latin America and South Africa, there is a close relationship between alcoholism and almost all cases of chronic calcifying pancreatitis. The other major cause of pancreatic inflammation, biliary tract disease, is rarely, if ever, a predisposing factor in the development of pancreatic lithiasis. It takes at least six years of chronic alcohol abuse to develop calcifications in the pancreas, and calculi are usually first noted in the fourth decade.[3] It is not known what predisposes some alcoholics to develop calcification. There appears to be no

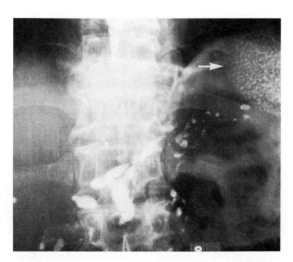

Figure 5–6. Thorotrast in peripancreatic lymph nodes. Very dense discrete opacities cross the midline in the upper abdomen. There is also Thorotrast in the spleen (arrow).

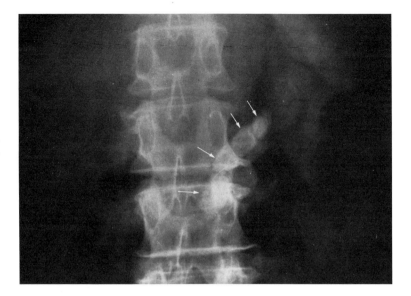

Figure 5–7. The arrows point to four faceted stones in the duct of Wirsung. The patient had a long history of alcoholic abuse.

correlation between the development of calculi and the type of alcohol consumed. Perhaps the propensity for both calculi formation and pancreatitis is related to the nutritional status of the alcoholic. At present, however, little has been established about the mechanism of chronic calcifying pancreatitis beyond the fact that there is a strong association with ethanol intake.

In less developed regions of the world, pancreatic calculi appear to be related to malnutrition. On a global scale, there may be more people with pancreatic stones as a result of protein deficiency than there are alcoholics with pancreatic stones. For example, pancreatic lithiasis is common in Marseilles, France, but its incidence is ten times higher in Kerala, India.[3] Calcification occurs at a younger age in patients with nutritionally induced chronic pancreatitis. In a series of 45 patients observed in western Nigeria, the average age of onset of calculi was 20 years. These patients rarely complained of abdominal pain but many had diabetes mellitus and their presenting problem was often steatorrhea.[15] In an investigation of 18 Indonesian adolescents and young adults with diffuse intraductal pancreatic calcification, none had a history of alcohol intake. Few complained of abdominal pain but 45 percent had diabetes and the majority presented with steatorrhea.[16] There was a recent report of a nonalcoholic patient in the United States who had celiac disease for several years and then developed pancreatic calculi.[17] The relationship between malnutrition and calcifying pancreatitis has not yet been given much attention in the western medical literature, but the suggestively large group of patients with this disease in poorer regions of the world should provide the impetus for further study (Fig. 10–22).

There is an association between hyperparathyroidism and chronic pancreatitis. In one study, seven of 37 patients with primary hyperparathyroidism had pancreatic stones.[18] In a later investigation, only nine of 155 patients had calcification in the pancreas.[19] The radiographic appearance of calcification induced by hyperparathyroidism is indistinguishable from that of the more common form of chronic calcifying pancreatitis.[20] Plain film recognition of pancreatic stones should raise the ques-

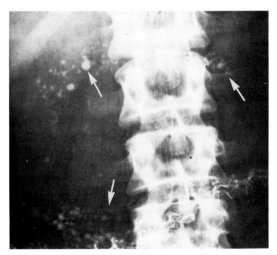

Figure 5–8. There is a pseudocyst of the pancreas which has displaced the head inferiorly and the body superiorly. The separation of calculi (arrows) suggests stretching of the pancreas.

tion of parathyroid disease. However, these cases represent a very small percentage of all those with pancreatic concretions.

A rarer cause of stones in the pancreas is cystic fibrosis. Here again, calcific densities are only occasionally found.[21,22] Almost always other clinical and radiographic features of this disease will be present (Fig. 10–23). Hereditary pancreatitis is a very rare but interesting entity that affects several Caucasian families in Appalachia. The disease, transmitted by an autosomal dominant gene, causes repeated episodes of abdominal pain. There is an increased risk for the development of pancreatic carcinoma.[23] Calcifications are usually fewer but larger than those found in other types of chronic pancreatitis. Calcifying pancreatitis has also been noted in one patient whose only pertinent history was trauma to the upper abdomen. Whether traumatic calcifying pancreatitis is a real entity remains an open question.[24]

There is a small group of patients who have calcifications without a history of pancreatitis and have no apparent clinical predisposition for the development of stones. Stobbe et al. studied 130 patients with pancreatic lithiasis. Twenty-two had stones in localized sections of the pancreas. Nineteen of them were over 70 years and none in the subgroup with focal stones ever had signs or symptoms of pancreatitis. Only one had a history of alcohol intake and none had evidence of hyperparathyroidism. At autopsy there were focal occlusions of distal pancreatic ducts with scarring and calculi.[25] The presence of asymptomatic pancreatic stones is still a poorly defined condition. Since usually only a few concretions are present, it is easy to dismiss or misdiagnose them on plain films. When there are isolated stones in the pancreatic tail, they may go unrecognized or be ascribed to the left adrenal gland, left kidney, or even costal cartilage (Fig. 5–9).

Solid Mass Calcification

The overwhelming majority of patients with pancreatic opacities have chronic calcifying pancreatitis, but there are a few other conditions in which calcifications occur. Cystadenomas and cystadenocarcinomas are rare pancreatic neoplasms, and the cell of origin for both tumors is uncertain. They may arise from pancreatic ductal epithelium or acinar tissue or may develop from displaced embryonic cells. Both are composed of multiple small cysts which do not connect with pancreatic ducts.[26] The cysts contain viscid or gelatinous material embedded in a vascular stroma, and they appear as

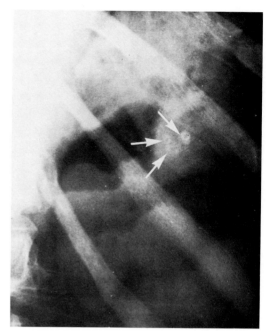

Figure 5–9. Several rounded calculi in the pancreatic tail (arrows). They look like phleboliths or isolated costal cartilage calcification. The patient had no history of pancreatic disease. CT confirmed their intrapancreatic location.

coarsely lobulated and rounded masses. Cystadenomas and cystadenocarcinomas are found primarily in middle-aged females. They are slow-growing and are found most often in the pancreatic tail. In approximately 10 to 20 percent of cases, tumor calcification is seen on plain films.[27] Clumps of separate and widely scattered radiodensities are found and occasionally the calcifications assume a radial or sunburst appearance.[28] In both cystadenomas and cystadenocarcinomas, ossification may be found in the stroma of the tumor. Hence, the pattern of calcification is usually that of a solid mass and the arcuate lines of calcium typical of other cysts are infrequently encountered here. The radially oriented clumps of calcification should not be confused with the concretions of chronic calcifying pancreatitis. In cystadenoma, the individual densities are larger and sparser than in pancreatitis, and they do not conform to the general outline of the pancreas (Fig. 5–10). Rarely, calcification in lymphangiomas of the pancreas may mimic cystadenoma.[8] Also, other large calcific masses such as retroperitoneal sarcomas or renal tumors may resemble the dense and irregular calcification of cystadenomas.

Calcification may be found in endocrine tumors of the pancreas. Of 23 malignant islet cell tumors studied by Imhof et al., two were calcified while coexistent pancreatic carcinoma.[34] In another report of 417 patients with adenocarcinoma of the pancreas, 1.4 percent had calcification consistent with chronic calcifying pancreatitis.[35,36] This is distinctly higher than the incidence of pancreatic calcifications in the general population. Although these investigations are not definitive, they suggest that patients with chronic calcifying pancreatitis appear to be at a greater risk for the development of carcinoma.

Cystic Calcification

Calcification in the wall of fluid-filled masses in the pancreas is rare and information on this subject is meager. Occasionally pseudocysts may calcify and the typical rimlike opacity found in other types of cystic lesions will be seen. Calcification may be thin and incomplete or thick and circumferential (Fig. 5–12). Most calcified pseudocysts occur in the tail of the pancreas. The differential diagnosis

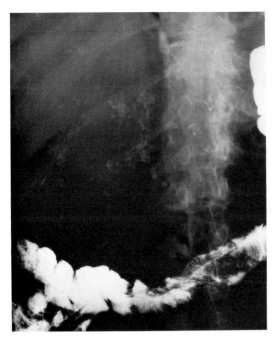

Figure 5–10. Cystadenoma of the pancreas. Scattered streaky calcification in a large mass which is displacing the barium-filled transverse colon downward. (Courtesy of Drs. L. Berliner and P. Redmond, Staten Island Hospital, Staten Island, New York.)

none of 71 benign islet cell tumors contained opacities visible on plain films.[29] In another study of ten cases of calcification in endocrine tumors of the pancreas, seven occurred in malignant masses.[30] Islet cell tumors of all types can calcify, and in most cases the calcifications appear as irregular, coarse, poorly defined densities. Occasionally sheets of calcification may occupy a section of the pancreas.[31] In three patients, similar calcifications were noted in liver metastases.[29] Calcifications in endocrine tumors of the pancreas are usually not as dense or as sharply margined as those seen in cystadenoma.

The incidence of adenocarcinoma of the pancreas has been increasing gradually in the past 20 years. In 1981 it was the fifth most common cause of cancer death in the United States.[32] Yet, in spite of its frequency, calcification in the primary tumor is exceedingly rare[33] (Fig. 5–11). The presumption should be that, in a patient with suspected adenocarcinoma, the calcification is not within the tumor but is a manifestation of some other process, most often chronic pancreatitis. However, patients with chronic calcifying pancreatitis may be more likely to develop adenocarcinoma. In one series of 677 patients with pancreatic calcification, 24 had

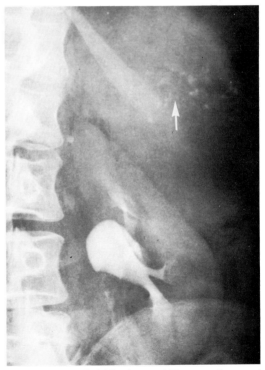

Figure 5–11. Calcifications within an adenocarcinoma of the tail of the pancreas. An oblique film obtained during an intravenous urography reveals scattered calculi in a large carcinoma of the pancreas (arrow). Histologic examination demonstrated calcium within the tumor. (Courtesy of Dr. Diane LoRusso, Rye, New York.)

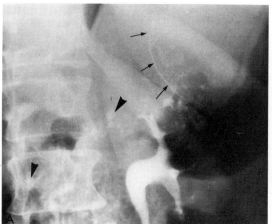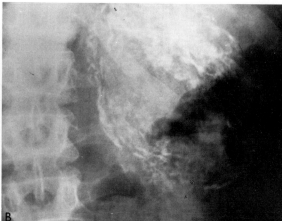

Figure 5–12. Two examples of calcified pancreatic pseudocyst. *A,* Thin-walled calcified pseudocyst of the pancreas (arrows). An oblique film from an intravenous urography also shows calculi in the pancreas (arrowheads). *B,* Thick-walled pancreatic pseudocyst. The margins are irregular because the cyst was partially drained. (Courtesy of Dr. Barry Siskind, Bronx, New York.)

includes renal or adrenal cysts, other retroperitoneal and mesenteric cysts, renal and splenic artery aneurysms, and a tortuous splenic artery. The coexistence of pancreatic concretions will raise the possibility of pseudocyst calcification, but a definite diagnosis will usually require CT scan. Milk of calcium in a pancreatic pseudocyst has also been reported.[37] Its radiographic appearance resembles milk of calcium in other cystic structures.

ADRENAL GLANDS

As in the pancreas, only a few diseases are associated with adrenal calcification. But, unlike the pancreas, where chronic calcifying pancreatitis is the leading cause of calcification and usually presents with a characteristic roentgenographic appearance, both clinically significant and innocuous adrenal entities may calcify with similar frequencies and may resemble each other on plain radiographs. There are no lesions with a pathognomonic pattern of calcification. Almost all calcifications will either be cystic or solid, or occasionally a combination of the two. Hence, the finding of calcification on plain films will often be followed by other studies before a diagnosis can be established. Nonetheless, the plain film can offer clues which will contribute to narrowing the range of diagnostic possibilities. The following discussion will focus primarily on adrenal calcification encountered in the adult. Adrenal calcification in the pediatric age group is considered in Chapter 10.

Solid Calcification in a Normal-Sized Gland

The adrenal gland rests on the superior medial border of the adjacent kidney. The right gland is usually more caudally situated than the left. Normally the adrenal glands are not longer than 3 cm. or wider than 2.5 cm. If the extent of solid calcification describes an area and configuration consistent with a normal-sized gland and there is no other evidence of glandular enlargement, then it is unlikely that the calcification is caused by a malignant neoplasm. In the adult, calcification in a normal-sized gland can be encountered in several conditions.

In many instances, adrenal calcification is observed as an incidental finding on abdominal plain films in individuals with no other evidence of adrenal disease. Many of these patients may have had abnormal birth histories with perinatal events that predispose to adrenal hemorrhage; i.e., forceful delivery, prematurity, and newborn infection.

Table 5–2. Calcification in a Normal-Sized Gland

1. Neonatal hemorrhage
2. Tuberculosis, with or without Addison's disease
3. Histoplasmosis
4. Myelolipoma
5. Adrenal adenoma
6. Adrenal cortical carcinoma
7. Pheochromocytoma

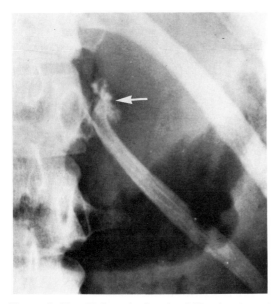

Figure 5–13. Unilateral adrenal calcification (arrow) in a normal-sized gland in a young adult with a history of difficult birth. There are no symptoms of adrenal disease or abdominal pain. The calcification most likely is a consequence of a neonatal adrenal hemorrhage.

While a few infants succumb to adrenal hemorrhage, many others will survive without symptoms of adrenal insufficiency. Either unilateral or bilateral calcifications have been shown to occur within eight days of hemorrhage and may persist into adulthood.[38,39] Adrenal calcification will be asymptomatic and go unnoticed until radiographs of the adrenal region are made at some later date (Fig. 5–13). Mottled calcification ranging from faint to dense may occupy a portion of the adrenal gland, or can extend throughout the entirety of the organ, and appear as a triangular clump of calcification[40] (Fig. 5–14).

Adrenal calcification can occur in Addison's disease. In a study of 120 patients with adrenal insufficiency, Jarvis et al. noted three forms of calcification: (a) gross mottled calcification of the gland, (b) multiple discrete deposits of calcium scattered throughout a normal-sized adrenal, and (c) a homogeneous increase in density of the gland. However, only 23 percent of this group had adrenal calcification, and in all cases the adrenal glands were not enlarged.[40] Hence, only a fraction of patients with Addison's disease have calcification, and since Addison's disease is rare, only a small percentage of patients with adrenal calcification suffer from adrenal insufficiency.[41]

In another study, 15 of 24 patients with adrenal calcification had evidence of tuberculosis, and seven had active disease. In this series there were nine patients with both Addison's disease and active tuberculosis, and seven of them had adrenal calcification.[42] It appears that patients whose adrenal disease is caused by tuberculosis have a greater chance of developing calcification. However, the frequency with which tuberculosis alone produces calcification is not known. Rarely, other granulomatous infections will be associated with adrenal calcification. Disseminated histoplasmosis may involve the adrenal glands along with other solid organs, but, unlike the liver and spleen, radiographically detectable calcification is seldom noted.[43]

Small areas of punctate or mottled densities in the adrenal glands may be seen in patients over 50 and can be a source of puzzlement on plain films. Usually they are either ignored or thought to represent a granuloma or old hemorrhage. Infrequently, they are investigated further and operative removal may be undertaken. Occasionally such

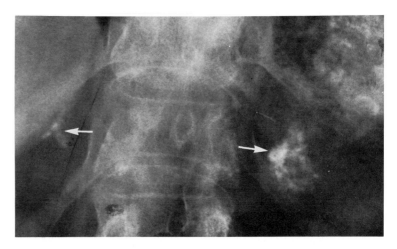

Figure 5–14. Bilateral adrenal calcification (arrows). There is no history of adrenal disease. While calcifications are often bilateral, they need not be symmetrical.

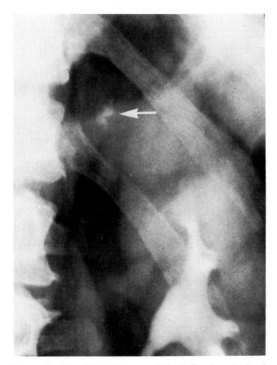

Figure 5–15. Myelolipoma of the left adrenal gland. Superior to the left kidney in a 62-year-old male are closely packed punctate calcifications (arrow). Because there was a coincident adrenal cyst, the left adrenal was removed and the calcification was shown to be within the myeloid stroma of the tumor.

calcifications are seen to lie within the substance of a myelolipoma, a benign tumefaction consisting of varying concretions of fat and bone marrow elements. Myelolipoma, also known as choristoma, is a well-defined encapsulated mass, generally no more than a few millimeters in size, but it can occasionally enlarge to 5 to 6 cm. in diameter.[39] It is not associated with endocrine abnormalities. When small, it may be unrecognized by most imaging modalities. Often, the only identifying feature will be punctate calcification. Usually it appears in the sixth and seventh decades, but the youngest reported case was in a 32-year-old.[44] Myelolipomas are thought to arise from either embryonic rests in the adrenal or to represent metaplasia of glandular elements into fat and marrow tissue.[45] Almost always, calcification occurs in areas of necrosis in the myeloid stroma.[46,47] The incidence of myelolipoma in older age groups is unknown, but it probably is not rare (Fig. 5–15).

Less commonly, focal areas of calcification may be seen in both benign and malignant tumors of the adrenal gland. The only clue to the presence of an enlarging mass on plain films may be a nidus of mottled or speckled calcification, and the extent of calcification may not correspond to the actual size of the tumor.[48,49] Occasionally, adenocarcinoma of the adrenal cortex or pheochromocytoma will manifest only as a small area of radiopacity.[50] While most often calcification in an apparently normal-sized gland indicates benign disease, in the appropriate clinical setting the possibility of a growing malignancy cannot be ruled out.

It is not always easy to sort out adrenal calcification from opacities in adjacent structures. Calcium deposition in costal cartilage may resemble adrenal calcification, and an attempt should be made to see if the calcification lies along the course of a rib in more than one projection. Calcification of the aorta or splenic artery can look like the flecks of calcification in adrenal masses. The tail of the pancreas lies close to and in front of the left adrenal, but since isolated pancreatic calcifications are rare, this is not often a cause of confusion. Parenchymal calcification localized in the superior margin of the kidney or renal capsule may be indistinguishable from adrenal calcification. Yet, despite the fact that many nearby structures may calcify, it is usually possible to recognize and localize small adrenal calcifications on plain films.

Solid Calcification in Enlarged Adrenal Gland

When extensive suprarenal calcification is seen on plain films, adrenal mass becomes a prime diagnostic consideration. Many solid adrenal masses of large size are cortical carcinomas with calcification deposited in areas of tumor degeneration and hemorrhage.[51-53] Calcification may be found diffusely in the tumor, but there is a propensity for calcium to localize in the more necrotic portions of the mass. Up to 31 percent of all adrenal cortical malignancies contain radiologically visible calcification which can be seen as speckled or mottled conglomerations, or as amorphous densities scattered throughout the mass.[41,54]

On the other hand, adrenal adenomas rarely calcify. For the most part, benign cortical tumors have a pattern of calcification identical with that seen in

Table 5–3. Solid Calcification in an Enlarged Adrenal Gland

Cortical carcinoma	Hibernoma
Adenoma	Hemangioma
Pheochromocytoma	Hematoma

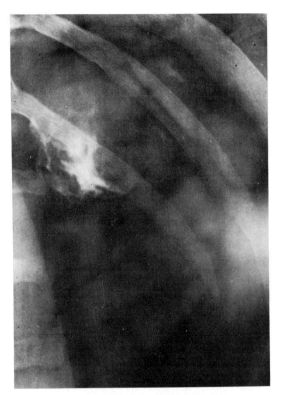

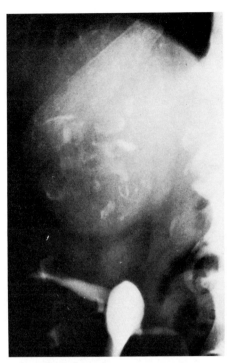

Figure 5–17. Calcification within an adrenal hematoma. There is curvilinear and amorphous calcification within a mass consisting mostly of old blood. A small adenoma was found at the periphery of the mass.

Figure 5–16. Benign adrenal adenoma. The irregular calcification is mostly in the inferior portion of the tumor. Carcinoma of the adrenal gland cannot be excluded on the basis of the radiographic appearance. (Courtesy of Dr. Arthur Diamond, Ranchos Palos Verdes, California.)

adrenal malignancies, but they uncommonly reach the size of cortical carcinoma[54] (Fig. 5–16). A rare benign tumor, a hibernoma, which is akin to myelolipoma but lacks marrow elements, may reach a large size and calcify with multiple punctate calcifications.[55] Hemangiomas of the adrenal can become large and contain phlebolithic calcifications.[55] Solid calcification may also be found in adrenal hematomas (Fig. 5–17).

Pheochromocytoma is a well-studied but uncommon tumor of the adrenal medulla. Calcification in pheochromocytomas is usually cystlike, but occasionally flecks or plaques of calcium may be present within the substance of the tumor. Sometimes the flecks may be multiple and oriented at different angles, giving the calcification a stellate appearance.[56] Between 10 and 20 percent of pheochromocytomas are bilateral, but bilateral calcification is very rare.[55]

Not all solid wall mass calcifications located in the region of the adrenal on plain films are adrenal tumors. On the right, solid calcification in the liver, superior pole of the right kidney, or the retroperitoneum may be confused with adrenal masses. On the left, cystadenomas in the pancreatic tail, renal tumors, carcinoma and leiomyoma of the stomach, solid calcification in the left lobe of the liver, and retroperitoneal masses enter into the differential diagnosis. Oblique films and contrast studies may help to localize lesions. However, because the suspicion of malignancy is so high, CT scanning or angiography must be relied upon for full characterization of a calcified mass in this area.

Cystic Lesions of the Adrenal Glands

Cystic lesions in the adrenal glands are infrequent. Unless they become large, they may not be detected on plain films except if they calcify. However, calcification in adrenal cysts is uncommon, occurring in approximately 15 percent of patients.[57] Cysts are found with equal frequency in either adrenal gland and are usually encountered in

Table 5–4. Adrenal Cysts that Calcify on Plain Films

1. Pseudocyst (cystic masses which result from hemorrhage or necrosis in a normal gland or adrenal neoplasm)
   a. Cystic adrenal hematoma
   b. Cystic benign tumor
   c. Cystic cortical carcinoma
   d. Metastases (melanoma)
2. True cysts with a calcified wall
   a. Epithelial-lined
   b. Endothelial-lined
3. Cystic pheochromocytoma
4. Parasitic cyst (*Echinococcus granulosus*)

the fifth and sixth decades. The incidence of adrenal cysts of all types is 50 percent higher in females.[58]

Pseudocysts are probably the most common adrenal cysts that calcify. Often part of the wall may be irregularly dense, suggesting residual adrenal tissue or part of the solid tumor from which the cyst arose.[59] It is important to remember that cystic calcification may be the first manifestation of a benign tumor or a malignancy (either a primary cortical carcinoma or a metastatic deposit, usually from melanoma).[60–62] Unless historical and clinical in-

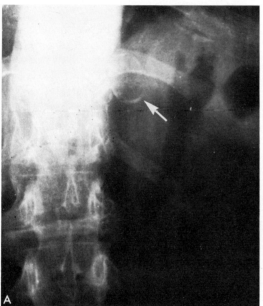
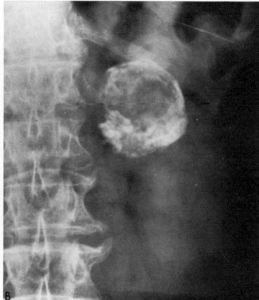
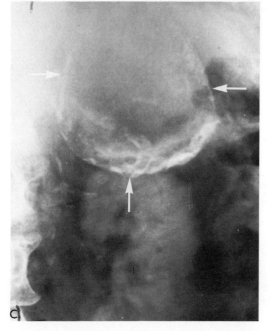

Figure 5–18. Three calcified cysts in the adrenal gland. *A,* Small cyst with smooth walls (arrow) simulates a calcified splenic artery aneurysm. *B,* Both cystic and solid calcifications are present in this calcified pseudocyst. *C,* Large adrenal cyst (arrows) above the left kidney. Its etiology was not determined.

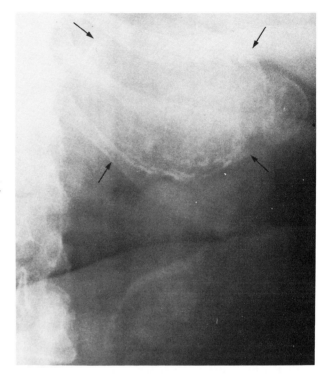

Figure 5–19. Calcified cyst (arrows) of *Echinococcus granulosus* in the left adrenal gland. (Courtesy of Dr. Irwin Bluth, Brooklyn, New York.)

formation indicates no recent growth of the cyst, it must be considered as a malignant neoplasm until proven otherwise. Almost always, true cysts cannot be differentiated from pseudocysts by plain film appearance (Fig. 5–18). True cysts may contain either an endothelial or an epithelial lining. Rarely, milk of calcium may occur in a benign adrenal cyst, and a diffuse opacity will be seen in the cyst which layers out on upright films.[63] Eggshell calcifications may be a feature of pheochromoctyoma.[64-66] The arclike circumferential calcifications often have a relatively small diameter, sometimes no more than 3 to 4 cm. On the right they resemble the rim calcification of solitary gallstones. Most cystic pheochromocytomas are probably pseudocysts which have resulted from hemorrhage and necrosis in the tumor.[67,68] *Echinococcus granulosus* cysts in the adrenals are rare; the more common sites for hydatid cysts in the upper abdomen are the liver, spleen, and kidney (Fig. 5–19).

Other abdominal cystic calcifications may simulate adrenal cysts. On the left, aneurysms of the splenic artery and the aorta, cysts of the spleen, pancreatic pseudocysts, and upper pole renal masses with rim calcification may look like adrenal cysts. On the right, calcification in hepatic artery aneurysms, gallbladder wall calcification, and cystic renal masses should be ruled out. Retroperitoneal and mesenteric cysts can be mistaken for adrenal cysts on either side.

RETROPERITONEUM

Many tumors arising from the connective tissue in the retroperitoneum may calcify. Most of these neoplasms are very uncommon and calcification is rarely found within them. Except for teratomas

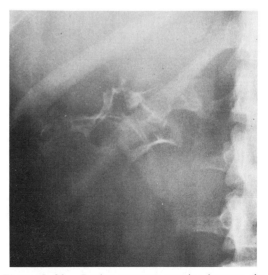

Figure 5–20. Benign teratoma growing between the right adrenal gland and the right kidney. Multiple foci of ossification occupy part of the mass.

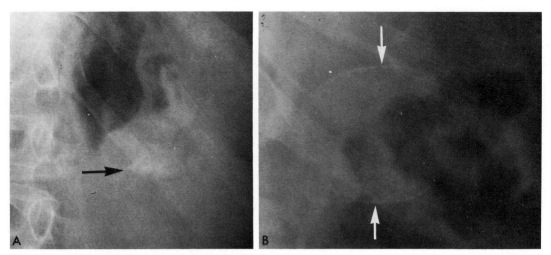

Figure 5–21. Retroperitoneal mesenchymoma calcifications. *A,* Faint solid calcification (arrow). *B,* A mass with cystic calcification (arrows).

there are no published series about calcification in individual tumors. Rather, the literature is limited to widely scattered case reports, and, for almost all retroperitoneal neoplasms, no discernible pattern of calcification has emerged.

However, there are a few exceptions. Teratomas often have a characteristic plain film appearance. While these tumors are most often seen in children, they can be encountered at any age. They frequently reach a large size, and typically they may grow anteriorly between the adrenal gland and the kidney. Teratomas may ossify and they often present on plain films as large masses containing bone and even teeth.[69] The size of the lesion and the extent of calcification and ossification are not predictors of biological activity. Both benign and malignant tumors may have similar plain film appearances (Fig. 5–20).

Mesenchymoma is a neoplasm containing two or more mesenchymal elements that usually do

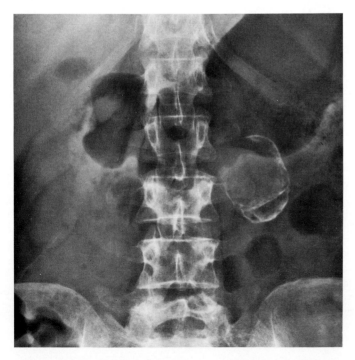

Figure 5–22. Cystic calcification in a retroperitoneal pheochromocytoma. (Courtesy of Dr. Morton Bosniak. Reprinted with the permission of the American College of Radiology from The Adrenal Retroperitoneum and Lower Urinary Tract, Yearbook Medical Publishers, Chicago, 1976.)

not exist together in one tumor. Within mesenchymomas can be found muscle, fat, blood vessels, cartilage, and bone. Calcification in these tumors tends to be diffuse and ill-defined.[55] Sometimes the calcifications are very faint and may be undetected on casual examination of a plain film of the abdomen. Mesenchymomas tend to grow rapidly, and calcification may appear abruptly as a result of hemorrhage or necrosis. Less often they may have cystic calcification and resemble large splenic aneurysms or cysts in the kidney, spleen, adrenal, or mesentery (Fig. 5–21). Mesenchymomas may be the retroperitoneal sarcoma that most frequently calcifies.

Approximately 10 percent of pheochromocytomas can arise outside the adrenal.[55] Calcified lesions have been noted in vesical and retroperitoneal pheochromocytomas. Just as in the adrenal, they may calcify as a ring of opacity and be indistinguishable from other cystic masses (Fig. 5–22).

REFERENCES

1. Minagi H, Margolin FR: Pancreatic calcifications. Am J Gastroenterol 57:139–145, 1972.
2. Lagergren C: Calcium carbonate precipitation in the pancreas, gallstones, and urinary calculi. Acta Chir Scand 124:320–325, 1962.
3. Sarles H, Sahel J: Pathology of chronic calcifying pancreatitis. Am J Gastroenterol 66:117–139, 1976.
4. Snell AM, Comfort MW: Incidence and diagnosis of pancreatic lithiasis. Am J Dig Dis 8:237–243, 1941.
5. McGeorge CK, Widmann BP, Ostrum H, et al: Diffuse calcification of the pancreas. Am J Roentgenol 78:599–606, 1957.
6. Peters BJ, Lubitz JM, Lindert MCF: Diffuse calcification of the pancreas. AMA Arch Intern Med 87:391–409, 1951.
7. Ring ER, Eaton SB Jr, Ferrucci JT, et al: Differential diagnosis of pancreatic calcification. Am J Roentgenol 117:446–452, 1973.
8. Hanelin LG, Schimmel DH: Lymphangioma of the pancreas exhibiting an unusual pattern of calcification. Radiology 122:636, 1977.
9. Okuda K, Ichinohe A, Kono K, et al: Minimal Thorotrast deposition in parapancreatic lymph nodes. Radiology 119:25–26, 1976.
10. Gillies CL: Pancreatic lithiasis with report of a case. Am J Roentgenol 41:42–46, 1939.
11. Johnson RB, Baker HW: Solitary calculus of the duct of Wirsung. Gastroenterology 27:849–860, 1954.
12. Tucker DH, Moore IB: Vanishing pancreatic calcifications in chronic pancreatitis. A sign of pancreatic carcinoma. N Engl J Med 268:31–33, 1968.
13. Baltaxe HA, Leslie EV: Vanishing pancreatic calcifications. Am J Roentgenol 99:642–644, 1967.
14. Donowitz M, Stein SA, Keohane MF: Vanishing pancreatic calcifications. A non-specific finding in chronic pancreatitis. JAMA 228:1575–1576, 1974.
15. Olurin EO, Olurin O: Pancreatic calcification: A report of 45 cases. Brit Med J 4:534–539, 1969.
16. Zuidema PO: Cirrhosis and disseminated calcification of the pancreas in patients with malnutrition. Trop Geogr Med 11:70–79, 1959.
17. Pitchumoni CS, Thomas E, Balthazar E, et al: Chronic calcific pancreatitis in association with celiac disease. Am J Gastroenterol 68:358–361, 1977.
18. Cope O, Culve PO, Mixter CG Jr: Pancreatitis. A diagnostic clue to hyperparathyroidism. Ann Surg 145:847–852, 1957.
19. Mixter CG Jr, Keynes WM, Cope O: Further experience with pancreatitis as a diagnostic clue to hyperparathyroidism. N Engl J Med 266:265–272, 1962.
20. Schmidt A, Creutzfeldt W: Calciphylactic pancreatitis and pancreatitis in hyperparathyroidism. Clin Orthop 69:135–145, 1970.
21. Singleton EB, Gray PM Jr: Radiologic evaluation of pancreatic disease in children. Semin Roentgenol 3:267–279, 1968.
22. Joffe N: Pancreatic calcification in childhood associated with protein malnutrition. Brit J Radiol 36:758–761, 1963.
23. Kattwinkel J, Lapey A, diSant'Agnese PA: Hereditary pancreatitis: three new kindreds and a critical review of the literature. Pediatrics 51:55–69, 1973.
24. Batson JM, Law DH: Chronic calcific pancreatitis in a child. Gastroenterology 43:95–98, 1962.
25. Stobbe KC, ReMine WH, Baggenstoss AH: Pancreatic lithiasis. Surg Gynecol Obstet 131:1090–1099, 1970.
26. Sawyer RB, Sawyer KC, Spencer JR: Proliferative cysts of the pancreas. Am J Surg 116:763–767, 1968.
27. Piper CE Jr, ReMine WH, Priestly JT: Pancreatic cystadenomata: Report of 20 cases. JAMA 180:648–652, 1962.
28. Haukohl RS, Melamed A: Cystadenomas of the pancreas. Am J Roentgenol 63:234–245, 1950.
29. Imhof H, Frank P: Pancreatic calcifications in malignant islet cell tumors. Radiology 122:333–337, 1977.
30. Jahnke RW, Gnekow W, Harell S: Non-beta cell islet tumor calcification associated with Zollinger-Ellison syndrome and multiple endocrine adenomatosis. Gastrointest Radiol 1:345–347, 1977.
31. Bozymski EM, Woodruff K, Sessions JR Jr: Zollinger-Ellison syndrome with hypoglycemia associated with calcification of the tumor and its metastases. Gastroenterology 65:658–661, 1973.
32. Beazley RM, Cohn I Jr: Pancreatic cancer. Cancer 31:346–358, 1981.
33. Kendig TA, Johnson RM, Shackford BC: Calcification in pancreatic carcinoma. Ann Intern Med 65:122–124, 1966.
34. Johnson JR, Zintel HA: Pancreatic calcification and cancer of the pancreas. Surg Gynecol Obstet 117:585–588, 1963.
35. Lundh G, Nordenstam H: Pancreas calcification and pancreas cancer: A discussion of two cases. Acta Chir Scand 136:493–496, 1970.
36. Paulino-Netto A, Dreiling PA, Baronofsky ID: The relationship between pancreatic calcification and cancer of the pancreas. Ann Surg 151:530–537, 1960.
37. Van Nostrand WR, Renert WD, Hileman WT: Milk-of-calcium of the pancreas. Radiology 110:323–324, 1974.
38. Gabrielle OF, Sheehan WF: Bilateral neonatal adrenal hemorrhage. Am J Roentgenol 91:656–658, 1964.
39. Martin JF: Suprarenal calcifications. Radiol Clin N Amer 3:129–138, 1965.
40. Jarvis JL, Jenkins D, Sosman MC, et al: Roentgenologic observations in Addison's disease. A review of 120 cases. Radiology 62:16–29, 1954.
41. McAlister WH, Lester PD: Diseases of the adrenal. Med Radiol Photogr 47:62–81, 1971.

42. Jarvis JL, Seaman WB: Idiopathic adrenal calcification in infants and children. Am J Roentgenol 82:510–520, 1959.

43. Schwarz E: Regional roentgen manifestations of histoplasmosis. Am J Roentgenol 87:865–874, 1962.

44. Giffen HK: Myelolipoma of the adrenals: Report of seven cases. Am J Pathol 23:613–619, 1947.

45. Tulcinsky DB, Deutsch V, Bubis JJ: Myelolipoma of the adrenal gland. Brit J Surg 57:465–467, 1970.

46. McAlister WN, Koehler PR: Diseases of the adrenal. Radiol Clin N Amer 5:205–220, 1967.

47. Costello P, Clouse ME, Kane RA, et al: Problems in the diagnosis of adrenal tumors. Radiology 125:335–341, 1977.

48. Vermess M, Schour L, Jaffe ES: Calcification in benign, non-functioning adrenal adenoma: Report of a case with selective adrenal arteriogram. Brit J Radiol 45:621–623, 1972.

49. Drucker WD, Longo FW, Christy MP: Calcifications in a benign non-functioning tumor of the adrenal. JAMA 177:577–579, 1961.

50. Pendergrass HP, Tristan TA, Blakemore WS, et al: Roentgen technics in the diagnosis and localization of pheochromocytoma. Radiology 78:725–737, 1962.

51. Colapinto RF, Steed BL: Arteriography of adrenal tumors. Radiology 100:343–350, 1971

52. Strittmatter WC, Brown CH, Tretbar HA: A large carcinoma of the adrenal. Radiology 68:230–232, 1957.

53. Boise CL, Sears WN: Calcification in adrenal neoplasms. Radiology 56:731–734, 1951.

54. McNulty JG, Lea Thomas M, Tighe JR: Angiographic diagnosis of benign adrenal adenoma. Am J Roentgenol 104:386–388, 1968.

55. Bosniak MA, Seigelman SS, Evans JA: The Adrenal Retroperitoneum and Lower Urinary Tract. Chicago, Year Book Medical Publishers, 1976, p. 138.

56. Mori Y, Kiyohara H, Miki T, et al: Pheochromocytoma with prominent calcification and associated pancreatic islet cell tumor. J Urol 118:843–844, 1977.

57. Palubinskas AJ, Christensen WR, Harrison JH, et al: Calcified adrenal cysts. Am J Roentgenol 82:853–861, 1959.

58. Parker JM: Calcified cyst of the adrenal gland. Milit Med 138:791–792, 1970.

59. Anderson MY, Roberts HG, Smith ET: Calcified cyst of the adrenal cortex without endocrine symptoms. Radiology 54:236–241, 1950.

60. Wood JC: A calcified adrenal tumor. Brit J Radiol 25:222–224, 1952.

61. Samuel E: Calcification in suprarenal neoplasms. Brit J Radiol 21:139–142, 1948.

62. Twersky J, Levin DC: Metastatic melanoma of the adrenal. Radiology 116:627–628, 1975.

63. Moss AA: Milk of calcium of the adrenal gland. Brit J Radiol 49:186–187, 1976.

64. Grainger RG, Lloyd GAS, Williams JL: Eggshell calcification: A sign of phaeochromocytoma. Clin Radiol 18:282–286, 1967.

65. Neilson J, Smith S McC: Eggshell calcification in phaeochromocytoma. J R Coll Surg Edinb 18:183–187, 1973.

66. Feist JE, Lasser EC: Pheochromocytoma with large cystic calcification and associated sphenoid ridge malformation. Radiology 76:21–26, 1961.

67. Meyers MA, King MC: Unusual features of pheochromocytoma. Clin Radiol 20:52–56, 1965.

68. Moser M, Sheehan G, Schwinger H: Pheochromocytoma with calcification simulating cholelithiasis. Radiology 55:855–858, 1950.

69. Jansson G: On roentgen diagnostics of adrenal tumors. Acta Radiol 27:526–530, 1946.

Chapter 6

GENITAL TRACT CALCIFICATION

Milton Elkin, M.D.

FEMALE GENITAL TRACT

Uterus

Leiomyomas

Except for pregnancy, most commonly, calcifications associated with the uterus occur in leiomyomas. This dystrophic calcification of solid mass type usually appears in mottled distribution with no well-defined curvilinear rim (Figs. 1–25, 1–27, 6–1). There are, however, instances of calcifications with a well-defined, thin dense rim with relatively little or even much internal calcification which can be mottled, whorled, or streaked (Figs. 1–35, 6–2). Sometimes early calcification in a uterine fibroid is ill-defined and punctate similar to that seen in malignant neoplasms (Fig. 6–3). The occasional case of leiomyosarcoma can also contain calcification, often indistinguishable from that of a benign uterine fibroid (Fig. 6–4).

Although uterine fibroids are apt to be multiple in a given patient, only a single tumor may calcify. Also the soft-tissue mass of an individual fibroid is frequently much larger than the volume of calcification, merely reflecting the fact that calcification may be limited to only a part of the tumor.

A small mottled zone of calcification or diffuse calcification of mottled or speckled type in a small fibroid can simulate calcification in a pelvic lymph node. Location may be of help in the differential diagnosis. Lymph nodes in the pelvis are distributed along the course of major vessels, such as the iliac arteries and their branches. Hence, in general, nodal calcification occupies a more lateral site in the pelvis than do calcified fibroids. Similarly, arterial calcifications and phleboliths are located laterally in the pelvis.

It is important to remember that large leiomyomas extend from the pelvis into the abdominal cavity, sometimes to the level of the kidneys or even higher. If such fibroids calcify completely or widely, it is easy to determine that the calcified structure most likely originates in the pelvis, and the type of the calcification indicates the correct diagnosis. However, if only a portion of the huge fibroid calcifies and that portion is in the abdomen, the nature of the abnormality may remain obscure unless note is made of the extent of the entire soft-tissue component of the leiomyoma. In addition, the position of the uterus varies with the degree of

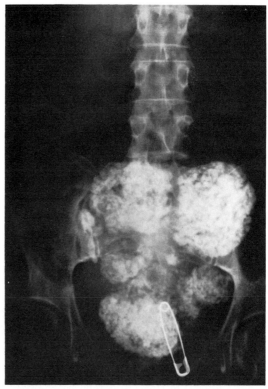

Figure 6–1 Multiple uterine leiomyomas with mottled calcifications and no well-defined rim.

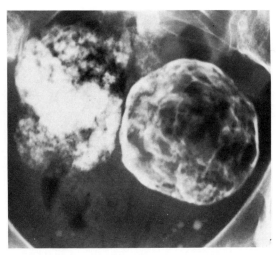

Figure 6–2. Uterine leiomyomas with different types of calcifications. The fibroid on the patient's right has coarsely mottled calcification with no rim. The fibroid on the patient's left has a well-defined dense rim with whorled internal calcification.

filling of the urinary bladder. A uterine fibroid, appearing in its expected location in the pelvis with the bladder empty, can be displaced into the abdomen by a distended bladder (Fig. 6–5).

Other Neoplasms

Other types of uterine neoplasms, of which the most common are squamous cell carcinoma of the cervix and adenocarcinoma of the endometrium, show calcification only very rarely. Infrequently, calcification appears in a malignancy of the uterus after radiation therapy.[1] The calcification is of the solid mass type, consisting of a speckled to coarsely nodular pattern, apparently occurring in zones of necrosis, ischemia, and hemorrhage. Very infrequently, calcification takes place in lymph nodes involved by metastasis from uterine carcinoma, following radiotherapy, or even without prior treatment.[2] Calcification of a fine punctate nature has been reported in malignant mixed uterine tumors.[3] These are neoplasms containing both sarcomatous and carcinomatous elements, accounting for about 6 percent of primary malignancies of the uterine corpus. The plain film finding of a localized zone of fine punctate calcification within an enlarging soft-tissue mass located centrally in the pelvis of a postmenopausal female should raise the suspicion of malignant mixed uterine tumor.

Of special interest is the occurrence of calcifications bilaterally in the soft tissues of the pelvis secondary to injections of radioactive gold (^{198}Au) into the parametrium as adjunctive therapy in patients with carcinoma of the cervix.[4] The calcification, first appearing five to ten years after treatment, is limited to the region of the gold injection, close to the lateral walls of the bony pelvis at the location of the iliac and hypogastric lymph nodes, and is most likely due to focal areas of tissue necrosis secondary to the radiation. The appearance varies from thin linear and laminated to thick globular calcifications, which progress in density and extent.

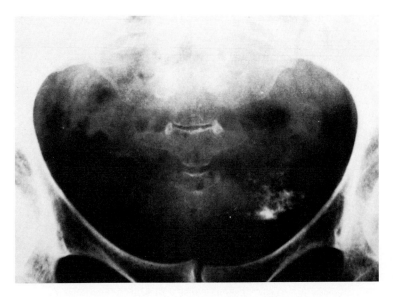

Figure 6–3. Ill-defined and punctate calcification in a uterine leiomyoma.

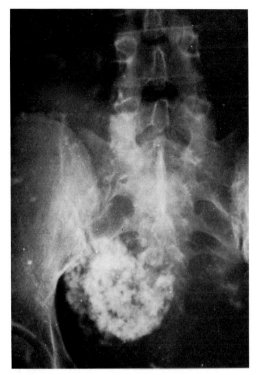

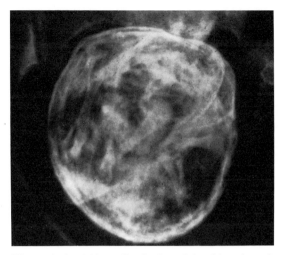

Figure 6–6. Lithopedion in the pelvis with major calcification of the membranes and well-formed fetal bones.

Pregnancy

Ossification in the normal fetus is so distinctive that it needs no discussion. Yet faint calcification in the fetus in early pregnancy can be confused with pelvic calcification of other types.

Lithopedion, the petrifaction or calcification of a retained, dead fetus, is an end result of an extrauterine pregnancy (Fig. 6–6). Three general patterns have been described.[5]

Figure 6–4. Large uterine leiomyosarcoma, with a collection of dense mottled calcifications in the pelvis, characteristic of leiomyoma. The diffusely scattered irregular calcifications in other parts of the tumor are not characteristic of leiomyoma and should raise the suspicion of malignant change.

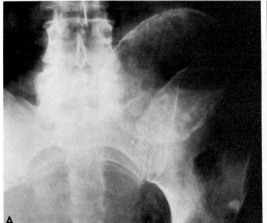
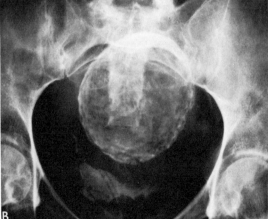

Figure 6–5. Change in position of uterine leiomyoma with extent of bladder distention. *A,* With a filled bladder, the calcified uterine leiomyoma is located in the lower abdomen. The patient is paraparetic, with bladder atony. *B,* With the bladder emptied, the leiomyoma is in the pelvis.

1. The membranes are calcified, forming a hard shell surrounding the fetus, which may be skeletonized but not involved in the process of calcification (lithokelyphos).

2. The membranes and the fetus are both calcified (lithokelyphopedion).

3. The fetus is infiltrated with calcium salts but calcification of the membranes is negligible (true lithopedion).

For the development of a lithopedion the patient must have had an extrauterine pregnancy that had not been diagnosed and thus not treated. The abdominal pregnancy must have survived for over three months; otherwise, it would have been absorbed.[6]

Usually the configuration of a fetal part can be recognized on the abdominal radiograph along with the calcification, leading to the appropriate diagnosis. If the abdominal pregnancy had been implanted on the omentum, the lithopedion may show marked mobility with changes in patient position. The location of the lithopedion can be highly unusual. An extrauterine pregnancy implanted on the liver can end up as a calcified mass in the right upper quadrant.

Fallopian Tubes

The occurrence of radiographically demonstrable calcification in the fallopian tubes is rare. A few cases of salpingolithiasis have been reported, as has calcification in the tubal lumen due to genital tuberculosis. Calcification in the walls of the uterine arteries may on the radiograph be misinterpreted as tubal calcification (Fig. 6–7).

Other Opacities

Contraceptive devices, of various shapes and radiopacity, are easily distinguishable. They come in so many different configurations that there is no point in listing names and shapes. Most important is the observation whether such a device has maintained its intrauterine location, as determined by its position in relation to the soft-tissue shadow of the uterus as well as by its configuration (e.g., the closeness of the bends of the loop type of device).

Ovary

Dermoid Cyst (Cystic Teratoma)

Although "cystic teratoma" is the preferable term since most contain derivatives of all three germ layers, "dermoid" and "dermoid cyst" are the more commonly used terms. They make up about 10 percent of all ovarian tumors and have a 10 to 20 percent incidence of bilaterality, occasionally being multiple in one or both ovaries.[7] Malignancy, usually squamous cell carcinoma, occurs in less than 1 percent of the lesions. In a review of 1,007 dermoid cysts, Peterson et al. reported that 80 percent were between 5 and 15 cm. in diameter, 13 percent less than 5 cm., and 7 percent larger than 15 cm.[8]

Dermoids are the most common ovarian lesions with radiographically demonstrable calcification, usually representing rudimentary teeth. Sometimes there is a single tooth and at other times several teeth, usually of distinctive enough shape to allow

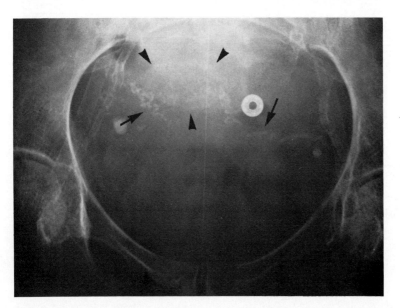

Figure 6–7. Marked vascular calcification in the pelvis. The markedly calcified uterine arteries (arrows) could be mistaken for fallopian tube calcification. The uterus is defined (arrowheads) by calcification of the intrauterine arteries.

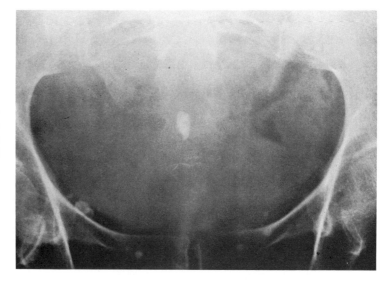

Figure 6–8. Dermoid cyst containing one tooth, having the appearance of an incisor. There is an ill-defined soft tissue mass without radiolucent contents.

the correct diagnosis (Figs. 1–31, 6–8, 6–9). The teeth are most frequently of incisor or molar type and may be contained in a rudimentary fragment of maxillary bone or mandible. The teeth may lie free within the cyst, but more often are embedded in the cyst wall, usually in a raised nipplelike tissue protuberance, the dermal plug. It has been reported that about 10 percent of ovarian dermoids show calcification of cyst type, i.e., curvilinear calcification in the entire cyst wall or a segment of the wall (Fig. 6–10). Calcification of either type, bone within the cyst or curvilinear calcific plaques in the wall, can be seen in about 50 to 60 percent of all dermoid cysts.[9]

The observation of a soft-tissue mass, within which the presumed tooth or teeth are situated, is helpful in the diagnosis, the mass appearing smoothly rounded and characteristically relatively radiolucent owing to its content of thick, lardaceous material formed by the sebaceous glands of the squamous epithelium lining the cyst wall (Fig. 6–11).

Sometimes the calcifications in dermoid cysts are structureless, not resembling teeth, and thus not suggestive of the specific diagnosis. The curvilinear type of calcification occurs in other types of cysts and is not specific for dermoids. The radiolucency of the contained sebaceous material can be seen in about 35 percent of cystic teratomas. Overall, in about 40 percent of dermoids the findings on

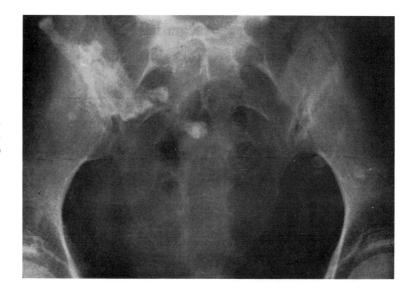

Figure 6–9. Dermoid cyst containing several teeth and a rudimentary mandible. There is no radiolucent mass.

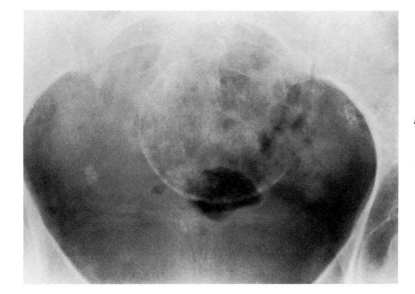

Figure 6–10. Dermoid cyst with curvilinear calcification in its wall. (Courtesy of Dr. Erich Leichter, Paterson, New Jersey.)

scout abdominal radiographs are characteristic enough to allow a specific diagnosis.

Papillary Serous Cystadenoma and Cystadenocarcinoma

Cystadenocarcinomas constitute 70 to 80 percent of ovarian malignancies; of these, 75 to 95 percent are serous, 10 to 25 percent are mucinous, and less than 5 percent are mixed. Of all cystic tumors of the ovary, 15 to 35 percent are papillary serous cystadenocarcinomas, these being the most common malignant ovarian lesions.[10,11] They are often bilateral. The peak age of incidence is 30 to 60 years.

Calcification can occur in the primary papillary serous cystadenocarcinoma (Fig. 6–12) as well as in metastases, most often of psammomatous type.[10-13] Psammoma bodies are small discrete calcifications, fairly uniform in size and distribution. They have also been called corpora amylacea or calcospherites, and are made up of calcium carbonate in a concentric organic framework. They are typically less dense than the calcifications of lymph nodes or leiomyomas. Psammoma bodies may be seen only in the metastases in patients

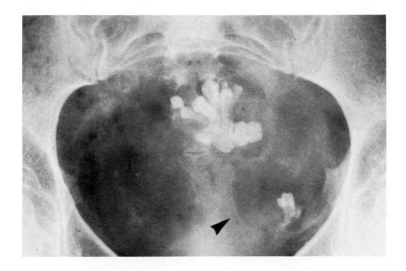

Figure 6–11. Two dermoid cysts with radiolucent (sebaceous) contents. The dermoid cyst on the patient's right contains multiple teeth and its border is not well defined. The dermoid cyst on the left contains a single tooth embedded in a small section of rudimentary jawbone; its border is well defined with visualization of a thin wall (arrowhead).

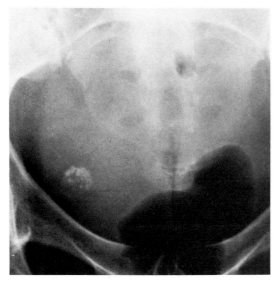

Figure 6–12. Serous cystadenocarcinoma of the ovary, containing psammomatous calcification. There is a large pelvic soft-tissue mass, containing a discrete collection of punctate calcifications.

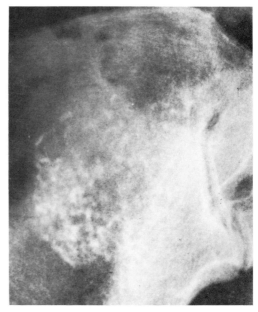

Figure 6–13. Metastasis to the peritoneum from serous cystadenocarcinoma of the ovary. The metastatic mass contains psammomatous calcification. There was no radiographically demonstrable calcification in the primary neoplasm.

without calcification in the primary neoplasm, producing finely speckled or granular amorphous calcifications in the liver, retroperitoneal or abdominal lymph nodes, or peritoneum (Fig. 6–13). Metastatic serosal implants can occur along the course of the colon, the cloud of faint calcification resembling barium in the colon remaining from a recent upper GI examination (Figs. 1–29, 6–14). A similar appearance resembling psammomatous calcification can be produced by other opacities in the colon. There is a report of a young woman with punctate calcifications in the pelvis representing opacities in the colon resulting from the ingestion of bone meal.[14]

Psammomatous calcification is said to develop also in benign serous cystadenoma; however, this

Figure 6–14. Papillary serous cystadenocarcinoma of the ovary with widespread metastases to the peritoneum and implants on the serosa of the colon, with psammoma bodies producing a cloud of faint calcification. (Courtesy of Dr. Arnold Geller, Riverside, California.)

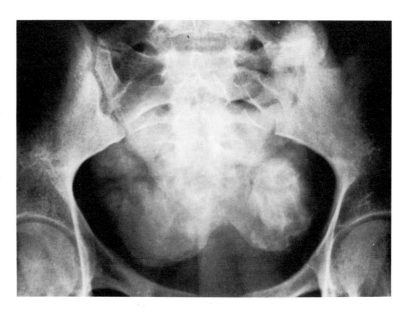

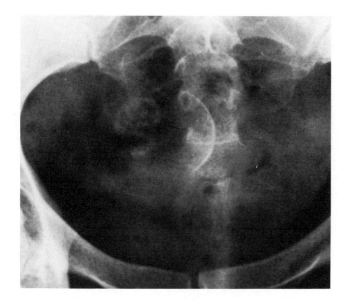

Figure 6–15. Calcification of cystic type involving a segment of the wall of a benign serous cystadenoma. (Courtesy of Dr. Paul Tartell, Queens, New York.)

must be extremely unusual, if it actually occurs. Rarely, benign serous cystadenoma has curvilinear wall calcification of cystic type (Fig. 6–15).

Mucinous Cystadenoma and Cystadenocarcinoma

Calcification is not a feature of these neoplasms. However, mucinous cystadenocarcinoma may rupture with implantation of cell nests on the peritoneum, resulting in pseudomyxoma peritonei. The accumulations of myxomatous material from these multiple implants can be associated with peripheral curvilinear calcifications of cystic type[13,15] (Figs. 3–18, 6–16).

Other Ovarian Neoplasms

Gonadoblastoma, a rare ovarian neoplasm composed of germ cells, cells of sex chord origin, and usually cells of mesenchymal origin, can show calcification of circumscribed mottled or punctate appearance.[16,17] The tumors can be bilateral. Although potentially malignant, most reported cases were benign. Gonadoblastoma, previously classified as an atypical dysgerminoma, occurs usually in patients under age 25 years and is usually hormonally active, with the clinical syndrome including primary amenorrhea, virilization, hirsutism, clitoral hypertrophy, and infantilism of the uterus. Another rare ovarian neoplasm, also hormonally active and also potentially malignant, the lipid cell tumor, can show a cluster of punctate calcifications

within its soft-tissue mass similar to that described for gonadoblastoma.[18]

There are rare case reports of calcification of solid mass type in other ovarian tumors, such as thecoma and fibroma (Fig. 6–17).

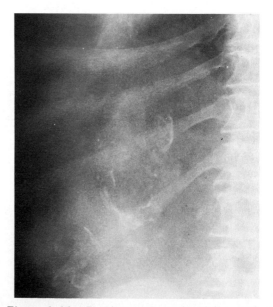

Figure 6–16. Pseudomyxoma peritonei in a patient with mucinous cystadenocarcinoma of the ovary. There are linear and curvilinear calcifications at the periphery of the peritoneal myxomatous collections.

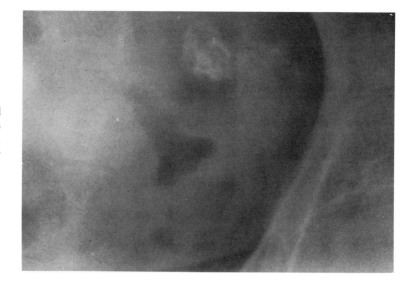

Figure 6–17. Amorphous and streaky calcification of solid mass type in a left parametrial tumor, which proved to be an ovarian fibroma.

Miscellaneous Ovarian Calcifications

Radiographically demonstrable calcification occurs rarely in corpora albicantia.[19,20] The calcifications can be of popcorn configuration resembling that of a uterine fibroid or appear as roughly round clusters of sharply defined nodules, the clusters measuring a few centimeters in diameter and the individual nodules a few millimeters. The individual calcific nodules may have lucent centers, simulating the appearance of small phleboliths. Among the dozen or so reported cases, a few have shown involvement of both ovaries with bilateral pelvic calcifications.

A rare cause of abdominal calcification is autoamputated ovary, i.e., an ovary that has undergone torsion, become infarcted, separated from its ligamentous moorings and subsequently calcified. The usual radiographic appearance is that of a coarsely stippled oval pelvic mass, a few centimeters in greatest diameter.[21,22] Being freely mobile, the calcification can appear at different locations on serial films, sometimes in the pelvis and sometimes in the lower abdomen. It is usually an incidental radiologic or surgical finding at any age group, although most often in children and young adults without a documented antecedent episode of abdominal pain. Pneumogynecography shows absence of one ovary and all or part of the ipsilateral fallopian tube.

Calcification of one or both ovaries, usually of mottled, solid mass type, can result from tuberculous infection.[23] The appearance resembles that of lymph node calcification, but the overall size is

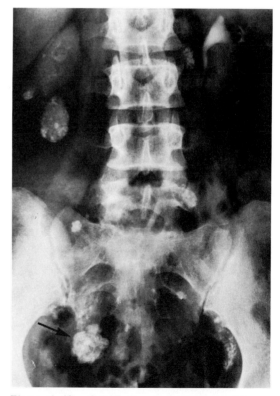

Figure 6–18. Calcification in genitourinary tuberculosis in a 62-year-old woman. Supine radiograph during urography shows a small, non-excreting right kidney with mottled areas of calcification. The right ovary is calcified (arrow). The other calcifications are in abdominal and pelvic lymph nodes.

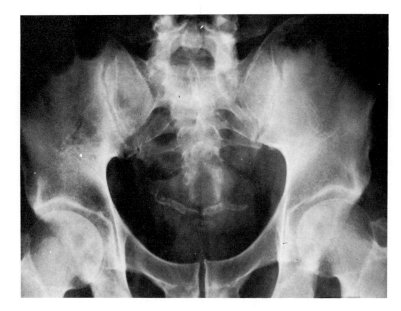

Figure 6–19. Calcification of the vasa deferentia in their ampullary segments in a 53-year-old diabetic man.

larger than that of the typical lymph node and the calcification is situated more medially than pelvic nodes (Fig. 6–18). Associated findings, such as tuberculous calcifications of the urinary tract, help in the diagnosis.

MALE GENITAL TRACT

Vas Deferens

Calcification of the vas deferens occurs most often in diabetic patients but sometimes in nondiabetics as a manifestation of aging or as a result of infection. The relationship to diabetes mellitus was first reported by Marks and Ham[24] from a hospital with a large population of diabetic patients; of nine patients with vasal calcification, six had diabetes. In a later report from the same hospital, of 60 patients with vasal calcification, 56 had diabetes.[25] Even though many diabetic patients were seen at that hospital, nondiabetic patients made up over 80 percent of patients examined in the x-ray department. In the 56 patients with diabetes, the diabetes had been acquired at an average age of 33.4 years,

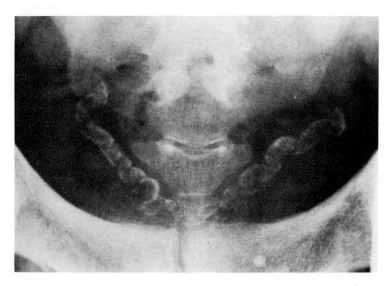

Figure 6–20. Prone projection of the abdomen of a 47-year-old diabetic man. There is calcification in the walls of the tortuous ampullary segments of the vasa deferentia as they descend toward the urethra.

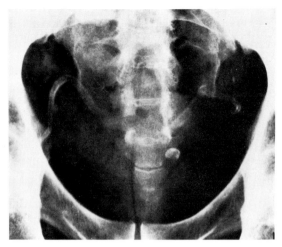

Figure 6–21. Bilateral calcification of the vasa deferentia in their ampullary segments as well as in the portions ascending from the inguinal canals, more pronounced on the patient's right.

and vasal calcification was first noted radiologically after an average duration of 18.3 years of diabetes. In general, it took longer for vasal calcification to develop in patients with onset of diabetes at an early age than in those with onset later in life, 22 years being the average duration of diabetes in patients with onset of the disease before age 40, and 13 years in patients with onset of diabetes after age 40. Other reports have confirmed the association of diabetes mellitus and calcification of the vas deferens.[26-28]

Calcification occurring in diabetics and in nondiabetic elderly patients is located within the muscular wall of the vas deferens and is considered degenerative in nature. Vasal calcification resulting from infection is intraluminal; among the causative infections are tuberculosis, gonorrhea, syphilis, and chronic urinary tract infections. It is usually not possible to distinguish radiologically the intramural from the intraluminal calcification.[29]

The vas deferens, ascending as the ductus deferens from the scrotum into the pelvic retroperitoneal space via the inguinal canal, may exhibit calcification of conduit type in any segment, but the most common site is its horizontal and descending ampullary segment. The calcification, most often bilateral and symmetrical, is typically manifest as two horizontal calcific tramlines just cephalad to the empty bladder or posterior to the distended bladder (Figs. 6–19, 6–20). On occasion the linear calcifications can be seen to continue toward the region of the inguinal canal (Fig. 6–21) or even into the scrotum. Infrequently, the calcification can be seen only in that portion of the vas deferens close to the scrotum (Fig. 6–22). Often the lines of calcific density are not continuous, there being very short intervening segments without visible calcification, suggesting that there are plaques of calcification (Fig. 6–23).

The radiologic appearance of calcification of the vas might be misinterpreted as calcification in an arterial wall. However, vasal calcification is usually denser and thicker than arterial calcification, and in the usual location and direction of vasal calcification there are no sizable arteries in the male.

Figure 6–22. Calcification of each ductus deferens in the scrotum of a 77-year-old nondiabetic man. There was no radiographically demonstrable calcification in other portions of the vasa deferentia.

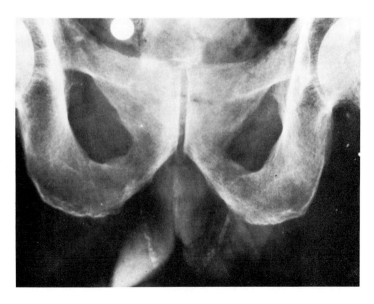

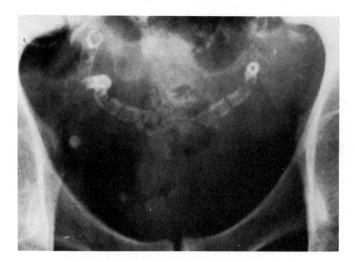

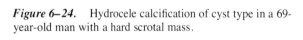

Figure 6–23. Calcification of the vasa deferentia in a 68-year-old diabetic man. Note the plaquelike appearance of the calcium deposition.

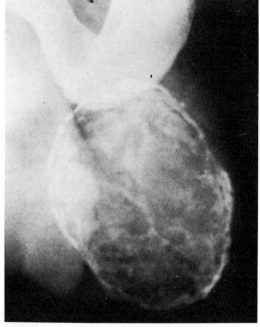

Figure 6–24. Hydrocele calcification of cyst type in a 69-year-old man with a hard scrotal mass.

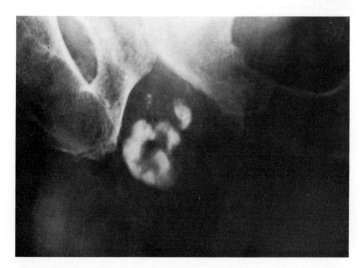

Figure 6–25. Testicular calcification presumably following infarction. An 86-year-old man with adenocarcinoma of the sigmoid was found to have a stony-hard left testicle, of which he was aware for at least ten years. He recalled an episode of severe testicular pain as a young man. Very likely he had suffered torsion of the testicle. There are several clumps of dense amorphous calcification of solid mass type in the testis.

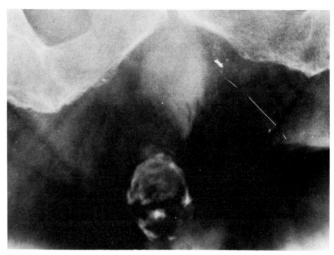

Figure 6–26. Most likely calcification of a hematoma in the scrotum. An elderly man had had bilateral orchiectomies several years before for treatment of carcinoma of the prostate. There are collections of amorphous calcification with an incomplete rim calcification of irregular thickness.

Seminal Vesicles

Calcification in the seminal vesicles is rare, occurring as small intraluminal concretions located posterior to the bladder and cephalad to the prostate. Very likely these calculi result from infection, such as tuberculosis and gonorrhea. The concretions may be so numerous as to produce a cloud of radiopacity defining the shape of the seminal vesicles.

Scrotum

Radiographically demonstrable calcification in the scrotum is infrequent. As already noted, calcification of the ductus deferens can occur in its intrascrotal portion. Hydroceles or spermatoceles can show curvilinear wall calcification of cyst type (Fig. 6–24). Dense, solid mass type calcification of oval shape can be due to tuberculosis of the testicle. A similar appearance can result from infarction of the testis secondary to torsion, reported most often in the newborn (Fig. 6–25). Very uncommon is postinfarction calcification in an undescended testicle, resulting in the radiographic finding of an irregularly calcified mass, a few centimeters in diameter, in the mid or lower abdomen.[30] Hematoma in the scrotum, such as that following orchiectomy, can be the cause for the development of a roughly rounded or oval dense calcification (Fig. 6–26). Also phleboliths can be seen in the scrotum (Fig. 7–29).

It is unusual for testicular tumors to show calcification. Streaky or lacelike calcification has been described in an occasional Leydig cell tumor and fine punctate calcifications have been reported in tera-

toma.[31] Several instances of calcified steatomata (sebaceous cysts) of the skin of the scrotum have been reported, appearing radiographically as dense, well-defined, round or oval calcifications of concretion type, a few millimeters to one centimeter or so in diameter.[32]

REFERENCES

1. Dolan PA: Tumor calcification following therapy. Am J Roentgenol 89:166–174, 1963.
2. Hutcheson J, Page DL, Oldham RR: Calcified lymph node metastases from carcinoma of the cervix. Cancer 32:266–269, 1973.
3. Schabel SI, Burgener FA, Reynolds J, Gephardt G: Radiographic manifestations of malignant mixed uterine tumors. J Canad Assoc Radiol 26:176–183, 1975.
4. Deeths TM, Stanley RJ: Parametrial calcification in cervical carcinoma patients treated with radioactive gold. Am J Roentgenol 127:511–513, 1976.
5. Hemley SD, Schwinger A: Lithopedion. Case report and survey. Radiology 58:235–238, 1952.
6. Oden PW, Lee HC: Lithopedion with calcified placenta. Case report. Va Med Mon 67:304–306, 1940.
7. Sloan RD: Cystic teratoma (dermoid) of the ovary. Radiology 81:847–853, 1963.
8. Peterson WF, Prevost EC, Edmonds FT, et al: Benign cystic teratoma of the ovary: Clinico-statistical study of 1007 cases with review of literature. Am J Obst Gynecol 70:368–382, 1955.
9. Cusmano JV: Dermoid cysts of the ovary: Roentgen features. Radiology 66:719–722, 1956.
10. Castro JR, Klein EW: The incidence and appearance of roentgenologically visible psammomatous calcification of papillary cystadenocarcinoma of the ovaries. Am J Roentgenol 88:886–891, 1962.
11. Teplick JG, Haskins ME, Alavi A: Calcified intraperitoneal metastases from ovarian carcinoma. Am J Roentgenol 127:1003–1006, 1976.
12. Lingley JR: The significance of psammoma calcification in the roentgen diagnosis of papillary tumors of the ovary. Am J Roentgenol 47:563–570, 1942.
13. Moncada R, Cooper RA, Garces M, Badrinath K: Calci-

fied metastases from malignant ovarian neoplasm. Review of the literature. Radiology 113:31–35, 1974.

14. Schabel SI, Rogers CJ: Opaque artifacts in a health food faddist simulating ovarian neoplasm. Am J Roentgenol 130:789–790, 1978.

15. Noonan CD: Primary and secondary malignancy of the female reproductive system. Radiol Clin N Amer 3:375, 1965.

16. Cooperman LR, Hamlin J, Ng E: Gonadoblastoma. A rare ovarian tumor related to the dysgerminoma with characteristic roentgen appearance. Radiology 90:322–324, 1968.

17. Seymour EQ, Hood JB, Underwood PB Jr, Williamson HO: Gonadoblastoma: an ovarian tumor with characteristic pelvic calcifications. Am J Roentgenol 127:1001–1002, 1976.

18. Villee DB: Case 22–1982: Case records of the Massachusetts General Hospital. N Engl J Med 306:1348–1354, 1982.

19. Buhrow CJ, Gary TM, Clark WE II: Ovarian corpora albicantia calcifications. A case report. Radiology 87:746–747, 1966.

20. Puckette SE Jr, Williamson HO, Seymour EQ: Calcification in an ovarian corpus albicans. Radiology 92:1105, 1969.

21. Lester PD, McAlister WH: A mobile calcified spontaneously amputated ovary. J Canad Assoc Radiol 21:143–145, 1970.

22. Nixon GW, Condon VR: Amputated ovary: a cause of migratory abdominal calcification. Am J Roentgenol 128:1053–1055, 1977.

23. Rozin S: The x-ray diagnosis of genital tuberculosis. J Obst Gynecol Brit Emp 59:59–63, 1952.

24. Marks JH, Ham DP: Calcification of vas deferens. Am J Roentgenol 47:859–863, 1942.

25. Wilson JL, Marks JH: Calcification of the vas deferens. Its relation to diabetes mellitus and arteriosclerosis. N Engl J Med 245:321–325, 1951.

26. Culver GJ, Tannenhaus J: Calcification of the vas deferens in diabetics. JAMA 173:648–651, 1960.

27. Camiel MR: Calcification of vas deferens associated with diabetes. J Urol 86:634–636, 1961.

28. Hafiz A, Melnick JC: Calcification of the vas deferens. J Canad Assoc Radiol 19:56–60, 1968.

29. King JC Jr, Rosenbaum, HD: Calcification of the vasa deferentia in nondiabetics. Radiology 100:603–606, 1971.

30. Cho SK, Hamoudi AB, Clatworthy HW Jr, Frye TR: Infarction of an abdominal undescended testis presenting as a calcified abdominal mass in a newborn. Radiology 110:173–174, 1974.

31. Loveday BO, Price JL: Soft tissue radiography of the testes. Clin Radiol 29:685–689, 1978.

32. Phillips EW: Calcified steatomata of the scrotum. Report of a case. Am J Roentgenol 92:388–389, 1964.

Chapter 7

CALCIFICATION IN ABDOMINAL ARTERIES AND VEINS

*Chusilp Charnsangavej, M.D.,
and Stephen R. Baker, M.D.*

ARTERIAL CALCIFICATION

Arterial calcification is a frequently encountered finding on plain films of the abdomen. With advancing age, the probability of calcium deposition in vascular walls increases, and in the elderly, calcification is common. Usually, arterial calcification is easily recognized. However, difficulties in interpretation arise when the focus of radiopacity is faint, small, or displaced from its usual position. It is these circumstances which demand careful inspection of plain films because the observation of vascular calcification may avoid the need for further imaging procedures, or at least direct the workup to more definitive examinations. For example, the presence of calcification in the wall of an aortic aneurysm on plain abdominal films can readily indicate the location and size of the aneurysm. Appreciation of the conduit morphology of vascular calcification can help distinguish arterial densities from other radiodensities.

General Features of Arterial Calcification

In almost all cases, arterial calcification involves the vessel wall; calcified intraluminal clots are rarely seen on plain films. The appearance of calcification depends on three factors: (1) the orientation of the vessel wall with respect to the x-ray beam, (2) the degree of calcium deposition, and (3) the location of calcification in the vessel wall.

When the artery is oriented perpendicular to the x-ray beam and is diffusely calcified, two parallel tracks of radiopacity can be observed (Fig. 1–11). They represent calcification at the sites in the vessel wall where the radiographic beam is directed tangentially. X-rays passing through the vessel on a tangent must traverse the greatest thickness of vascular wall, and this section of the wall will appear more dense on radiographs. Hence, while all the vessel may be calcified, often only marginal lines of calcification are appreciated. On the other hand, when the lumen is parallel to the x-ray beam, the artery is viewed en face. The radiographic beam then passes through all parts of the vascular wall equally, and a calcified vessel will appear as a ring of calcification (Fig. 1–12). In either case, calcification may be irregular and nonuniform, reflecting the inhomogeneous nature of calcium deposition in arterial walls.

The pattern of calcification in extensively calcified aneurysms is relatively independent of position in regard to the x-ray beam. This is particularly true in saccular aneurysms, which assume a spherical configuration, and present with arcuate lines of radiodensity. Usually, the curvilinear calcification of aneurysms may not describe a complete circle, the area of absent calcification representing the orifice of the neck of the aneurysm (Fig. 7–1). In fusiform aneurysms, two convex outward tracks of calcification are observed (Fig. 7–2). Most often, aneurysms are larger than calcified vessels of normal caliber.

Dilated arteries as well as those of normal caliber may lengthen and become tortuous. Thus, while arterial calcification is most often found at an expected anatomic site, it may also be seen on plain films away from its usual position. For example,

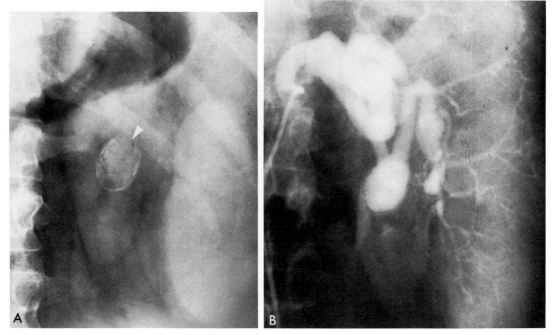

Figure 7–1. Calcified saccular aneurysm of the splenic artery. *A,* A plain film demonstrates a ring of calcification with an area of interruption (arrowhead) corresponding to the site where the normal artery enters the aneurysm. *B,* An angiography film demonstrates the normal artery entering the aneurysm at the site of the disrupted calcification.

the abdominal aorta below the renal arteries can extend to the right side of the lumbar spine, or far from the spine to the left, or caudal to its normal bifurcation at L3–L4.

The recognition of arterial calcification is usu-ally easy if the calcification is extensive. However, if calcium deposition is focal and limited, it may often be missed or misinterpreted. Vascular calcification is oriented along the course of a vessel and a single calcific deposit reflects that orientation (Fig.

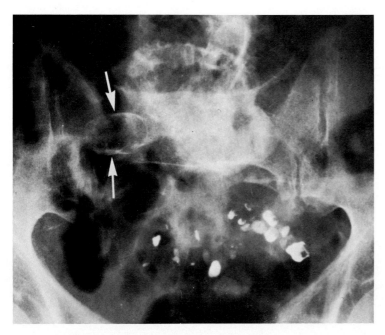

Figure 7–2. Calcified fusiform aneurysm of the common iliac artery. The elliptical lines of calcification (arrows) lie along the course of the right common iliac artery.

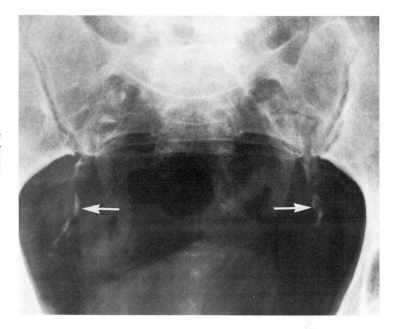

Figure 7–3. Calcification of the internal iliac arteries. Irregular plaques of calcification are aligned in the direction of the internal iliac arteries (arrows).

7–3). Commonly, it may appear as a thin line or streaks of density, but in the internal or common iliac arteries focal calcification may be more irregularly shaped. Limited vascular calcification can occur in any vessel but is most common in the aorta, internal and common iliac arteries, renal arteries, and splenic artery.

Patterns of Calcification

Calcification can occur in either the medial or intimal layer of the artery, and both types have specific radiographic and pathologic features.[1,2]

Intimal calcification results from deposition of calcium in atherosclerotic plaques. Its presence indicates significant arterial disease and suggests the likelihood of vascular narrowing, especially in medium and small arteries. Atherosclerotic plaques are usually nonuniform and patchy. Consequently, calcium deposits are focal and irregular. Almost all cases of asymmetric calcifications, whether in renal arteries (Fig. 1–17), iliac arteries, or aorta (Fig. 1–13), represent intimal calcification. Calcified atheromatous plaques can be very extensive, resulting in thick, roughened, and irregular calcification aligned along the course of the artery. Most frequently, this pattern is seen in the abdominal aorta and the splenic artery.

In medial calcification, first described by Mönckeberg, the calcification is found entirely within the tunica media of the artery, sparing both internal and external elastic membranes.[3,4] Cal-

cium salts initially deposit extracellularly between smooth muscle cells and progressively involve the entire medial layer. Medial calcification occurs primarily in the small and medium-sized muscular arteries, and is most often encountered in arteries of the pelvis, particularly the internal iliac artery and its branches (Fig. 7–4). Unlike intimal calcification, which generally is seen in elderly patients, medial calcification often occurs in the third, fourth, and fifth decades, particularly in diabetics. In fact, the recognition of medial calcification in the pelvic arteries in a young adult should alert one to the possibility of diabetes mellitus, even in the absence of clinical symptoms. With the exception of occasional cases of medial calcification in the renal arteries, involvement of other vessels outside the pelvis is unusual.[3,5]

Radiographically, medial calcification is detected by smooth continuous accumulations of calcium without focal irregularities (Fig. 7–4). The width of the band of calcification is unvarying and the density of the deposits is uniform throughout the length of the vessels. Medial calcification, in itself, does not imply vascular narrowing and is not related to atherosclerosis. However, atherosclerosis may superimpose on vessels with medial calcification.

Calcification of the Abdominal Aorta

Aortic calcification occurs mostly as a result of atherosclerosis.[6,7] It may be of little clinical signif-

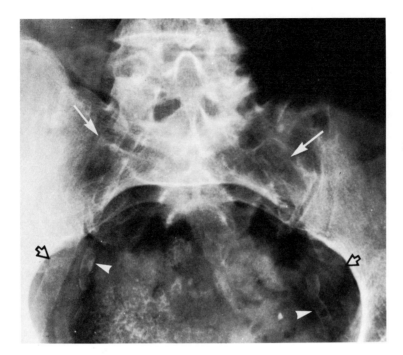

Figure 7–4. Medical calcification of the common (arrows), internal (white arrowheads), and external iliac arteries (open black arrowheads). Note the smooth, uniform linear calcification.

icance, cause no symptoms, and is not necessarily associated with calcification in other arteries. However, calcifications in the distal abdominal aorta and the common iliac arteries are often seen together.

The incidence of abdominal aortic calcification advances with age. Rare under 40, its presence increases steadily with each decade. In younger patients, calcification may be due to aortitis of various etiologies, renal failure, or hyperparathyroidism.[8–11] In one study of 610 consecutive patients over 15 years of age seen in the emergency room at a university hospital, abdominal aortic calcification was found in 20 percent of all patients and 40 percent of those over age 45.[12] In a survey of garment workers over age 40 in New York City, Epstein et al. found calcification in the abdominal aorta in 26 percent of patients.[13] This is similar to a finding from Iceland of 33 percent incidence in individuals over 40.[14]

Calcification in the aorta may be more common in women, but the evidence is conflicting.[12,15,16] Some investigators point to a slight female preponderance, but others have found the same incidence in both sexes. Elkeles attributed the higher frequency of aortic calcification in elderly females to the increased presence of osteoporosis in postmenopausal women.[15] He proposed that calcium lost from osteoporotic bones could be deposited in the damaged intima of the aorta. Anderson noted a correlation between osteoporosis and aortic calci-

fications in both sexes and concluded that the apparent association is largely accounted for by the accelerated occurrence of both conditions with aging.[16]

The percentage of patients with a calcified abdominal aorta varies with ethnicity and geography.[13,17,18] The greatest incidence has been found in Caucasians in North America and in Europe. It is less common in blacks residing in either North America or Africa, and very infrequent in some populations of Asia, South America, and Africa. Dietary and socioeconomic differences may explain the discrepancies in incidence, but no specific causes or factors have been isolated.

Perhaps tobacco consumption plays a role because atherosclerosis and calcification in the aorta occur more frequently in smokers.[19–21] Auerbach and Garfinkel found advanced calcification in the aorta in 85 percent of patients over 55 who smoked one pack or more per day in comparison to only 63 percent in nonsmokers of a similar age.[19] The precise mechanism by which smoking affects the aortic wall is not known. However, animal experiments suggest that a constituent of tobacco smoke may impede the normal migration of cholesterol from the intima into the vascular lymphatics, thereby promoting plaque formation.

There is an association between aortic calcification and some systemic diseases. The incidence of calcification in the aorta and iliac arteries is higher in hypertensive and diabetic patients.[1] Epstein et al. found that individuals with diabetes had approximately twice as much aortic calcification as nondiabetics.[13] Unlike the pelvic vessels, aortic calcification in diabetics is mostly in the intima. Meema et al. found a high incidence of aortic calcifications in patients aged 15 to 30 with chronic renal disease.[11] On the other hand, there may be a negative correlation between abdominal aortic calcification and cancers of the stomach, breast, and prostate.[22-25] The reason for the relative protection of the aorta in patients with these malignancies is unclear.

Radiographic Findings in Abdominal Aortic Calcification

The appearance of calcification in the abdominal aorta varies with the extent of the atherosclerotic process. Calcification is best detected when the x-ray beam hits the atherosclerotic plaque tangentially. Thus, on the anteroposterior projection of the abdomen, calcification in the lateral walls is demonstrated, while on lateral views the anterior and posterior walls can be seen (Fig. 7–5). Calci-

fication is more frequent below the renal arteries and may often extend into both common iliac arteries. In advanced cases, the calcification can outline the entire aorta. Almost always, the distribution of calcification is irregular and patchy in appearance. If calcification is focal, it may not be appreciated on an anteroposterior projection owing to the overlying lumbar vertebrae. Oblique or lateral views which separate the aorta from the spine may then be helpful in revealing calcified plaques (Fig. 7–5). Rarely, calcification may be smooth and uniform, and in this instance one should consider Takayasu's aortitis, or aortitis due to connective tissue disorders.[8,9,26]

Rarely, clot within the lumen of the aorta can calcify.[27,28] Occurring either in aneurysms or in vessels of normal caliber, calcium may deposit through the entirety of a clot causing it to appear on plain films as a uniform density with a granular or mottled internal architecture (Fig. 7–6). Since the aorta usually overlies the spine and clot calcification is rarely very dense, it may not be recognized on supine films. Steep oblique and lateral films are often required to demonstrate this phenomenon.

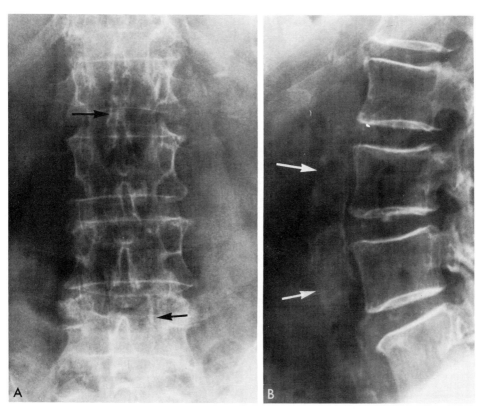

Figure 7–5. Calcification in the abdominal aorta. *A,* AP projection. The wall calcifications (arrows) are seen only faintly because of overlying vertebrae. *B,* Lateral projection. The calcifications are better demonstrated.

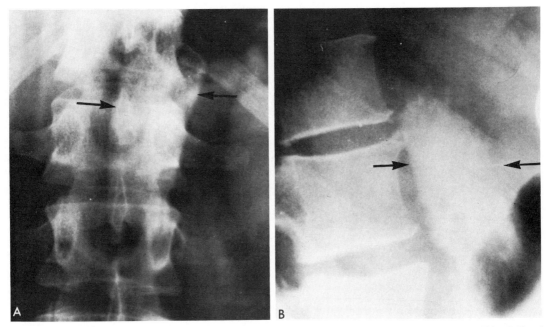

Figure 7–6. Calcification in a clot in the abdominal aorta. *A,* Plain film of the upper abdomen. Solid calcification in the area of the upper abdominal aorta (arrow), overlying the spine. *B,* Lateral projection. Intraluminal clot calcification (arrows). (Reprinted with permission of Cardiovascular and Interventional Radiology.[27])

Calcification in Abdominal Aortic Aneurysms

Atherosclerosis is the most common cause of abdominal aortic aneurysms. The incidence of aneurysms in autopsy series approximates 0.5 percent.[29] More than 95 percent of atherosclerotic aneurysms occur in patients between 60 and 80 years old, and its incidence is four times more common in men than in women. Calcification in the walls of the aneurysm is frequently seen on plain films. Steinberg and Stein found calcification on abdominal films in 55 percent of patients with documented aortic aneurysms.[30] The calcification may be of two types. In the majority, scattered plaques of calcification are noted (Fig. 7–7), but in approximately 10 percent, long curvilinear lines are seen. Preliminary abdominal radiographs will not always reveal the extent of an aneurysm or delineate its size, but in many cases they can play an important role in first ascertaining the diagnosis.

Radiographic Findings

The diagnosis of calcified abdominal aortic aneurysms on plain films depends upon the size and configuration of the aneurysm, the extent of calcification, and the degree of tortuosity of the

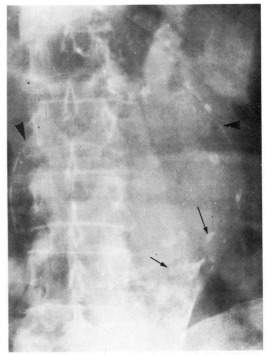

Figure 7–7. Calcification in the wall of a large saccular abdominal aortic aneurysm (arrowheads). Note the scattered plaques of more dense calcification (arrows) at the lower margin of the aneurysm and in the aorta below the aneurysm.

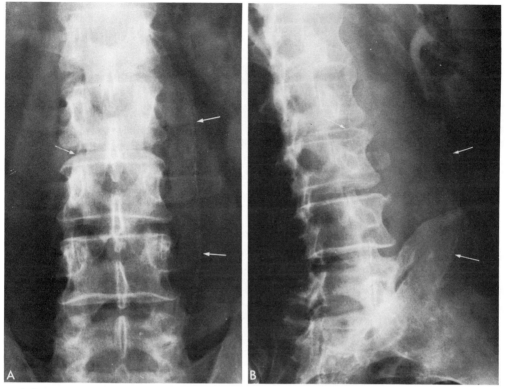

Figure 7–8. Fusiform abdominal aortic calcification. *A*, The walls of the aneurysm are calcified and can be identified on AP film (arrows). *B*, Oblique view demonstrates the anterior extent of the aneurysm (arrows).

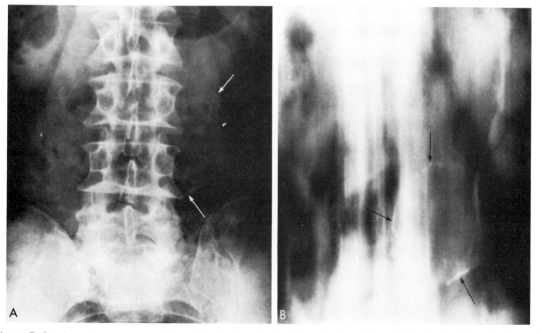

Figure 7–9. Saccular aneurysm of the abdominal aorta. *A*, AP projection. The calcification is faint and obscured by bowel gas (arrows). *B*, Tomogram of the abdomen. The calcified aneurysm (arrows) is clearly identified.

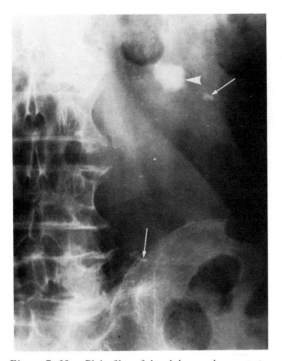

Figure 7–10. Plain film of the abdomen demonstrates a large mass to the left side of the lower lumbar vertebrae. Small calcific densities are aligned along the margin of the mass (arrows). This is a large saccular aneurysm with calcification in the wall. Also noted is a stone in the pelvis of the left kidney (arrowhead).

aorta. Large and extensively calcified saccular aneurysms are usually easily recognized, and their size can be determined on plain films of the abdomen. Fusiform aneurysms can be diagnosed accurately when both walls of the aneurysms are identified (Fig. 7–8). However, when only one wall of the aneurysm is identified, size may not be gauged on a single supine film. In this situation, oblique and lateral views of the abdomen usually are helpful in establishing the diagnosis. If the calcification is focal or faint, or obscured by bowel gas, tomography can be used to localize the aneurysm (Fig. 7–9) and determine its size. Abdominal aortic aneurysms frequently are associated with tortuosity and elongation of the abdominal aorta. Thus, calcification in these aneurysms can be identified far away from the midline on the left or on the right side of the lumbar spine (Figs. 7–10, 7–11).

Calcification in the Common Iliac Artery

The common iliac arteries are the second most frequent site for abdominal arterial calcification. Primarily a consequence of atherosclerosis and often associated with lower abdominal aortic calcification, common iliac artery calcification, when extensive, is usually easy to recognize because it presents as well-defined parallel lines of radiodensity following the course of the artery. If calcifi-

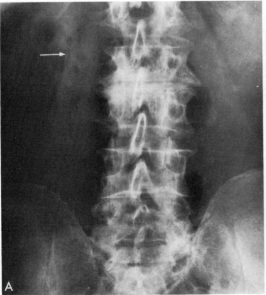
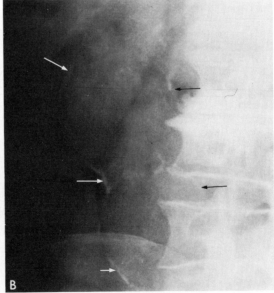

Figure 7–11. Multiple saccular aneurysms in the abdominal aorta, and a horseshoe kidney. *A,* AP projection. A small linear calcification is identified (arrows) just medial to the right kidney hilus. *B,* Right posterior oblique projection. A saccular aneurysm of the abdominal aorta is clearly identified (arrows). The aneurysm is displaced to the right because of the tortuosity of the aorta.

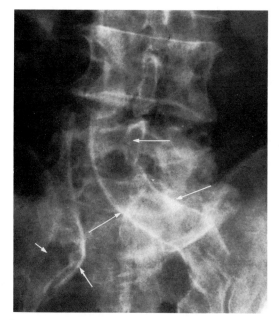

Figure 7–12. Calcified tortuous common iliac arteries. Parallel tracks of calcification (arrows) in both common iliac arteries.

cation is limited, it may be mistaken for bony densities because the common iliac arteries overlie the lower lumbar vertebrae and sacrum. When there is tortuosity and elongation of the aorta and common iliac arteries, the course of the iliac arteries may assume a more vertical or horizontal course. Consequently, the axis of calcified plaques in these vascular walls have an altered orientation in accordance with the direction of the vessels (Fig. 7–12). Occasionally it may be difficult, if not impossible, to distinguish between a focal calcification in the common iliac artery and a ureteral calculus, particularly when the calcification is projected over the sacrum. If the long axis of the calcification can be observed, it will most often point in the direction of the conduit with which it is associated. Thus, calcification in the common iliac artery will tend to line up along an axis extending toward the aorta, while a ureteral calculus is more vertical or slightly divergent from the aorta. Also, ureteral stones may move on successive films whereas vascular calcifications are fixed.

Calcification in Aneurysms of the Common Iliac Artery

After the aorta, the common iliac artery is the next most frequent site for aneurysmal dilatation in the abdomen. These aneurysms are usually fusiform and may be continuous with a dilated distal aorta. Often calcifications assume an elliptical shape, with the orientation of the ellipse along the expected axis of the artery (Fig. 7–2). Calcified saccular common iliac artery aneurysms may occur occasionally. At times they can simulate cystic masses in the pelvis or lower abdomen. A helpful distinguishing feature of calcified aneurysms in the common iliac arteries is the usual associated presence of extensive vascular disease in the aorta and other iliac vessels.

Calcification in the Internal Iliac Artery

The internal iliac or hypogastric artery is a common location for calcification in middle-aged and elderly individuals. Calcification can be due to atherosclerosis and will be seen as irregular plaques of radiodensity (Fig. 7–3). In diabetics, it can be of the medial type, presenting as smooth continuous parallel lines of radiodensity in both internal iliac arteries and their branches (Fig. 7–13).

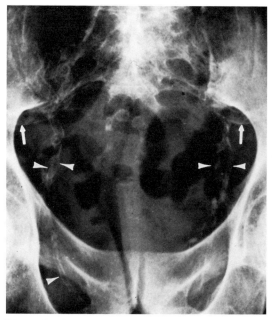

Figure 7–13. Internal iliac artery calcification. Multiple branches of the internal iliac artery are calcified. The superior gluteal artery (arrows) runs horizontally over the iliac bone. The obturator and internal pudendal arteries (arrowheads) follow a similar course and reach the obturator foramen.

The internal iliac artery arises from the common iliac artery and courses vertically at the superior lateral portion of the pelvis, then divides into posterior and anterior divisions. In the posterior division, the most frequently calcified vessels are the gluteal arteries, which are easy to recognize because they extend laterally as they supply the gluteus muscles. Parallel linear tracks of calcification with multiple branches running across the iliac bone are characteristic of this vascular calcification. From the anterior division arise the internal pudendal, obturator, uterine, and cystic arteries. The internal pudendal and obturator arteries follow a similar path along the lateral wall of the pelvis and then turn medially and inferiorly. Calcifications in both vessels are recognized as tracks of density originating from the hypogastric artery, passing along the lateral wall of the pelvis, and branching in the region of the obturator foramen.

In males, opacification of the vas deferens may simulate calcification in arteries. Both structures are conduits and the pelvic portion of the spermatic cord has a caliber similar to that of the iliac arteries. Moreover, the pattern of calcification may be identical. The vas, however, follows a course different from that of either the internal iliac artery or its branches (Fig. 7–14). If a section of a calcified pelvic conduit is long enough so that its orientation can be determined, it is usually possible to distinguish between the vas deferens and nearby vessels.[31-33]

Uterine Artery Calcification

The uterine artery, a branch of the anterior division of the internal iliac artery, initially follows the lateral pelvic wall and then traverses medially and anteriorly along the broad ligament to the lateral margin of the uterus, where it may again turn in a longitudinal direction. Most often, calcification is recognized along the transverse portion of the artery. Linear and narrow tubular radiodensities extending horizontally for 3 to 4 cm. from the lateral pelvic wall just above the ischial spines are characteristic of uterine artery calcification[34,35] (Fig. 1–16). The artery may deviate from the horizontal plane if the uterus is situated away from the midline. The general direction of the uterine artery is straight, but slight undulations are to be expected. Rarely, marked tortuosity of the intrauterine portion of the artery may occur, and the calcified wall can be seen as an irregular ill-defined

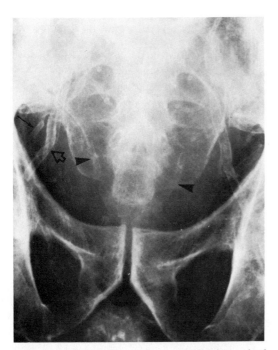

Figure 7–14. Internal iliac artery calcification and calcified vas deferens. The intrapelvic portion of the vas deferens runs laterally and superiorly from the seminal vesicles (arrowheads), then descends at the lateral pelvic wall (arrow) down to the scrotum. The descending portion of the vas may be mistaken for a branch of the internal iliac artery (open arrow), which runs in a similar direction.

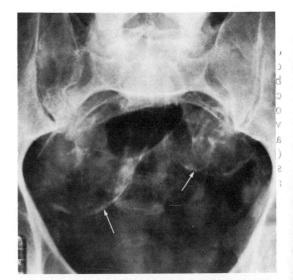

Figure 7–15. Saccular aneurysms of the internal iliac arteries. Curvilinear calcification convex outward in both internal iliac arteries (arrows). (Courtesy of Dr. Lawrence Oliver, Reading, Pa.)

structure simulating psammomatous calcification in ovarian neoplasms.[36] Generally, however, uterine artery calcification has a distinctive appearance.

Isolated calcification of the external iliac artery is less frequent than hypogastric artery calcification. Opacification of the walls of this vessel usually occurs along with internal and common iliac artery calcification (Fig. 7–4). Both the medial and intimal layers can be calcified.

Aneurysms of Pelvic Arteries

Aneurysms of the internal and external iliac arteries or their branches are rare. Since they are usually well-defined saccular aneurysms (Fig. 7–15), they may resemble other rounded calcifications in the pelvis such as mucocele of the appendix, mesenteric cysts, benign ovarian cysts, and cystic-appearing leiomyomas of the uterus.

Calcification of the Splenic Artery

The splenic artery ranks third in incidence of all abdominal arterial calcifications. Arising from the celiac axis and passing horizontally behind and adjacent to the pancreas, the splenic artery runs toward the hilus of the spleen where it divides into several intrasplenic branches. The artery passes behind the stomach and may indent upon the posterior gastric wall below the cardia (Fig. 7–16).[37] Calcification in the splenic artery can be seen as disconnected arcs of parallel curvilinear lines of radiodensity. The pattern of calcification of the artery on plain films depends upon the extent of radiopacity, the degree of tortuosity, and the orientation of the vessel with respect to the x-ray beam. When the artery is both very tortuous and calcified, it may appear as a disordered assemblage of irregular streaks. Sometimes, a markedly convoluted artery may have a regular pattern of twists and turns, giving it an appearance of a folded hose (Fig. 7–17). On the other hand, the finding of straight line calcification is rare because the splenic artery will usually elongate before it is calcified.

Splenic Artery Aneurysms

Splenic artery aneurysms are not uncommon.[38–40] In one series, they have been noted in 0.8 percent of all autopsies.[41] They may be present in up to 10 percent of patients over 60 years.[41] Under age 50, they are two to three times more common in females than males, but in older age

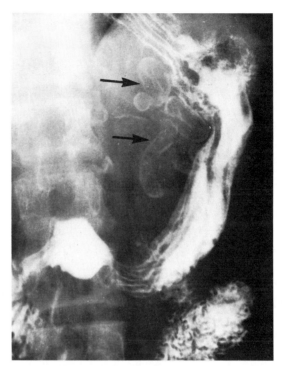

Figure 7–16. Calcified splenic artery (arrows) with impression upon the posterior wall of the stomach. Note the marked tortuosity of the splenic artery.

groups there is an equal sex ratio. Usually, these aneurysms are asymptomatic, but occasionally patients may complain of left upper quadrant fullness or pain, and in approximately 50 percent of cases there may also be significant splenomegaly. Splenic artery aneurysms are apt to rupture; pregnant women are especially susceptible to this complication.[42]

Aneurysms appear anywhere along the course of the artery and may result from atherosclerosis, trauma, or infection.[43,44] In the aged, atherosclerosis is the leading cause and aneurysmal calcification is usually noted along with intimal calcification in other parts of the artery (Fig. 7–18). A congenital defect in the vascular wall appears to account for a significant minority of cases in younger females. Occasionally, aneurysms occur in patients with portal hypertension and splenomegaly.

At any place in the splenic artery, aneurysmal dilatation may be mistaken for a markedly tortuous artery of normal caliber. An annular calcification is a constant finding in calcified aneurysms (Fig. 7–18). In most cases, the circle of calcification will be open at the junction of the normal artery and the aneurysm (Fig. 7–1).

Many other calcified cystic structures may re-

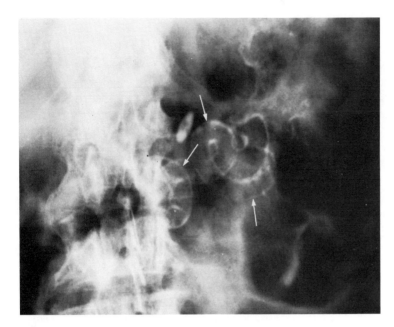

Figure 7–17. Tortuous and calcified splenic artery (arrows) with multiple twists and turns, an appearance suggesting a folded hose.

semble splenic artery aneurysms.[45] The differential diagnosis can be narrowed by dividing the artery into three segments. Near the origin of the splenic artery, calcified cystic lesions of the superior and medial aspects of the left kidney, aneurysms in the main left renal artery, cystic retroperitoneal tumors, left adrenal cysts, calcified echinococcal cysts in the lateral segment of the left lobe of the liver, and rarely pancreatic pseudocysts should be ruled out. In the middle third of the artery, renal cysts, renal artery aneurysms, mesenteric or omental cysts should also be excluded. In the peripheral third, splenic cysts should also be considered along with cystic lesions in the lateral margin of the left kidney. Splenic artery aneurysms may be complex and consist of more than one annular rim of calcification (Fig. 7–19). This is an important point in distinguishing between aneurysms and splenic cysts because intrasplenic cysts are usually unilocular. Aneurysms arising from any portion of the splenic artery can be differentiated from cystic lesions in adjacent structures with the help of lateral and oblique films (Fig. 7–20). However, often the differentiation between aneurysms and other lesions cannot be made on plain radiographs alone, and contrast studies including computed tomography and angiography may be necessary to secure a diagnosis.

Calcification in the Renal Artery

The renal arteries arise from the abdominal aorta at L1 and run horizontally and posteriorly toward the hilum of the kidney, where they then divide into segmental branches which radiate through the renal parenchyma. Calcification can occur anywhere in the main artery. On supine films, opacities in the proximal right renal artery may be hid-

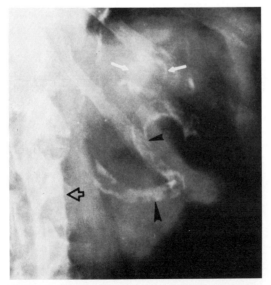

Figure 7–18. Intrasplenic artery aneurysm. The rim calcification (arrows) represents an intrasplenic aneurysm. The main splenic artery is markedly calcified (arrowheads), as is the abdominal aorta (open arrow).

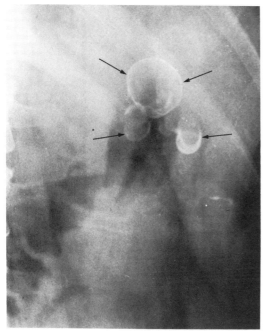

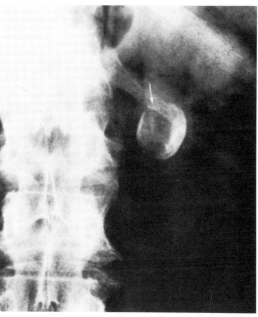

Figure 7–19. Multiple saccular aneurysms of the splenic artery. Note the several circular calcifications (arrows) in the splenic hilus. Multiple annular calcification is more suggestive of aneurysm than of cysts.

Figure 7–21. Calcified renal artery aneurysm. The location of this calcification is near the hilus of the kidney. The area of interruption of circular calcification (arrow) indicates the entrance of the normal artery into the aneurysm: the "broken wreath" sign.

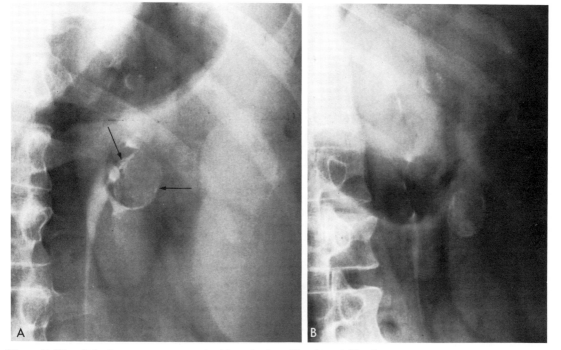

Figure 7–20. Splenic artery aneurysm. *A,* AP projection. Circular calcification (arrows) superimposed on the renal hilus. This can be mistaken for a calcified renal mass or renal artery aneurysm. *B,* Left posterior oblique projection. The calcification is clearly located anterior to the kidney. There is also splenomegaly.

den by the vertebra. Placing the patient in the right posterior oblique position can bring out the calcification as the artery moves away from the spine.

The orientation of calcification in the renal arteries is an important distinguishing feature. Renal artery calcification is directed horizontally, unlike ureteral calculi, which follow the vertical course of the ureter. Often, multiple segmental renal arteries are calcified and have a distinctive radiographic appearance as they cross the renal pelvis to enter the parenchyma[46,47] (Fig. 1–15). For the most part, calcification in main renal arteries is a consequence of atherosclerosis and is accompanied by aortic

calcification. If only segmental arteries are involved, it may be a result of either atherosclerosis or diabetes.

Renal Artery Aneurysms

Renal artery aneurysms are relatively rare, occurring in only 0.01 percent of autopsies. However, extensive calcification may be found in 25 percent of these lesions. Again the leading cause is atherosclerosis, but trauma and infection may also be responsible for aneurysmal dilatation of a renal

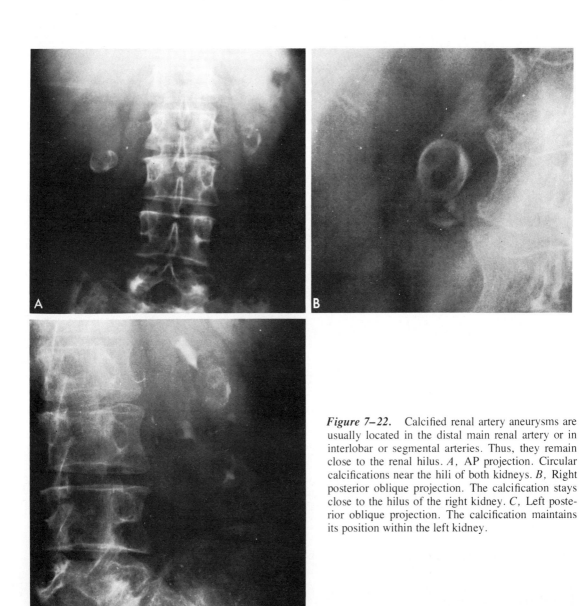

Figure 7–22. Calcified renal artery aneurysms are usually located in the distal main renal artery or in interlobar or segmental arteries. Thus, they remain close to the renal hilus. *A,* AP projection. Circular calcifications near the hili of both kidneys. *B,* Right posterior oblique projection. The calcification stays close to the hilus of the right kidney. *C,* Left posterior oblique projection. The calcification maintains its position within the left kidney.

artery. The aneurysms are most often saccular and, when calcified, show an incomplete rim of density (Fig. 7–21). They are most often between 1 and 3 cm. in diameter, but larger lesions may occur. Both the main artery and its branches can be involved but usually the aneurysm is located near the renal hilus (Fig. 7–22).[48] Right renal artery aneurysm should be distinguished from a round gallstone or a urinary calculus. Stones have a complete margin of radiodensity and may be laminated. Aneurysms of hepatic and gastroduodenal arteries may be included in the differential diagnosis, but they are much less common. On the left, splenic and renal artery aneurysms can look exactly alike on supine films. A left posterior oblique film may be helpful because the splenic artery should move anteriorly while the renal artery will stay close to the spine and within the renal hilus.

Calcification in Other Abdominal Arteries

Superior Mesenteric Artery

In patients with extensive atherosclerosis, the superior mesenteric arteries may calcify.[49] It pre-

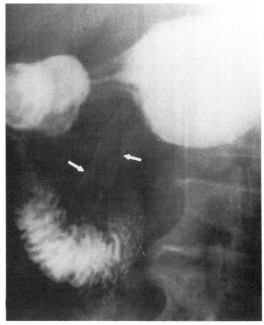

Figure 7–24. Superior mesenteric artery calcification. Note the relationship between the artery (arrows) and the third portion of the duodenum on this right posterior oblique projection.

sents as a tubular calcification on either side of the spine, coursing longitudinally from L1 inferiorly (Fig. 7–23). It is almost always associated with marked aortic calcification, and it can be differentiated from the aorta by its narrowed caliber. In diabetics, medial calcification may appear in the superior mesenteric artery.[3] On lateral or oblique films, the superior mesenteric artery runs slightly oblique to the course of the aorta and in front of the third portion of the duodenum (Fig. 7–24).

Calcified aneurysms of the superior mesenteric artery are rare.[50] As in other saccular aneurysms, circular rim calcification is present. On plain films they resemble the radiographic appearance of renal, pancreatic, or mesenteric cysts.

Hepatic Artery

Calcification in the hepatic artery is also rare. Often diabetes is a predisposing cause. The hepatic artery is usually located to the right side of T12 or L1, coursing obliquely toward the hilum of the liver. Aneurysms of this vessel are also very uncommon.[51-54] They appear more frequently in the extrahepatic portion of the hepatic artery and can be recognized as a rounded calcification in the right upper quadrant on an abdominal film.

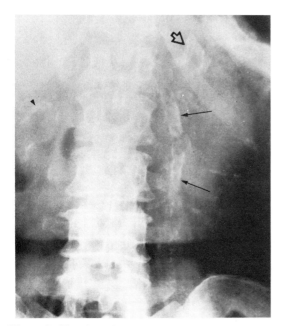

Figure 7–23. Superior mesenteric artery calcification. There is a tubular calcification to the left of the midline (arrows) running in a cephalocaudad direction. Also noted are calcifications in the right renal artery (small arrowhead) and splenic artery (large arrowhead).

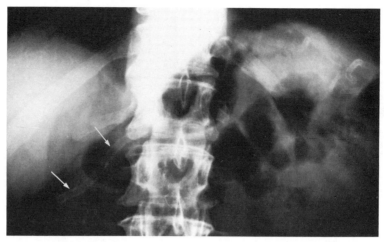

Figure 7–25. Gastroduodenal artery calcification (arrows).

Gastroduodenal Artery

The gastroduodenal artery is a branch of the common hepatic artery, running caudally and then horizontally across the lumbar spine at the greater curvature of the stomach, where it becomes the gastroepiploic artery. Calcification of this artery usually is associated with diabetes and presents as uniform tracks of calcification along the expected course of the artery (Fig. 7–25). Calcification of aneurysms of the gastroduodenal artery and its branches (pancreaticoduodenal arcades) has been reported in association with stenosis or occlusion of either the celiac axis or superior mesenteric artery.[55,56] The pancreaticoduodenal arcades and gastroduodenal artery can become the major collateral supply to the liver, spleen and bowel. Increased flow through these arteries probably promotes the development of the calcified aneurysm (Fig. 7–26).

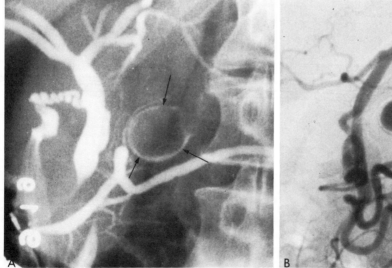
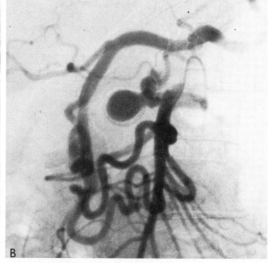

Figure 7–26. Calcified aneurysm of a branch of the dorsal pancreatic artery in a patient with stenosis of the celiac artery. *A,* An endoscopic retrograde cholangiopancreaticogram. This round calcification (arrows) was also noted on the plain film of the abdomen. The pancreatic duct and common bile duct are normal. *B,* A superior mesenteric arteriogram demonstrates a calcified aneurysm arising from the dorsal pancreatic artery. (Courtesy of Dr. Ronald Schliftman, White Plains, N.Y.)

VENOUS CALCIFICATION

Calcification in Phleboliths

Phleboliths are by far the most commonly encountered calcifications in the pelvis. By age 40, one or more phleboliths can be found in at least 35 percent of patients. Frequently they are multiple and bilateral. Although they generally have an easily recognizable shape, they can be confused with ureteral stones or calcifications in a pelvic mass. Because they are asymptomatic and have not been shown to be associated with other diseases, they are usually regarded as innocuous and inconsequential and are often not mentioned on radiographic reports. At times, however, the location and movement of phleboliths may provide practical clinical information, and a knowledge of their radiologic characteristics can be important in assessing the presence or growth of masses and in evaluating the nature of pelvic opacities.

Pathogenesis

Von Rokitansky in 1852 was the first to describe pelvic phleboliths in dissections of periprostatic veins in males. In 1881 Von Recklinghausen stated they were harmless entities. Nevertheless, in the early 1900's it was felt by some physicians that phleboliths were the cause of pelvic pain and were often associated with tumors. Thus, at that time, operations were often performed to remove them.[57] In 1908 Orton discussed their radiologic appearance and in the following year, Clark proved that phleboliths were intravenous concretions by demonstrating, in autopsy studies, their disappearance on pelvic radiographs after the veins were dissected.[58,59]

Phleboliths are concretions of thrombi attached to the walls of veins. They consist of thickly packed laminae of platelets sandwiched between a reticulum of red blood cells and fibrin.[60] Calcification usually takes place after the phleboliths have fully formed. Culligan analyzed 20 venous stones and found they were remarkably similar in chemical constituents. Approximately 50 percent by weight was calcium carbonate with lesser amounts of ammonium phosphate and magnesium ammonium phosphate. Twelve to 20 percent of the stones' mass consisted of organic matter.[61]

Shenult has shown that, in the adult, pelvic veins are valveless and poorly supported in loose connective tissue. Sudden intermittent increase in intra-abdominal pressure, such as with straining at stools may damage the venous wall and predispose to thrombosis.[57] Burkitt offered epidemiologic data supporting the notion that episodic marked increases in intra-abdominal pressure lead to the formation of pelvic vein thrombi. Phleboliths are most frequent in people living in industrial countries and uncommon in rural people living in developing nations and eating a traditional diet. For example, the incidence of phleboliths is 48 percent in adults in the United Kingdom but only 11.5 percent in Fiji.[62] Genetic factors do not seem significant; blacks and whites in the United States have a similar prevalence. Burkitt suggested that a diet low in fiber, the diet of many people in developed countries, leads to constipation and thus to straining at stools. Interestingly, phleboliths have not been described in veterinary radiology, possibly because the pelvic veins are not subjected to intermittent elevations of pressure in four-footed animals.[60]

That phleboliths may be the result of decreased consumption of cereals and fiber requires confirmation. We charted the number and position of phleboliths in 200 patients over age 40 undergoing barium enema examinations. There is strong evidence that colonic diverticulosis may be a consequence of a long history of constipation.[63] However, in our series, there was no difference in the incidence of phleboliths in patients with diverticula and in those with normal colons. In this sample, pelvic phleboliths also appeared unrelated to a past history of appendicitis, being as common in normal patients as in those who had previous appendectomy. Contrary to past assumptions, there appears to be no relationship between phleboliths and a history of urinary tract disease.[64] Hence, while there are interesting clues to the cause of pelvic venous concretions, their pathogenesis is by no means fully understood.

Most studies have indicated that phleboliths increase in prevalence up to the fifth decade of life. We have not observed them in patients under 16 but they are not a rare phenomenon by the third decade.[60] In some series, phleboliths continue to increase in prevalence to old age, but other investigations have noted a leveling off in the fifth and sixth decades with no further increases in later years.[60,63] One study evaluating 1,555 consecutive pelvic radiographs found phleboliths in 50 percent of males and in only 40 percent of females.[61]

Butzler, however, observed a definite female prevalence.[65] More recent investigations have shown an equal sex prevalence.[60,64] In pelvic radiographs of patients over 40 that we have examined, concretions were present in 48 percent of 71 males and 54 percent of 131 females, a difference of 6 percent, which is not statistically significant.

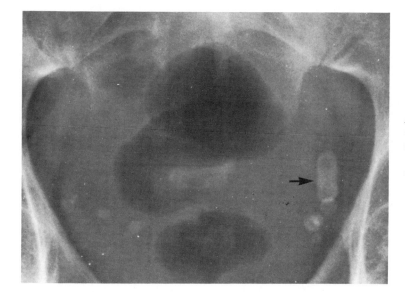

Figure 7–27. Fused phleboliths. Oblong density (arrow) with smooth margins and two areas of internal lucency located along the course of a pelvic vein.

Radiographic Appearance

Phleboliths are dense, oval to round, and well-defined. Usually there are no discontinuities in their outer margin, but often there is a concentric or slightly eccentric lucency. Sometimes the lucency may be large and only a thin rim of calcification will be seen. Generally they are 1.5 to 5 mm. in diameter, but larger concretions occur occasionally. The larger stones may represent fused phleboliths and may contain multiple lucencies suggesting the mottled appearance of solid masses (Fig. 7–27). A fused phlebolith can simulate the pattern of calcification seen in leiomyoma of the uterus,

but this appearance of phleboliths is uncommon. Usually between one to six phleboliths are present, but on occasion up to two to three dozen pelvic concretions may be noted. When there are numerous phleboliths in the pelvis they are almost always bilateral and tend to be arrayed in gently curving chains that follow the course of the distal ureters (Fig. 7–28).

In males, phleboliths are found in perirectal and perivesical veins.[66] In females they occur also in veins in the broad ligament, where they are situated near the termination of the vein and hence are laterally placed. Occasionally, phleboliths are located in a more medial position but are still off the

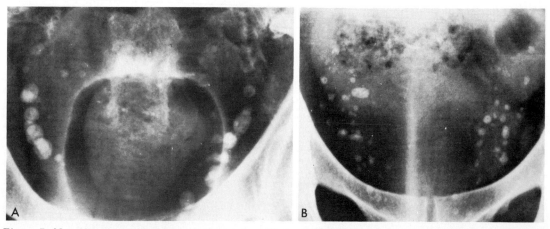

Figure 7–28. Numerous phleboliths. *A,* Bilateral, multiple phleboliths arranged in chains directed obliquely inferiorly. *B,* Multiple phleboliths in perivesical veins and veins of the broad ligament. More than one chain of phleboliths is present on each side.

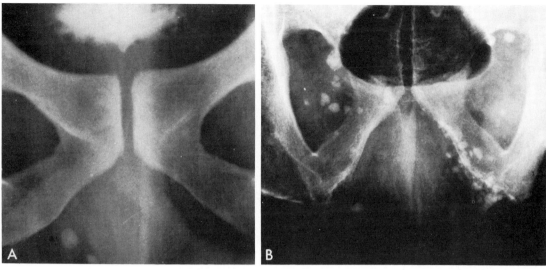

Figure 7–29. Phleboliths in scrotal veins. *A,* Two scrotal vein phleboliths below the right inferior pubic ramus. *B,* Many scrotal vein phleboliths on the left and one on the right.

midline. The great preponderance of phleboliths lie at or just below a line drawn from the ischial spine to the fourth sacral segment. When there are many phleboliths, the majority are below that line and their course proceeding caudally will be from lateral to medial. Often phleboliths may be noted slightly below the superior margin of the symphysis pubis. In men, phleboliths may occasionally be present in scrotal veins, sometimes in large numbers (Fig. 7–29).

Occasionally, a pelvic radiograph will reveal one or several concretions in the superior pelvis, often without phleboliths present inferiorly. If the concretion is outside the genitourinary tract, it may be in a phlebolith located in a gonadal vein (Fig. 1–9). These concretions tend to be multiple and are seen along the course of the vein as it ascends in the abdomen adjacent to the ureter (Fig. 7–30).

It is often difficult to distinguish between a lower ureteral calculus and a phlebolith in its usual position. Ureteral calculi are often angulated, and usually lack a central lucency. However, their appearance may exactly mimic a phlebolith. One way of differentiating between the two is to obtain serial films a few hours or a day apart. Ureteral calculi may move in either an antegrade or retrograde fashion while phleboliths are usually fixed in position (Fig. 7–31). However, if there is no movement of the ureteral stone it may be impossible to distinguish the two types of concretions even on repeated plain films.

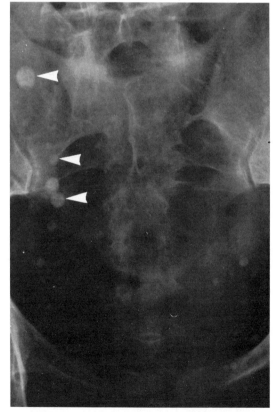

Figure 7–30. Multiple phleboliths in the right ovarian vein (arrowheads). They may simulate ureteral stones on a plain film.

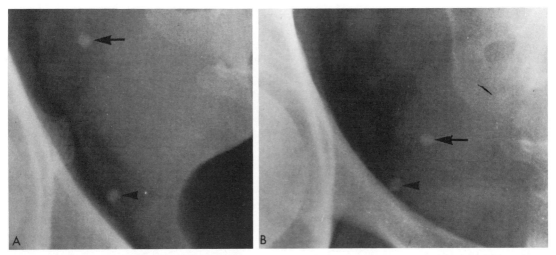

Figure 7–31.   A phlebolith and a ureteral calculus may look similar on pelvic films. *A,* The initial films shows a ureteral calculus (arrow) superior to a phlebolith (arrowhead). *B,* A film taken the next day demonstrates movement of the ureteral stone inferiorly (arrow), while the phlebolith is fixed (arrowhead).

Abnormal Position of Phleboliths

Careful attention to the position of phleboliths may be rewarding in determining the presence of pelvic masses or ascertaining the nature of previous surgery. Normally, phleboliths situated in perivesical veins may be displaced slightly inferiorly and laterally if the bladder enlarges to a great degree (Fig. 7–32). Occasionally, perirectal phleboliths will be deviated laterally in the presence of rectal distention.[66] However, these movements are usually minimal. Greater motion may be observed in the presence of masses. In fact, when a phlebolith is displaced, its migration may be all that is necessary to monitor the growth or shrinkage of tumefactions (Fig. 1–44).[66–69]

Periurethral masses can elevate phleboliths as well as displace them to either side. Prolapse of the uterus can move phleboliths inferiorly, sometimes displacing them below the superior margin of the pubic bone (Fig. 7–33).

The veins of the pelvis are connected across the midline through the periprostatic and inferior vesical plexuses. However, crossing veins are usually small and are not the site of roentgenographically visible phleboliths. Hence, a phlebolith in the midline should always be regarded as abnormal. It may be caused by mass displacement, and, in females,

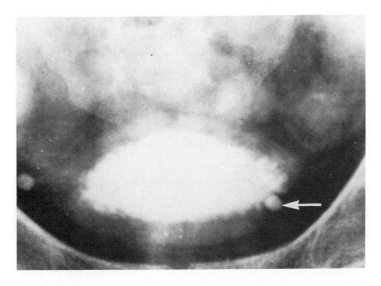

Figure 7–32.   The intimate relationship of the bladder to a perivesical vein phlebolith (arrow). Distention of the bladder can push phleboliths inferiorly and laterally.

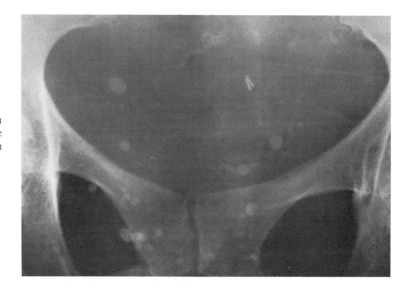

Figure 7–33. A woman with uterine prolapse. Phleboliths have moved below the superior margin of the pubic bone.

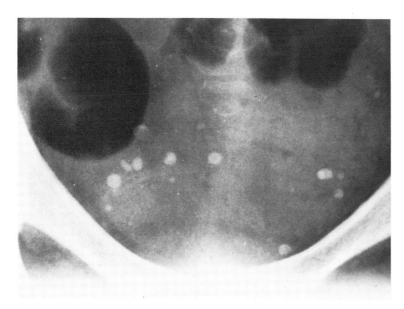

Figure 7–34. After a simple hysterectomy, phleboliths in broad ligament veins may be brought closer together. Observe the abnormal arrangement of phleboliths. They are aligned horizontally and one is situated at the midline.

Figure 7–35. Three phleboliths on the right and calcification in an ovarian dermoid on the left (arrow). While simulating a phlebolith, the superior location of the dermoid calcification is atypical for phleboliths, in view of the absence of other phleboliths on the same side. An adjacent lucency represents fat in the dermoid.

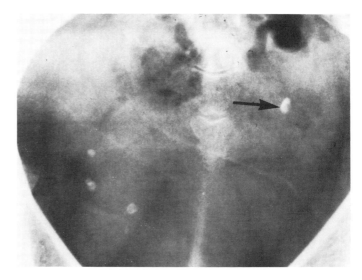

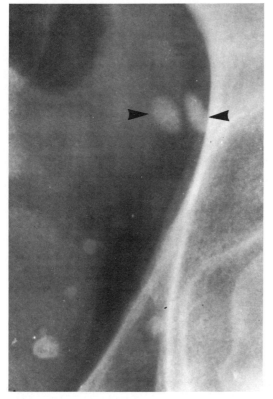

Figure 7–36. Two opaque pills (arrowheads) and phleboliths. Pills lack both a central lucency and a marginal rim of enhanced density.

it may be a consequence of surgery (Fig. 7–34). After hysterectomy, phleboliths at the termination of veins in the broad ligament may be pulled medially. Rarely, abnormally sited phleboliths may indicate a hemangioma (Fig. 4–28). Radiologically visible phleboliths have been noted in many abdominal locations in hemangiomas. Although uncommon tumors in the pelvis, hemangiomas should be considered when phleboliths are seen at the midline in the absence of previous operation, or when multiple phleboliths are seen on only one side of the midline.[70]

Simulators of Phleboliths

Not all concretions with central lucencies in the pelvis are phleboliths. Many other densities simulating venous stones can be mistaken for them. Besides ureteral calculi, concretions such as appendicoliths in low-lying appendices can be seen in the pelvis (Fig. 4–18). Bladder stones, rectal stones, calcified appendices epiploica, and calculi passing through the gastrointestinal tract may also be present in the pelvis. Ossification and tooth formation in ovarian dermoids can also look like phleboliths (Fig. 7–35).

From time to time foreign bodies may be mistaken for phlebolithic concretions. Radiopaque pills may resemble venous calculi but their homogeneous mass and absence of central lucency and their

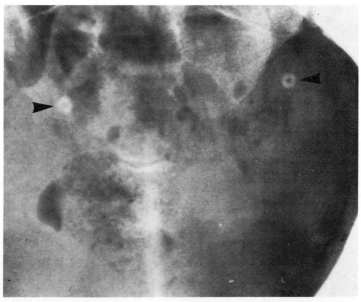

Figure 7–37. Bilateral fallopian tube occlusion rings (arrowheads) placed at the site of tubal ligation. The central lucency and complete border of increased density in these devices give them the appearance of phleboliths.

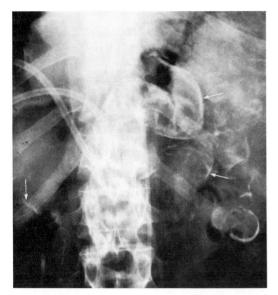

Figure 7–38. Calcification in the portal vein and splenic vein. Linear calcification in the portal vein (vertical arrow) and extensive calcification in the splenic vein (horizontal arrow) as a result of portal vein thrombosis. There are large collaterals in the splenic vein and esophageal veins. (Courtesy of Dr. John Adler. Reprinted with the permission of Radiology.)

movement on sequential films are points of differentiation (Fig. 7–36). Fallopian tube occlusion rings are implanted devices used in tubal ligations. They consist of siliconized synthetic rubber impregnated with barium sulfate, which makes them appear as annular opacities on plain radiographs. Often, they can closely simulate phleboliths (Fig. 7–37).

Other Venous Calcifications

Aside from pelvic phleboliths, calcification is seldom noted in abdominal veins on plain films. Veins are not subjected to either high pressure or large pulsatile flow and are therefore relatively protected from the risk of intimal injury. Consequently, venous walls, with the exception of portal veins, are rarely sufficiently damaged to be the site of intimal calcification. Mostly, calcification occurs in intraluminal clots in obstructed vessels.

Calcification in the Portal Vein

Portal venous calcification is seen usually in association with portal hypertension and thrombosis

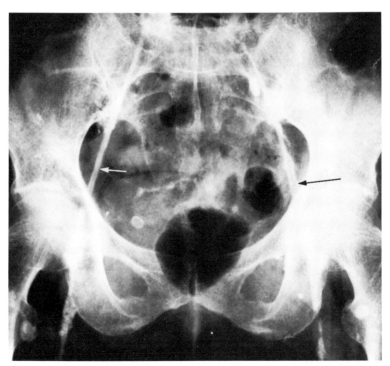

Figure 7–39. Iliac vein calcification. Thick linear calcification in the iliac veins (arrows) extending from the femoral veins to the inferior vena cava. The patient had chronic venous thrombosis. (Courtesy of Dr. G.A. Goodman, Reading, Pa. Reprinted with the permission of the British Journal of Radiology.)[83]

of the portal vein. Two types of calcific deposits can be appreciated on plain films, intraluminal and wall calcification. Calcific deposits in thrombi in the portal vein present as solid or linear calcification running diagonally in the right upper quadrant toward the hilum of the liver.[71-75] Infrequently, the calcified thrombus may extend into the splenic vein and a contiguous horizontal density will be seen passing across the abdomen into the left upper quadrant (Fig. 7–38).[76-79] Calcification of the wall of the portal vein occurs less frequently and is usually focal and linear. At times calcification of a section of the vein may be confused with calcification in the wall of a nondilated hepatic artery. Since veins are generally wider than corresponding arteries, venous calcification is broader than that encountered in adjacent arterial walls.

Calcification in the Inferior Vena Cava

Inferior vena caval calcification in adults is exceedingly rare.[80] Most examples have occurred in children who have a calcified thrombus in the intrahepatic portion of the inferior vena cava, which is the narrowest region of the inferior vena cava.[81] an opacified thrombus appears as a well-defined bullet-shaped opacity seen just to the right of T12 or L1 (Fig. 10–21).

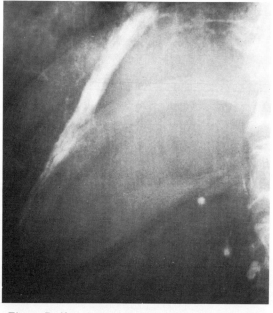

Figure 7–40. Dense calcification in a thrombosed hepatic vein.

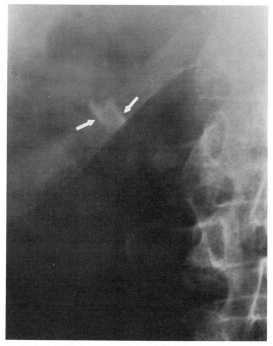

Figure 7–41. Localized calcification in a thrombosed segmental renal vein (arrows) draining the upper pole of the right kidney.

Calcification of the Iliac Vein

Like the inferior vena cava, the iliac veins are rarely the site of thrombus calcification, although thrombi are not unusual within the lumen of these vessels. Calcifications in the iliac veins occur as thick linear densities in the lateral portion of the pelvis converging toward the inferior vena cava (Fig. 7–39).[82,83] They should be distinguished from calcifications in the sacrotuberous ligament, which have a similar appearance but a different location in the pelvis.

Calcification in Other Veins

Calcification may occur in other abdominal veins. For example, hepatic vein calcification may be seen as a linear density overlying the liver shadow, running diagonally toward the right atrium (Fig. 7–40). Localized calcifications in segmental renal veins have also been observed (Fig. 7–41).

REFERENCES

1. Lindbom A: Arteriosclerosis and arterial thrombosis in the lower limb. A roentgenological study. Acta Radiol (Suppl) 80:1–80, 1950.
2. Orr DP, Myerowitz RL, Herbert DL, et al: Correlation of

radiographic and histologic findings in arterial calcification. Invest Radiol 13:110–114, 1978.

3. Lachman AS, Spray TL, Kerwin DM, et al: Medial calcinosis of Mönckeberg. A review of the problem and a description of a patient with involvement of peripheral visceral and coronary arteries. Am J Med 63:615–622, 1977.

4. Silbert S, Lippmann HT, Gordon E: Mönckeberg's arteriosclerosis. JAMA 151:1176, 1953.

5. Donner MW, McAfee JG: Roentgenographic manifestation of diabetes mellitus. Am J Med Sci 239:622–641, 1960.

6. Eggen DA, Strong JP, McGill HC: Calcification in the abdominal aorta. Arch Pathol 78:575–583, 1964.

7. Hyman JB, Epstein FH: A study of the correlation between roentgenographic and post-mortem calcification of the aorta. Am Heart J 48:540–543, 1954.

8. Reid MM, Fannin TF: Extensive vascular calcification in association with juvenile rheumatoid arthritis and amyloidosis. Arch Dis Child 43:607–610, 1968.

9. Choube BS: Extensive aortic calcification in a case of primary arteritis. Angiology 23:618–634, 1972.

10. Ibels LS, Alfrey AC, Heffer WE, et al: Arterial calcification and pathology in uremic patients undergoing dialysis. Am J Med 66:790–796, 1979.

11. Meema HE, Oreopoulos DB, de Veber GA: Arterial calcifications in severe chronic renal disease and their relationship to dialysis treatment, renal transplant, and parathyroidectomy. Radiology 121:315–321, 1971.

12. Boukhris R, Becker KL: Calcification of the aorta and osteoporosis. JAMA 219:1307–1311, 1972.

13. Epstein FH, Boas EP, Simpson R: The epidemiology of atherosclerosis among a random sample of clothing workers of different ethnic origins in New York City. J Chron Dis 5:300–325, 1957.

14. Petersen GF: Atherosclerosis of the abdominal aorta, a roentgenologic study. Acta Radiol 37:356–363, 1952.

15. Elkeles A: A comparative radiological study of calcified atheroma in males and females over 50 years of age. Lancet 2:714, 1957.

16. Anderson JB, Barnett E, Nordin BEC: The relation between osteoporosis and aortic calcification. Brit J Radiol 37:910–912, 1964.

17. Burhenne HJ, Strasser E: A simple radiographic method and epidemiological study of atherosclerosis. Radiology 97:180–182, 1970.

18. Tejada, C, Strong JP, Montenegro MR, et al: Distribution of Coronary and Aortic Atherosclerosis by Geographic Location, Race, and Sex. (in) McGill HC: The Geographic Pathology of Atherosclerosis. Baltimore, Williams and Wilkins Co 1968, pp 49–66.

19. Auerbach O, Garfinkel L: Atherosclerosis and aneurysm of aorta in relation to smoking habits and age. Chest 78:805–809, 1980.

20. Lawton G: Cigarette consumption and atherosclerosis: Their relationship in the aorta and iliac and femoral arteries. Brit J Surg 60:873–876, 1973.

21. Sackett DL, Winkelstein W Jr: The relationship between cigarette usage and aortic atherosclerosis. Am J Epidemiol 86:264–270, 1967.

22. Elkeles A: Calcified atherosclerosis and cancer. Brit J Cancer 13:403–407, 1959.

23. Elkeles A: Gastric ulcer in the aged and calcified atherosclerosis. Am J Roentgenol 91:744–750, 1964.

24. Fotopoulos JP, Crampton AR, Burkhead HC: Calcification of the abdominal aorta as an aid in diagnosis of gastric carcinoma vs benign ulcer. Radiology 79:637–643, 1962.

25. Winkelstein W Jr, Lilienfeld R, Pickren JW, et al: The relationship between aortic atherosclerosis and cancer. Brit J Cancer 13:606–613, 1959.

26. Lande A, Berkman YM: Aortitis. Pathologic, clinical and arteriographic review. Radiol Clin North Am 14:219–240, 1976.

27. Charnsangavej C: Intraluminal calcification and occlusion of the abdominal aorta above the renal arteries. Cardiovasc Intervent Radiol 4:242–244, 1981.

28. Lipchik EO, Rob CG, Schwartzberg S: Obstruction of the abdominal aorta above the level of the renal arteries. Radiology 82:443–445, 1964.

29. Estes JE Jr: Abdominal aorta aneurysm: A study of one hundred and two cases. Circulation 2:258–264, 1950.

30. Steinberg I, Stein HL: Visualization of abdominal aortic aneurysm. Am J Roentgenol 95:684–695, 1965.

31. Wilson JL, Marks JH: Calcification of the vas deferens; its relation to diabetes mellitus and arteriosclerosis. N Engl J Med 245:321–325, 1951.

32. Hafiz A, Melnick JC: Calcification of the vas deferens. J Canad Assoc Radiol 19:56–60, 1968.

33. King JC Jr, Rosenbaum HD: Calcification of the vasa deferentia in non diabetes. Radiology 100:603–606, 1971.

34. Camiel MR, Berkan HS, Alexander LL: Roentgen visualization of uterine artery calcification. Radiology 88:138–139, 1967.

35. Fisher MD, Hamm R: Uterine artery calcification: its association with diabetes. Radiology 117:537–538, 1975.

36. Schabel SI: Diffuse arterial calcification of the uterus. An unusual radiographic appearance. Brit J Radiol 49:797–798, 1976.

37. Rosenberg MA, Elkin M: Gastric deformity from extrinsic pressure by calcified splenic artery. Radiology 69:735–738, 1957.

38. Owens JC, Coffey RJ: Aneurysm of the splenic artery, including a report of 6 additional cases. International Abstracts of Surgery 97:313–335, 1953.

39. Spittel JA Jr, Fairbairn JF, Kincaid OW, et al: Aneurysm of the splenic artery. JAMA 175:452–456, 1961.

40. Berger JS, Forsee JH, Furst JN: Splenic artery aneurysm. Ann Surg 137:108–110, 1953.

41. Feldman M: Aneurysm of the splenic artery: An autopsy study. Am J Dig Dis 22:48–50, 1955.

42. Lennie RA, Sheehan HL: Splenic and renal aneurysm complicating pregnancy. J Obstet Gynecol 49:426–430, 1942.

43. Culver GJ, Pirson HS: Splenic artery aneurysm. Radiology 68:217–223, 1957.

44. Yang J, Spinuzza SJ, Gilchrist RK: Aneurysm of splenic artery with calcification. Arch Surg 87:676–681, 1963.

45. von Ronnen JR: The roentgen diagnosis of calcified aneurysms of the splenic and renal arteries. Acta Radiol 39:385–400, 1953.

46. Azimi F, Cameron DD: Calcification of the intrarenal branches of the renal arteries. Clin Radiol 28:217–219, 1977.

47. Seshanarayana, KN, Keats TE: Intrarenal arterial calcification: Roentgen appearance and significance. Radiology 95:145–147, 1970.

48. Salik JO, Abeshouse BS: Calcification, ossification and cartilage formation in the kidney. Am J Roentgenol 88:125–143, 1962.

49. Redman HC: Arterial calcification simulating aneurysm. JAMA 208:865–868, 1969.

50. Weidner W, Fox P, Brooks JW, et al: The roentgen diagnosis of aneurysms of the superior mesenteric artery. Am J Roentgenol 109:138–142, 1970.

51. Malloy HR, Jason RS: Aneurysm of the hepatic artery. Am J Surg 57:359–363, 1942.
52. Jarvis L, Hodes PJ: Aneurysm of the hepatic artery demonstrated roentgenographically. A case report. Am J Roentgenol 72:1037–1040, 1954.
53. Quinn JL III, Martin JP: Hepatic artery aneurysm, case report. Am J Roentgenol 87:284–287, 1962.
54. Bruwer AJ, Hellenbeck GA: Aneurysm of hepatic artery: Roentgenologic features in one case. Am J Roentgenol 78:270–272, 1957.
55. Mora JD: Celiac axis artery stenosis with aneurysmal calcification of collateral supply. Austral Radiol 20:252–254, 1976.
56. West JE, Bernhardt H, Bowers RF: Aneurysm of pancreatico-duodenal artery. Am J Surg 115:835–839, 1968.
57. Shenult P: The origin of phleboliths. Brit J Surg 59:695–700, 1972.
58. Orton GH: Some fallacies in the x-ray diagnosis of renal and ureteral calculi. Brit Med J 2:716–719, 1908.
59. Clark GD: Peri-ureteric pelvic phleboliths. J Urol 80:913–921, 1909.
60. Dovey P: Pelvic phleboliths. Clin Radiol 17:121–125, 1966.
61. Culligan JM: Phleboliths. J Urol 15:175–188, 1926.
62. Burkitt DP, et al: Pelvic phleboliths: Epidemiology and postulated etiology. N Engl J Med 296:1387–1391, 1977.
63. Burkitt DP: Hemorrhoids, varicose veins, and deep vein thrombosis: Epidemiologic features and suggested causative factors. Canad J Surg 18:483–488, 1975.
64. Green M, Thomas ML: The prevalence of pelvic phleboliths in relation to age, sex, and urinary tract infections. Clin Radiol 23:492–494, 1972.
65. Butzler O: Zur differential Diagnose der Phlebolithen und Ureterokonkremente im Röntgenbild des kleinen Becken. Fortschr Röentgenstr 49:253–262, 1934.
66. Steinbach HL: Identification of pelvic masses by phlebolith displacement. Am J Roentgenol 83:1063–1066, 1960.
67. Dodd GD, Rutledge F, Wallace S: Postoperative pelvic lymphocysts. Am J Roentgenol 108:312–323, 1970.
68. Fenlon JW, Augustin C: The significance of pelvic phlebolith displacement. J Urol 106:595–598, 1971.
69. Kolman MA: Radiologic soft tissues in the pelvis: Another look. Am J Roentgenol 130:493–498, 1977.
70. Grieco RV, Bartone NF: Roentgen visualization of phleboliths in hemangioma of the gastrointestinal tract. Am J Roentgenol 101:406–408, 1967.
71. Moberg G: Calcified thrombosis in portal system diagnosed by roentgen examination. Acta Radiol 24:374–383, 1943.
72. Smallwood, RA, Davidson JS: Calcification in the portal system. Gastroenterol 54:265–269, 1968.
73. Sherrick DW, Kincaid OW, Gambill EE: Calcification in the portal venous system. Unusual radiologic sign of portal venous thrombosis. JAMA 187:861–862, 1964.
74. Haddow RA, Kemp-Harper RA: Calcification in the liver and portal system. Clin Radiol 18:225–236, 1967.
75. MacKenzie RL, Tubbs HR, Laws JW, et al: Obstructive jaundice and portal vein calcification. Brit J Radiol 51:953–955, 1978.
76. Adler J: Venous calcifications associated with cavernous transformation of the portal vein: Computed tomographic and angiographic correlations. Radiology 132:27–28, 1979.
77. Blendis LM, Laws JW, Williams R, et al: Calcified collateral veins and gross dilatation of the azygos vein in cirrhosis. Brit J Radiol 41:909–912, 1968.
78. Magovern GJ, Muehsam GE: Calcification of the portal and splenic veins. Am J. Roentgenol 71:84–88, 1954.
79. Bleich AR, Kipen CS: Venous calcification in Banti's syndrome. Radiology 50:657–660, 1948.
80. Gammill SL, Nice CM Jr: Calcification in the inferior vena cava. Radiology 92:1288–1290, 1969.
81. Singleton EB, Rosenberg HS: Intraluminal calcification of the inferior vena cava. Am J Roentgenol 86:556–560, 1961.
82. Banker VP: Calcified external iliac vein thrombosis. Radiology 117:311–314, 1975.
83. Goodman GA: Intraluminal iliac venous calcification. Brit J Radiol 48:457–459, 1975.

Chapter 8

CALCIFICATION IN ABDOMINAL LYMPH NODES

Richard A. Rosen, M.D.

Abdominal lymph node calcifications are among the most frequently observed opacities on plain films of the abdomen. Most often, nodal calcifications are easily recognized, but occasionally they can be mistaken for other radiopacities such as ureteral stones, appendicoliths, and uterine leiomyoma. The appearance of nodal calcifications may be variable, but nearly always they exhibit the morphologic features of a solid mass.

ANATOMY

Inguinal nodes receive lymphatics draining the lower extremity and are situated medial to the origin of the common femoral artery. Pelvic nodes which drain the rectum, bladder, and adnexal organs are arrayed in chains next to and aligned with the internal, external, and common iliac arteries.[1] The para-aortic nodes are the major nodes of the retroperitoneum and flank the aorta and inferior vena cava. Lymphatics running from the left ovary and left testicle drain into nodes near the left renal hilus. In the upper abdomen are found perigastric, peripancreatic, perisplenic, and porta hepatis nodes.[2] Mesenteric lymph nodes are related to the small and large bowel and extend in a wide diagonal band from the left upper quadrant near the ligament of Treitz to the right lower quadrant, where they are most numerous (Fig. 8–1).

CALCIFIED MESENTERIC NODES

Calcification may occur in any abdominal nodal chain, but by far the most common are mesenteric lymph nodes. In nearly every instance, mesenteric node calcification is caused by tuberculous myco-

bacteria.[3] Previously, when intestinal tuberculoisis was common, involvement of mesenteric lymph nodes was nearly universal (Fig. 8–2). With the elimination of bovine tuberculosis as a clinical problem in most developed countries, the incidence of lymph node calcification has decreased.[4,5] Yet, calcified lymph nodes are still recognized on plain films of the abdomen in patients with no history of intestinal disease.[6,7] Mycobacteria enter intestinal lymphatics after passing through bowel mucosa and are deposited in mesenteric nodes.[8] Both animal and human studies have revealed that bacteria can pass through epithelial cells in the intestinal wall and cause no residual damage.[9,10,11]

Today, most mycobacteria entering the gastrointestinal tract originate from pulmonary foci. Nearly everyone who has had a clinical or subclinical tuberculous infection has swallowed mycobacteria. Most of the bacilli pass through the intestinal tract, but some penetrate the mucosa and eventually collect in lymphoid tissue. Almost all patients with calcified mesenteric nodes have had a pulmonary tuberculous infection.[12] Some may have residual evidence of disease in the lungs but chest x-rays will often not reveal changes of tuberculosis, especially when the initial infection occurred early in childhood. Moreover, not everyone with calcified mesenteric lymph nodes will be a positive reactor to tuberculin. It is well recognized that a response to tuberculin will diminish with time.[13] In many patients with calcified mesenteric nodes, the first exposure of intestinal lymphoid tissue to mycobacteria may have occurred several decades in the past.

Mycobacteria may cause caseation necrosis and hyaline degeneration of lymphoid tissue. Both processes promote the deposition of calcium salts.[13] Only a portion of a node may calcify, but usually

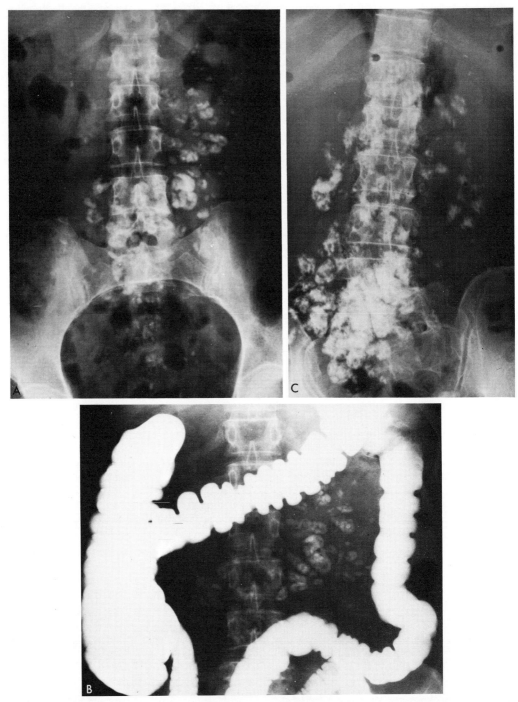

Figure 8–1. *A,* Widespread, predominantly mesenteric node calcification. *B,* Calcified mesenteric nodes. A film from a barium enema shows the relationship of mesenteric nodes to the colon. *C,* Another patient with extensive mesenteric node calcification.

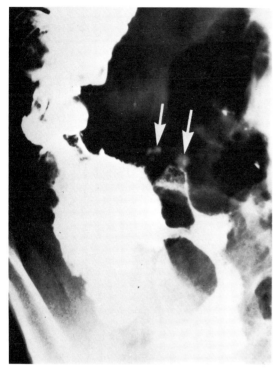

Figure 8–2. Calcified nodes (arrows) in the mesentery of a patient with ileocecal tuberculosis. Note the strictures in the cecum and terminal ileum. Nowadays, most calcified mesenteric nodes are unassociated with active intestinal disease.

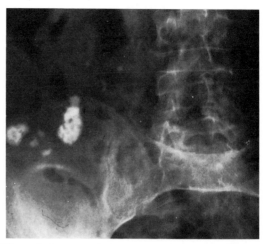

Figure 8–3. A typical appearance of mesenteric nodes. There are nodes of varying size with dense calcification. The larger nodes have curvilinear margins and multiple lucencies in the center and periphery.

enter draining lymphatics.[8,16] However, calcified lymph nodes may be seen elsewhere in the mesentery, even in the absence of right lower quadrant calcification. Mesenteric nodes may change in location on sequential examinations, the amount of movement related to the distance from the root of the mesentery.[6] To a limited extent, they can also change their position relative to each other (Fig. 8–7).

most of it will become radiodense. Typically, the calcification will be sharply defined with a curvilinear margin that is no more opaque than the interior of the node (Fig. 8–3). Occasionally, calcified nodes may appear as elongated, triangular, or roughly rectangular densities (Fig. 8–4). If multiple nodes are seen, they may vary in the extent of opacity, with some brightly calcified nodes next to others that are more faint (Fig. 8–5). Small rounded lucencies are almost always present and are located in both the center and the periphery, giving the node a mottled appearance. Rarely, a lymph node will have a homogeneous lucent center and an annular rim of calcification.[5,14]

Calcified nodes differ greatly in size. A few may reach 7 cm. in their longest axis, but usually they vary between 1 and 3 cm. in diameter[15] (Fig. 8–6). The most frequent location of calcified mesenteric nodes is in the right lower quadrant because the lymphoid tissue is most prominent here and intestinal contents move slowly in the cecum, permitting more bacteria to penetrate the mucosa and

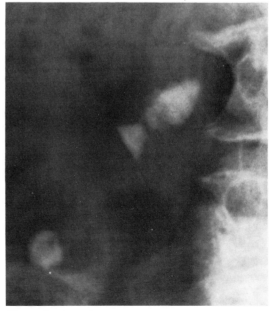

Figure 8–4. Triangular, ovoid, and rounded calcified mesenteric nodes.

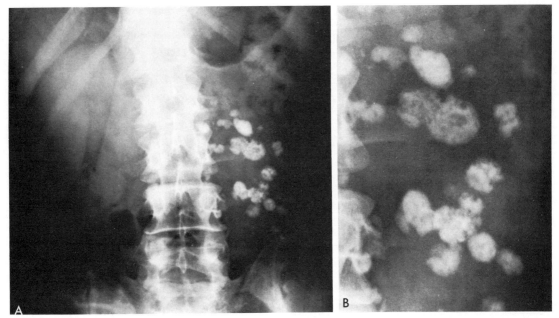

Figure 8–5. *A,* Many calcified mesenteric nodes but none are in the right lower quadrant. *B,* Detail of *A.* The nodes have differing degrees of radiopacity.

PARA-AORTIC NODE CALCIFICATION

Calcification in para-aortic nodes is uncommon. Occasionally it occurs in asymptomatic patients with no previous history of therapy. When seen in conjunction with calcified mesenteric nodes, para-aortic node calcification may be an indication of active or healed disseminated tuberculosis[17] (Fig. 8–8). However, when only para-aortic nodes are

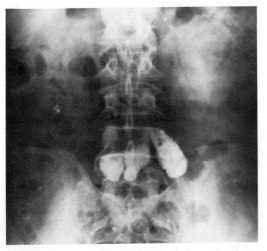

Figure 8–6. Large mesenteric nodes. The largest measures 7 cm.

radiodense, the etiology is often obscure. The most common cause of isolated para-aortic node calcification is infiltration with tumor. Metastatic adenocarcinoma of the colon and serous cystadenocarcinoma of the ovary are the two most common tumors that cause calcified nodes in this region.[18–25] In colon cancer, calcification occurs in areas of degenerating tissue, but in serous cystadenocarcinoma of the ovary, calcification is laid down intracellularly in psammoma bodies in a growing tumor (Fig. 8–9). In both malignancies, nodal calcification may occur before calcification in the primary site. Other carcinomas in which calcified para-aortic metastases have been demonstrated include cervix,[26,27] testes,[27] stomach,[28,29] breast,[27] thyroid,[27] and kidney.[18] Occasionally lymphomas may calcify before therapy is instituted.[30,31] Bone formation in nodes occurs in metastatic osteosarcoma,[32] adenocarcinoma of the colon,[33] and testicular teratocarcinoma,[34] where nodes in the left renal hilus may ossify (Fig. 8–10). Rarely, calcification occurs in para-aortic nodes in silicosis, almost always in association with extensive mediastinal nodal calcification (Fig. 8–11).

Calcified metastatic nodes tend to be larger than those involved with tuberculosis because of the enlargement of the node by tumor.[35] Initially they are faintly calcified but may increase in density and extent later on.[36] They appear as speckled, stippled, or finely mottled opacities.[37,38] Occasionally ring or plaque-like calcification may occur.[27,38]

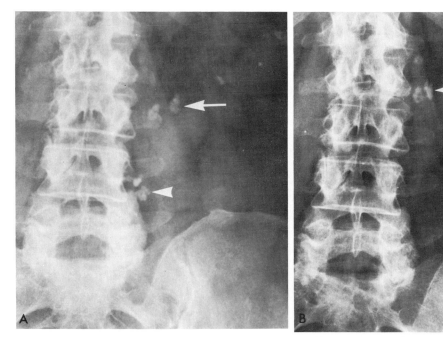

Figure 8–7, A and B. Calcified mesenteric node movement. The two upper nodes (arrows) move relative to each other on films taken at different times. The lower nodes (arrowheads) change their position also.

Calcification may be found in nodes infiltrated with Hodgkin's lymphoma or cervical cancer after chemotherapy or radiotherapy has been instituted.[39–41] The alkaline pH within nodes contain-

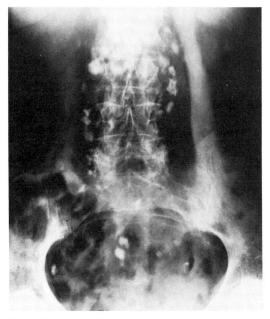

Figure 8–8. Calcification in mesenteric and para-aortic nodes in a patient with a history of tuberculosis.

ing metastasis, a consequence of cellular destruction, favors calcium deposition.[28] After therapy, calcification may occur rapidly, sometimes as early as five weeks, and almost always within a year[27] (Fig. 8–12). This is in contrast to intervals of between ten and 36 months following exposure to mycobacteria before nodal opacification appears.[8]

Increased lymph node density is not always due to calcification or ossification. It can be simulated by contrast material remaining after lymphangiography. Residual contrast nearly always is confined to para-aortic and pelvic nodes (Fig. 8–13). Sometimes contrast in nodes resembles calcification secondary to treatment of Hodgkin's disease or other neoplasms. Contrast tends to diminish or even disappear over a period of time, and this may be a useful finding if a sequence of films is available. On occasion, however, lymph node calcification can also gradually disappear.[13,42]

Increased deposition of hemosiderin can sometimes be detected on plain films as faint opacities in para-aortic nodes. Patients with thalassemia who have received multiple blood transfusions for a long time may have enlarged nodes in the upper lumbar and lower thoracic area, which can be seen on plain films. The nodes are generally moderately enlarged and only slightly more dense than the surrounding soft tissues. Almost always, the liver and spleen are also enlarged[43] (Fig. 8–14).

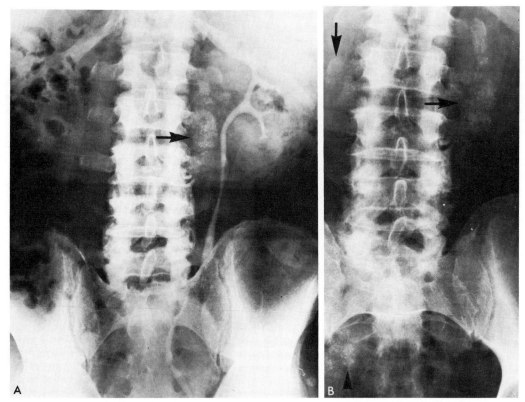

Figure 8–9. Lymph node calcification; metastases from rectal carcinoma. The primary tumor was removed but there was no history of radiotherapy or chemotherapy prior to the onset of calcification. *A,* Calcification of left para-aortic nodes (horizontal arrow) on film from an intravenous urography. *B,* Follow-up examination reveals right para-aortic nodal calcification (vertical arrow) and iliac node calcification (arrowhead). (Courtesy of Dr. Ronald Schliftman, White Plains, New York.)

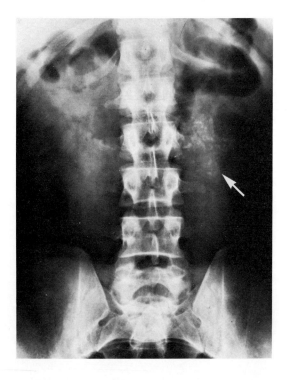

Figure 8–10. Metastatic teratorcarcinoma of the testes. Only the mass adjacent to L2 (arrow) was seen on plain films; at surgery an ossified lymph node metastasis just below the left renal hilus was found. The patient had received no therapy prior to this film.

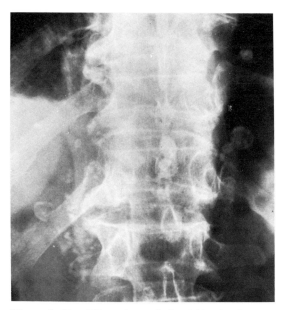

Figure 8–11. Bilateral egg-shell calcification in para-aortic lymph nodes in a patient with silicosis. There were similar changes in mediastinal and hilar nodes.

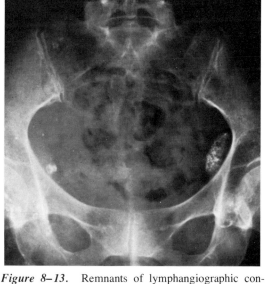

Figure 8–13. Remnants of lymphangiographic contrast material in pelvic nodes. Note the similarity of the nodal opacification to that seen in Figure 8–17.

CALCIFICATION IN PORTA HEPATIS AND PERIPANCREATIC NODES

Calcification may be rarely encountered in nodes in the porta hepatis and near the pancreas. Usually they calcify in response to mycobacteria[17] (Fig. 8–15). Metastatic deposits in porta hepatis nodes may also calcify. Peripancreatic nodes will opacify after the administration of Thorotrast, but there is

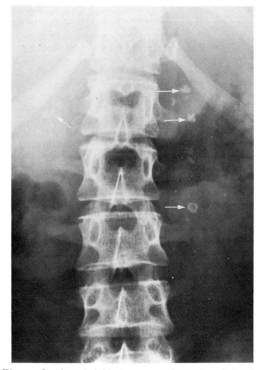

Figure 8–12. Calcified para-aortic nodes following radiotherapy for Hodgkin's disease (horizontal arrows). Calcified gallstones are present on the right (oblique arrows).

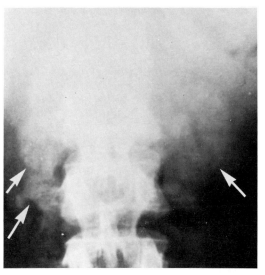

Figure 8–14. Hemosiderin-laden lymph nodes. Arrows point to enlarged para-aortic nodes infiltrated with iron. The nodes are enlarged.

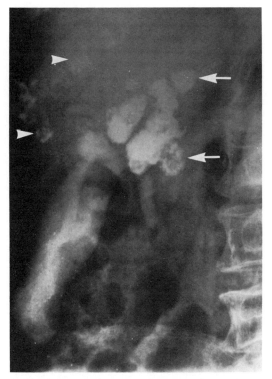

Figure 8–15. Large calcified porta hepatis nodes (arrows) in a patient with a history of tuberculosis. The arrowheads point to costal cartilage calcification. The gallbladder is opacified by contrast material.

little likelihood this will be confused with any other entity. Thorotrast nodes are very radiodense and there is always increased density in the liver and spleen. Occasionally, lymphatic channels near peripancreatic nodes will also opacify[44] (Fig. 5–6).

CALCIFICATION IN PELVIC AND INGUINAL NODES

Isolated calcification of inguinal nodes is rare but may be seen in tubercular or gonococcal infection (Fig. 8–16). Pelvic node calcification is also very uncommon. Nodal opacification can occur in tuberculosis after extension from foci in the adnexa or adjacent muscle and bone (Fig. 8–17),[45] in metastatic colon carcinoma (Fig. 8–9B), and after treatment of cervical malignancy. Lymphangiographic contrast can persist in pelvic nodes and may resemble calcification (Fig. 8–13).

SIMULATORS OF CALCIFICATION IN NODES

Many of the entities discussed in this monograph may mimic calcification in lymph nodes.

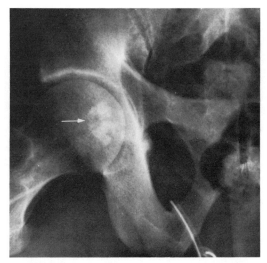

Figure 8–16. Inguinal node calcification (arrow) in a patient with gonorrhea.

Among these are stones in the urinary, biliary and gastrointestinal tract and solid masses in the buttocks and uterus. Differentiation of these densities from lymph nodes is usually not difficult. The anatomic distribution of nodal calcification is generally readily discernible, employing either a supine abdominal film alone or with the addition of oblique and lateral projections. Oblique films demonstrate the anterior position of gallbladder calculi as well as the posterior locations of urinary tract calcifications and the far posterior and lateral positions of opacities in the buttocks. The solid mass configuration of most lymph node calcifications can dis-

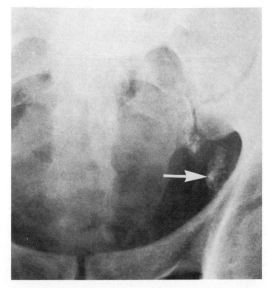

Figure 8–17. Calcified left pelvic node (arrow) in a patient with tuberculosis.

tinguish them from the ringlike or laminated appearance of concretions in the urinary tract, gallbladder, or appendix. Rarely, diffuse mesenteric nodes may be simulated by clumps of nonconjugated Telepaque in the bowel. They will disappear on later films, while nodal calcification is much more permanent (Fig. 4–5). Calcification in the pancreas is recognized by its characteristic location, crossing the midline and extending to the left upper quadrant. Uterine leiomyomas have a solid mass morphology and tend to be larger than nodes. However, occasionally it may be impossible to differentiate them from mesenteric or pelvic lymph nodes on plain films.

REFERENCES

1. Auchincloss H: A clinical study of calcified nodes in the mesentery. Ann Surg 91:401–415, 1930.
2. Walker JT: On the relation of calcified abdominal glands to urinary surgery. Lancet 2:1213–1217, 1922.
3. Corner EM: The surgical treatment of tuberculous glands in the mesentery. Lancet 2:1825–1827, 1905.
4. Schechter S: Calcified mesenteric lymph nodes: their incidence and significance in routine roentgen examination of the gastrointestinal tract. Radiology 27:485–493, 1936.
5. Pauson M (ed.): Gastroenterologic Medicine, Philadelphia, Lee & Febiger, 1969.
6. Morson BC, Dawson IMP: Gastrointestinal Pathology, Oxford, Blackwell Scientific Publications, 1979, p 276.
7. Pfuetze KH, Radner DB (eds.): Clinical Tuberculosis, Springfield, Illinois, Charles C Thomas, 1966, p 317.
8. Wilson GS: The Hazards of Immunization. London, Athlone Press, 1967, pp 67–68.
9. Branson WPS: In Corner, EM: The surgical treatment of tuberculous glands in the mesentery. Lancet 2:1825–1827, 1905.
10. Dobroklonski V: In Golden R, Reeves RJ: The significance of calcified abdominal lymph nodes. Am J Roentgenol 22:305–317, 1929.
11. Barrowman JA: Physiology of the Gastrointestinal Lymphatic System. Cambridge, Cambridge University Press, 1978, pp 54–56.
12. Symmers W: The Lymphoreticular System in Systemic Pathology by Thirty-eight Authors, Edinburgh, Churchill Livingstone, 1978.
13. Rich AR: The Pathogenesis of Tuberculosis, Springfield, Illinois, Charles C Thomas, 1951.
14. Dunham EC, Smythe AM: Tuberculosis of abdominal lymph nodes, diagnosis by means of the roentgen ray. Am J Dis Child 31:815–831, 1926.
15. Nolan DJ, Norman WJ, Airth GR: Traction diverticula of the colon. Clin Radiol 22:458–461, 1971.
16. Phillips S: Current Problems in Tuberculosis. Springfield, Illinois, Charles C Thomas, 1966, p 88.
17. Opie EL: Active and latent tuberculosis in the Negro race. Am Rev Tuberculosis 10:265–274, 1924.
18. Fred HL, Eiband JM, Collins LC: Calcifications in intra-abdominal and retroperitoneal metastases. Am J Roentgenol 91:138–148, 1964.
19. Lingley JR: The significance of psammoma calcification in roentgen diagnosis of papillary tumors of the ovary. Am J Roentgenol 91:138–148, 1964.
20. Moncada R, Cooper RA, Garces, M: Calcified metastases from malignant ovarian neoplasm. Radiology 113:31–35, 1974.
21. Stiedl RA: Extensive calcified retroperitoneal lymph node metastases from a primary carcinoma of the cecum. Radiology 89:263–264, 1967.
22. Ghahremani GG, Straus FH II: Calcification of distant lymph node metastases from carcinoma of the colon. Radiology 99:65–66, 1971.
23. Zboralske FF, Amberg JR, Subby WL: Calcified mucinous adenocarcinoma of the colon. Am J Gastroenterol 38:675–681, 1962.
24. Hermann G, Rozin R: Calcification in gastrointestinal carcinomata. Clin Radiol 15:139–141, 1964.
25. McNair M, Trapnell DH: Calcification in lymph node metastases from adenocarcinoma of the colon. Brit J Radiol 44:468–470, 1971.
26. Hutcheson J, Page DL, Oldham RR: Calcified lymph nodes. Brit J Radiol 48:396–400, 1975.
27. Dolan PA: Tumor calcification following therapy. Am J Roentgenol 89:166–174, 1963.
28. Batlan LE: Calcification within the stomach wall in gastric malignancy. Am J Roentgenol 72:788–794, 1954.
29. Butler RL, Cotran R: Petrified stomach. N Engl J Med 261:84–86, 1969.
30. Case 42242, Case Records of the Massachusetts General Hospital. N Engl J Med 254:1139–1141, 1956.
31. Fisher AMH, Kendall B, Van Leuven BD: Hodgkin's disease: a radiological survey. Clin Radiol 13:115–127, 1962.
32. Le Treut A, Dilhuydy MH, Denepoux R: Ossified lymph nodes metastatic from osteosarcoma. J Radiol Electrol Med Nucl 55:317–320, 1974.
33. Senturia HR, Schechter SE, Hulbert B: Heterotopic ossification in an area of metastasis from rectal carcinoma. Am J Roentgenol 60:507–510, 1948.
34. Valentin E: In Dunham, EC, Smythe AM: Tuberculosis of abdominal lymph nodes, diagnosis by means of the roentgen ray. Am J Dis Child 31:815–831, 1926.
35. Calmette A: Channels of tuberculous infection. Brit J Tuberc 3:199–201, 1909.
36. De Giuli E: Lymph node calcification after radiotherapy in 2 cases of seminoma testis. Tumori 63:543–548, 1977.
37. Oh KS: Mottled areas of intra-abdominal calcification. JAMA 208:521–523, 1969.
38. Syman SM, Weber AL: Calcification in intrathoracic nodes in Hodgkin's disease. Radiology 93:1021–1024, 1969.
39. McLennan TW, Castellino RA: Calcification in pelvic lymph nodes containing Hodgkin's disease following radiotherapy. Radiology 115:87–89, 1975.
40. Bertrand M, Chen JTT, Libshitz HI: Lymph node calcification in Hodgkin's disease after chemotherapy. Am J Roentgenol 129:1108–1110, 1977.
41. Korek-Amorosa J, Scheinman HZ, Clemett AR: Hypercalcemia and extensive lymph node calcification in a patient with Hodgkin's disease prior to therapy. Brit J Radiol 47:905–907, 1974.
42. Wright C, Payling, Heard BE: The lungs. In Systemic Pathology by Thirty-eight Authors, vol 1. Edinburgh, Churchill Livingstone, 1976, pp 269–428.
43. Winchester PH, Cerwin R, Dische R: Hemosiderin laden lymph nodes. Am J Roentgenol 118:222–226, 1973.
44. Gondos B: Late clinical and roentgen observations following Thorotrast administration. Clin Radiol 24:195–203, 1973.
45. Halbrecht I: Diagnosis, pathogenetic role and treatment of the sequels of female genital tuberculosis. In Rippmann ET, Wenner R (eds): Latent Female Genital Tuberculosis. Basel, S Karger, 1966, pp 232–238.

Chapter 9

MISCELLANEOUS ABDOMINAL RADIOPACITIES

Richard A. Rosen, M.D.

There is a heterogeneous group of radiodensities that lie outside abdominal organs and vessels. Calcification and other opacities may be found in the peritoneum, in muscles and ligaments, within subcutaneous tissue, and on the skin. The list of miscellaneous conditions that may be seen on plain films is long. In this chapter, the focus will be on only those entities that are common or have distinctive radiographic appearances.

PERITONEAL CALCIFICATION

Tuberculosis

Inflammation of the peritoneum by tuberculosis may cause calcification. Tuberculous foci vary in size and may remain separate or coalesce into thick plaques.[1,2,3] Fibrotic reaction within the peritoneum mats down the mesentery and the intestines and helps to localize and isolate the infection into several pockets.[4] When the tuberculous lesions caseate, they can calcify, and the distribution of calcification reflects the extent of peritoneal involvement.[5,6] Sheetlike deposits or thick masses up to 10 cm. in diameter may be seen along with smaller, scattered calcific conglomerations.[7] Since one of the sources of peritoneal infection is tuberculous mesenteric lymphadenopathy, radiodense nodes may be present as well.[8] Intraperitoneal calcification is usually more extensive and diffuse than nodal calcification and can be found at the periphery of the peritoneum (Fig. 9–1).

PERITONEAL TUMORS

Both primary and metastatic intraperitoneal neoplasms may calcify. In the rare mesothelioma of

the peritoneum diffuse calcifications sometimes occur.[9,10] More commonly, calcification is found in metastases to the peritoneum. Serous cystadenocarcinoma of the ovary and adenocarcinoma of the colon are the primary sites with the greatest predilection for peritoneal calcification (Fig. 1–29). Usually the metastatic deposits are faint densities with ill-defined margins. Denser calcifications are

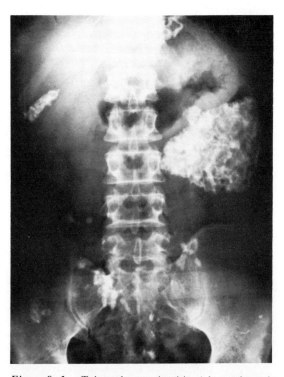

Figure 9–1. Tuberculous peritonitis. A large plaque in the left midabdomen as well as multiple nodular densities scattered elsewhere in the peritoneum. (Courtesy of Dr. Robert Mindelzun, Palo Alto, California.)

172

typical for intraperitoneal undifferentiated carcinoma.

In pseudomyxoma peritonei, the peritoneal cavity is studded with mucin-containing globules varying from a few millimeters to several centimeters in diameter. They result from the rupture of an appendix containing carcinoma or from peritoneal seeding from an ovarian mucinous cystadenocarcinoma.[11-13] While it has been stated that pseudomyxoma peritonei can be a complication of benign lesions of the ovary and appendix, the only well-documented cases have been in patients with malignancy.[1] Innumerable small rounded calcifications of varying diameter will be seen. A few cysts may be irregularly marginated and some may contain central calcification. There may also be small solid collections of calcium interspersed between the cysts.[12] The calcific lesions of pseudomyxoma peritonei may involve all the peritoneum or can be found in localized collections often superimposed on the liver or spleen (Fig. 3–18).

Paraffinoma or oleoma may simulate pseudomyxoma peritonei. During the first two decades of this century, surgeons instilled paraffin and similar materials into the peritoneum with the intent of preventing the formation of adhesions after abdominal operation. It soon became clear, however, that the opposite effect ensued and patients were left with fibrous bands surrounding the instilled material. Since paraffin will assume a globular shape when introduced into the peritoneum, the fibrous adhesions are also curvilinear. When they calcify they appear as ringlike collections similar to the densities noted in pseudomyxoma peritonei.[14,15] Recognition of the consequences of the intraperitoneal placement of paraffin caused abandonment of the procedure.

CALCIFICATION IN APPENDICES EPIPLOICAE

The appendices epiploicae are fatty collections attached to the colon and are located at the anterior and posterior-inferior teniae coli. There are approximately 100 appendices epiploicae arrayed along the course of the colon.[16-18] They range between 0.5 and 5.0 cm. in diameter but some may be

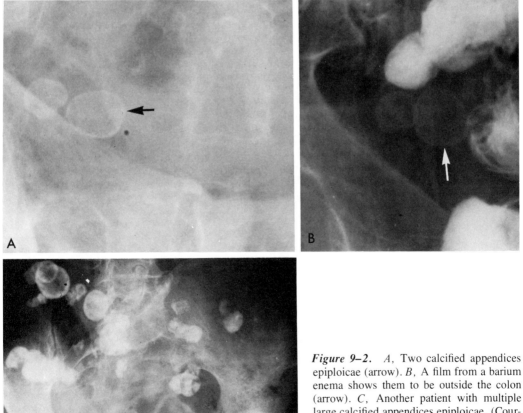

Figure 9–2. *A,* Two calcified appendices epiploicae (arrow). *B,* A film from a barium enema shows them to be outside the colon (arrow). *C,* Another patient with multiple large calcified appendices epiploicae. (Courtesy of Dr. Marcel Dolberg, Jerusalem, Israel.)

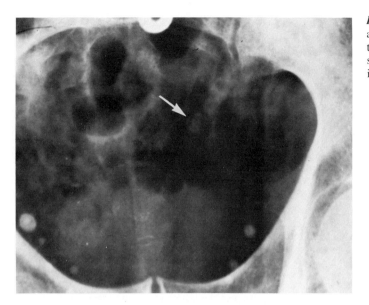

Figure 9–3. Faint rounded calcification above the bladder (arrow). The calcification was removed incidentally at bladder surgery and was found to be an intraperitoneal nodule of fat necrosis.

as large as 10 cm.[19] Torsion of these bodies compromises blood flow and leads to infarction. A devitalized appendix epiploica may calcify and detach from its colonic moorings, becoming free in the peritoneal cavity.[20] While torsion causes pain, mobile detached appendices epiploicae are asymptomatic.[21] They are usually round or oval densities

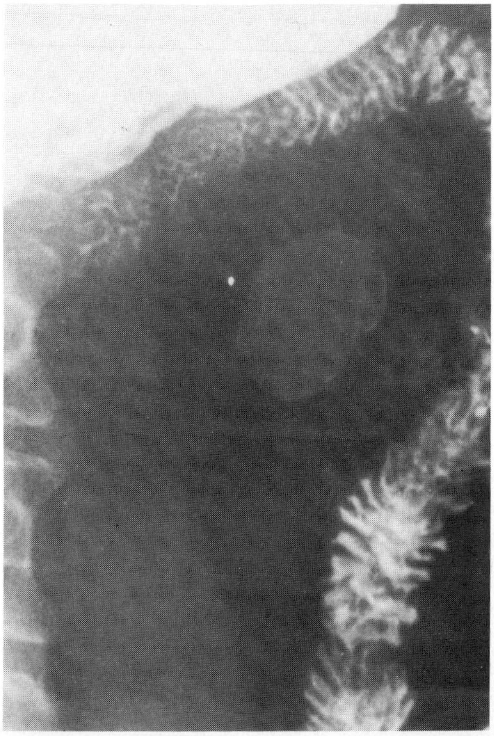

Figure 9–4. Calcified mesenteric cyst. A film from a small bowel series shows a cystic calcification in the mesentery.

with radiolucent centers and thin calcified margins. When they are no longer attached to the colon they tend to migrate to the pelvis, the most dependent part of the peritoneal cavity.[22] They may be suspected on plain abdominal radiographs by their characteristic annular or elliptical marginal calcification, their movement on successive films, and their location outside the gastrointestinal and genitourinary tracts (Fig. 9–2). Rarely, omental fat deposits may also calcify and lie free in the peritoneal cavity and look like appendices epiploicae (Fig. 9–3).

Calcifications occur in cysts in the mesentery and omentum, the cysts resulting from inflammation, trauma or congenital rests. Typically, they resemble other cysts with curvilinear marginal calcification (Fig. 9–4).[23,24] Mesenteric and omental cysts can move on sequential films but on a single abdominal radiograph they may not be differentiable from cysts in adjacent organs. Lateral and oblique projections demonstrate that they are anterior to the pancreas, kidney, spleen, and adrenal glands.

CALCIFICATION AND OTHER OPACITIES IN SOFT TISSUES OF THE ABDOMEN

Traumatic Calcification—Buttock Cysts

Calcification in the buttocks is often seen on abdominal films. Poorly absorbed or irritative material introduced by injections into the buttocks can cause local damage with the formation of calcified sterile abscesses. Recent evidence suggests that these calcifications occur nearly always in lipomatous tissue and not in deeper muscle layers.[25] In the past, heavy metals injected for the treatment of syphilis were the chief cause of these opacities. While arsenicals and bismuth may remain and appear dense on radiographs, most opacities in the buttocks after luetic therapy are calcifications and not the heavy metals themselves. Serial observations of children who received these injections demonstrated resorption of the metallic densities over several months with the later appearance of discrete calcification at the same site. Calcifications have been noted after the subcutaneous administration of quinine,[26, 27] which led to the popular description of buttocks calcification as ''cinchona cysts.''[28] The formation of sterile abscesses may occur with penicillin preparations, a fact which explains the continued recognition of these calcifications long after the discontinuance of heavy metal and quinine injections.[29]

The patterns of traumatic buttock calcification are varied. The two most common manifestations

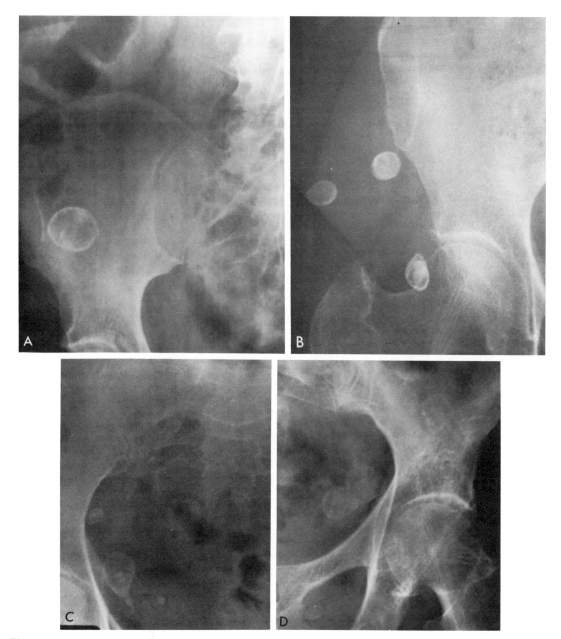

Figure 9–5. Buttocks calcification—ovoid configuration. *A,* A single calcification. *B,* Multiple calcifications. *C,* Buttock cyst with a ''tail.'' *D,* Bilobed buttock cyst.

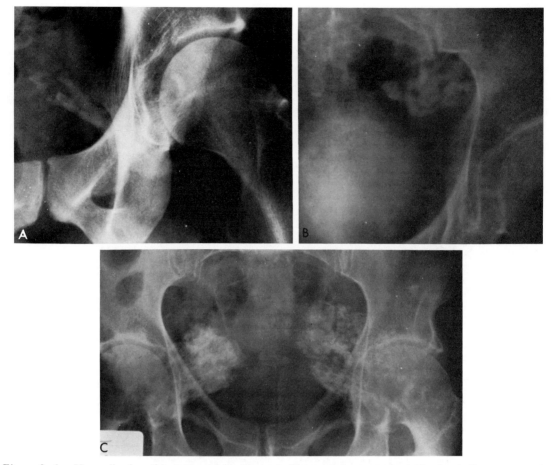

Figure 9–6. Unusually shaped buttocks calcifications. *A,* The medial aspect of calcification is linear, suggesting two needle tracks. *B,* Vermiform appearance, simulating a calcified guinea worm. *C,* Bulky calcifications similar to those seen in patients with scleroderma.

are rounded to oval opacities or linear densities which are oriented along needle tracks (Fig. 9–5). Occasionally, calcifications have a solid mass morphology with a dense center and irregular margination (Fig. 9–6). The calcifications are often located in the upper outer quadrant of the buttocks since this is the preferred location for injections, but they may also be seen above or below the bony pelvis, superimposed upon it, or lateral to it (Fig. 9–7). This does not necessarily indicate faulty technique but generally reflects the configuration of the buttocks at the time of the radiographic exposure. Often in patients with bulky soft tissues, the buttocks project above the iliac crest. In patients who have lost weight rapidly, calcifications will sometimes move medially or inferiorly. Because calcification overlying the pelvis may be confused with intra-abdominal entities such as appendicoliths or urinary stones, a steep oblique or lateral film may be required to locate the calcification posterior to the pelvic wing.

OSSIFICATION IN SCARS

Scars may ossify after upper abdominal operations, especially following gastric surgery. Observed almost exclusively in men who have had vertical supraumbilical incisions, the ossifications occur in both subcutaneous and deeper layers of the scar. Usually ossified scars are asymptomatic but they may cause pain which is accentuated by bending forward and relieved by assuming the erect position.[30–32] Since they are found at or near the midline on supine films they may simulate paraspinal masses, but lateral films will clearly demonstrate their anterior location (Fig. 9–8). However, if they are first encountered on oblique films, they can project over the gallbladder and bile ducts and be a source of confusion (Fig. 9–9). Much less common are calcifications and ossifications in rectus sheath hematomas. Ossification in the rectus muscle is always found below the umbilicus and may occur in both sexes.[33–36] Postoperative ossi-

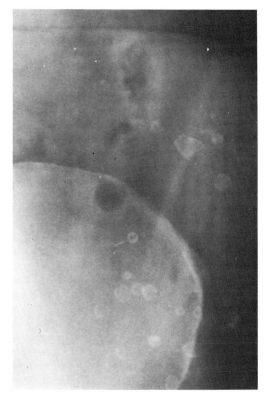

Figure 9–7. Buttocks calcifications both overlying and superior to the iliac wing.

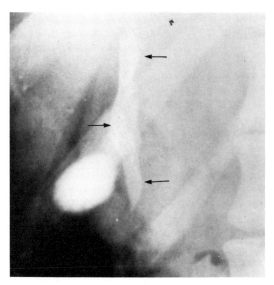

Figure 9–9. Ossification in a scar. On the right posterior oblique view taken during oral cholecystography the scar (arrows) appears near to the opacified gallbladder and may be mistaken for a contrast-filled common bile duct.

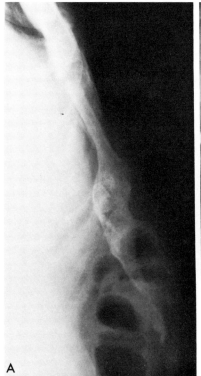

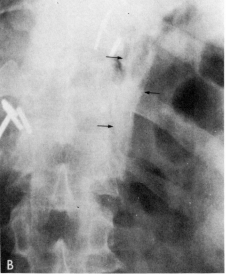

Figure 9–8. Scar ossification. *A,* Subxiphoid ossification is well seen on the lateral film. *B,* Another patient, frontal projection, shows a less well-defined density to the left of the spine (arrows).

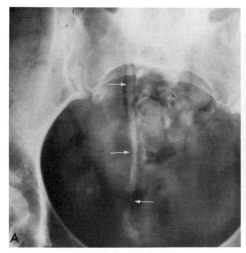
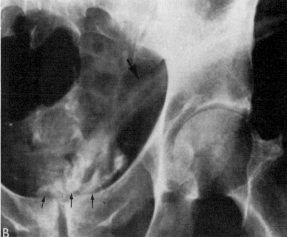

Figure 9–10. Suprapubic scar ossifications. *A,* Linear scar following bladder surgery (arrows). (Courtesy of Dr. Murray K. Dalinka, Philadelphia, Pennsylvania.) *B,* Infracystic ossification (small arrows), following the placement of a suprapubic drainage tube (large arrow).

fication may also be observed above the symphysis pubis in patients who have had bladder surgery (Fig. 9–10).

OTHER TRAUMATIC CAUSES OF CALCIFICATION

Extensive calcification may occur after trauma to the spine. Usually the relationship between the calcification and the vertebrae is obvious. However, if there is extensive bleeding, the calcifications may extend for several centimeters from the midline (Fig. 9–11). Ossification may also occur in intramuscular hematomas in hemophiliacs.[38,39] The usual site is in the pelvis within the iliopsoas muscle (Fig. 9–12).

INFLAMMATION

Calcified Psoas Abscesses

Nearly all cases of psoas muscle calcification represent tuberculous abscesses. Usually it is the result of an extension of a tuberculous infection from the kidney or spine. Calcification reflects the extension of the abscess along the psoas fascia. Since the infection may spread unhindered beneath the psoas fascia, it usually presents as broad sheets of density oriented along the course of the muscle (Fig. 9–13). Sometimes the calcification extends all the way to the lesser trochanter.[40–42] Less commonly the abscess may be localized and have a curvilinear margin resembling a calcified cyst.

CYSTICERCOSIS

Cysticerci are the embryo state of *Taenia solium*, the pork tapeworm. The contamination of food by pig feces permits man to ingest the em-

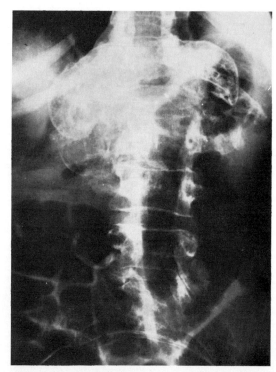

Figure 9–11. Massive calcified paraspinal hematoma. The formation of the hematoma followed a decompression laminectomy involving a hemangiomatous vertebra.

Figure 9–12. Peripheral ossifica-
tion in hemophilia. (Courtesy of Dr.
Murray K. Dalinka, Philadelphia,
Pennsylvania.)

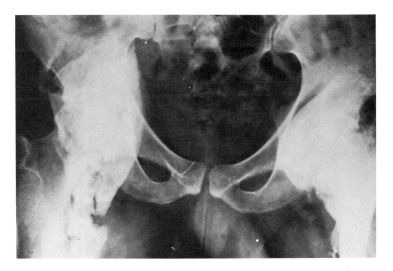

bryo, which migrates through the blood stream and
then encysts in the brain and in the lymphatics of
skeletal muscle.[43] Embryos are trapped at these
sites, and when they die they calcify. Encysted
embryos have the shape of rice grains, up to one
centimeter long. They are aligned along the course
of the muscle in which they are situated. Often they

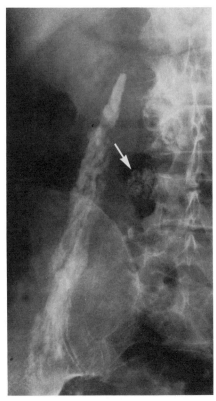

Figure 9–13. Tuberculous psoas abscess. Note the
calcified para-aortic node (arrow).

can be extremely numerous and may be found in
both abdominal and peripheral musculature. The
observation of rice grain type calcification in the
muscles and brain is pathognomonic for cysticercosis (Fig. 9–14).[44,45]

GUINEA WORM INFESTATION

Dracunculus medinensis, the guinea worm, is a
nematode found in Africa and Asia. The adult female can reach 35 to 120 cm. in length and usually
resides in subcutaneous tissue but can burrow more
deeply, even reaching the retroperitoneum.[46,47]
Wherever it is located, the worm may calcify, and
in the abdomen it is frequently coiled. Calcification rarely equals the length of the worm and is
often fragmented.[48-50] The radiographic appearance of intra-abdominal dracunculus infestation
depends upon the length and continuity of the calcification and the degree of coiling of the worm.
Plain film recognition is important because, while
the infestation is often asymptomatic, there appears to be an increased risk for the development
of malignancies at the site of the worm (Fig. 9–
15).[51]

Abdominal calcification in other parasitic diseases is rare. *Armillifer armillatus* was previously
discussed in relation to hepatic and peritoneal calcification (Fig. 3–12), but the typical C-shaped
opacities representing the encysted worm also occur in paravertebral muscles and in the anterior abdominal wall.[43,46] Filarial parasites such as *Onchocerca volvulus* and *Wuchereria bancrofti* have
punctate calcifications that are usually too small to
be seen on plain films of the abdomen.[52-56] Similarly, *Trichinella spiralis* will calcify in muscles
but cannot be identified on radiographs because of
its minute size.[43,57]

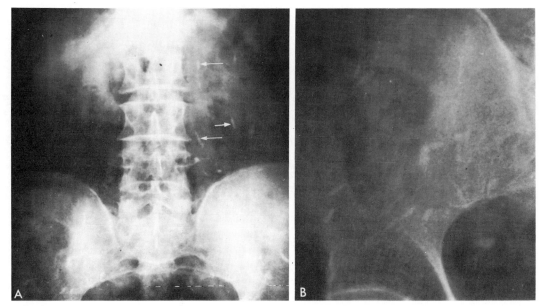

Figure 9–14. Cysticercosis. *A*, Linear calcifications oriented along muscle planes in the upper abdomen (arrows). *B*, Coned-down view of the pelvis in the same patient. The calcifications resemble needle tracks.

CALCIFICATION IN TUMORS

Calcified neoplasms in the soft tissues of the abdominal wall are uncommon. Angiomas, fibro-mas, and lipomas may occasionally contain sufficient calcium to be observed on plain films.[58] For masses on the anterior abdominal wall, cross-table lateral projections may best demonstrate calcification. Occasionally, tumors arising in bone cause

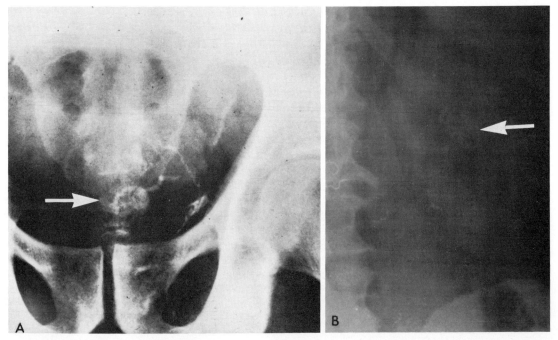

Figure 9–15. Dracunculosis. *A*, Coiled worm in the pelvis (arrow). *B*, Coiled worm overlying the left kidney (arrow). (Both cases courtesy of Dr. Marcel Dolberg, Jerusalem, Israel.)

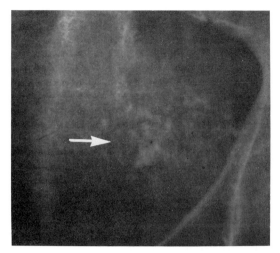

Figure 9–16. Pelvic chondrosarcoma. There are speckled calcifications (arrow) in the pelvic soft tissues but no bony changes.

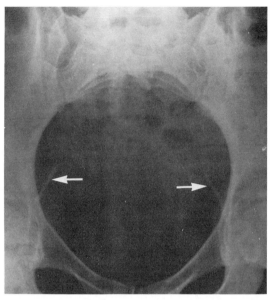

Figure 9–18. Bilateral sacrospinous ligament ossification (arrows).

little osseous change and are recognized primarily by increased densities in the soft tissues. Pelvic chondrosarcoma may present only as an irregular soft tissue calcification without demonstrable bony destruction and can simulate the mottled calcification of uterine leiomyomas (Fig. 9–16). Projections of benign and malignant tumors of the iliac bone may also extend into the pelvis and may resemble calcified or ossified soft tissue masses (Fig. 9–17).

LIGAMENT OSSIFICATION

The ligaments in the pelvis may occasionally ossify. Their predictable course and location usually make their recognition easy on plain films. The two most common ossified ligaments are the sacrotuberous ligament running from the ischial tuberosity to the sacrum and the sacrospinous ligament, which connects the lateral sacrum with the ischial spine (Figs. 9–18, 9–19). Ossifications may be unilateral or bilateral and may involve only a portion of the ligament. When they are associated with diffusely dense bones, fluorosis must be considered.[59] However, ossified ligaments in the pelvis are nearly always innocuous findings of no clinical significance.

Figure 9–17. Large osteochondroma (arrows) arising from the anterior lateral surface of the right iliac wing and projecting into the pelvis.

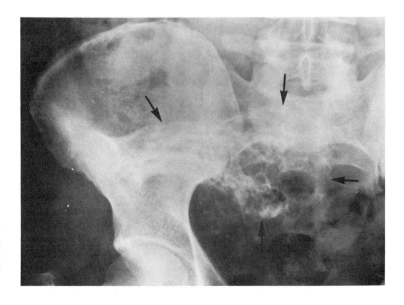

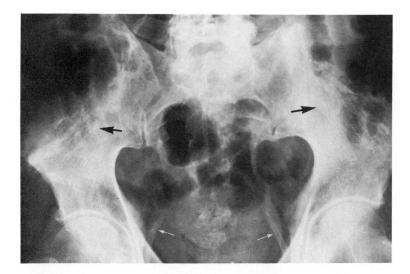

Figure 9–19. Bilateral sacrotuberous ligament ossification (white arrows). The black arrows point to linear buttocks calcification.

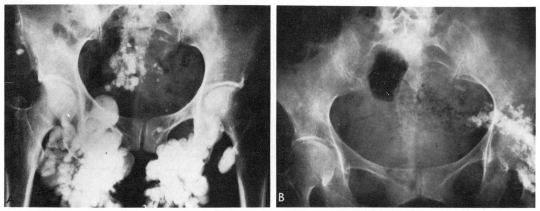

Figure 9–20. Two examples of calcification in scleroderma. *A,* Massive bilateral nodular calcifications. (Courtesy of Dr. Hugh Eisen, Hollywood, Florida.) *B,* Unilateral calcifications which are similar to those following buttocks injections.

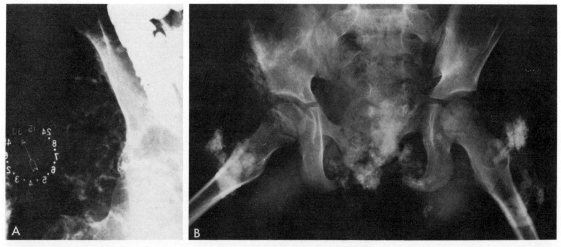

Figure 9–21. Dermatomyositis. *A,* Coned-down view of the right iliac bone during a barium enema examination. There is reticulated soft tissue calcification lateral to the bone. (Courtesy of Dr. Stanford Goldman, Baltimore, Maryland.) *B,* Bilateral multifocal nodular calcification. (Courtesy of Dr. Murray K. Dalinka, Philadelphia, Pennsylvania.)

CALCIFICATION IN DISEASES OF UNKNOWN ORIGIN

Bilateral diffuse calcifications in the soft tissues near the joints are frequently associated with collagen diseases, especially scleroderma and dermatomyositis.[60] While calcification in scleroderma appears more frequently in the extremities, it can occur in the soft tissues of the buttocks and near the hip joints.[61,62] Calcifications tend to be nodular and homogeneous and are usually small but sometimes become massive (Fig. 9–20). Diffuse calcification of the abdominal wall is found in dermatomyositis, where the pattern of calcifications resembles scleroderma. Occasionally, however, a reticulated or sheetlike appearance may be seen (Fig. 9–21).[63,64]

Relapsing febrile nonsuppurative panniculitis, or Weber-Christian disease, is a rare and poorly understood entity in which the formation of tender subcutaneous and mesenteric nodules occurs. Necrosis of subcutaneous fat may produce irregular and elongated calcifications (Fig. 9–22).[64–66]

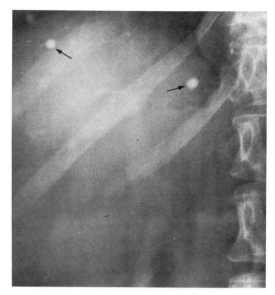

Figure 9–23. Several calcified granulomas in the base of the lung (arrows) resemble intra-abdominal concretions.

DENSITIES THAT SIMULATE INTRA-ABDOMINAL CALCIFICATION

In the upper abdomen, calcified costal cartilage may mimic intra-abdominal calcification. Nearly always, costal cartilage calcification is recognized by its continuity with a rib. Calcification increases with age and is more frequent in women.[67,68] The typical pattern in men is parallel tracks extending from the costochondral junction. In women, a single central line either near or at a distance from the costochondral junction is often found.[69,70] However, calcification may be unilateral and irregular and may exactly simulate concretions, conduits, or solid masses (Figs. 1–33,1–38). Calcified granulomas in the lung bases may be mistaken for stones in the abdomen (Fig. 9–23). Also, masses on the skin may appear opaque when they project from the abdominal wall and are outlined by air (Fig. 9–24).

FOREIGN BODIES

A diverse group of foreign bodies may be introduced into the abdominal wall or peritoneum. If their placement has been purposeful, the plain film serves to record their presence and location (Fig. 9–25).[71] Sutures, drains, and fabrics are easily recognized. With time, permanently in dwelling material such as tantalum mesh, used in hernia and abdominal wall repairs several decades ago, may fragment because of metal fatigue (Fig. 9–26).[72–74] The presence of discontinuities in the mesh serves to differentiate it from retained surgical sponges, which can be seen because of radiopaque threads woven into them or because of the precipitation of calcium salts on their surface (Fig. 9–27). Sometimes foreign bodies not placed by design may lie

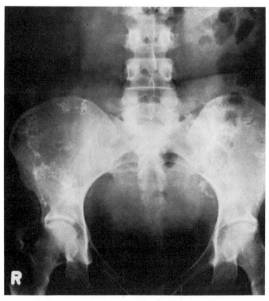

Figure 9–22. Weber-Christian disease. Reticular-appearing soft tissue calcification overlying the iliac bones. (Courtesy of Dr. George Stein, Philadelphia, Pennsylvania.)

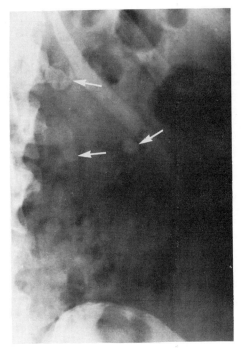

Figure 9–24. Neurofibromas (arrows) projecting from the skin stand out clearly on plain films even though they are not calcified.

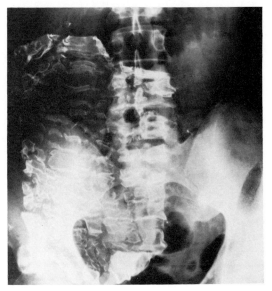

Figure 9–26. Large abdominal wall defect covered by tantalum mesh which has fragmented.

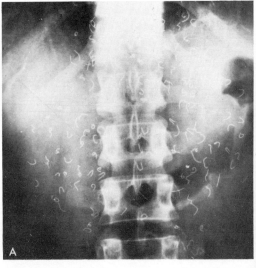

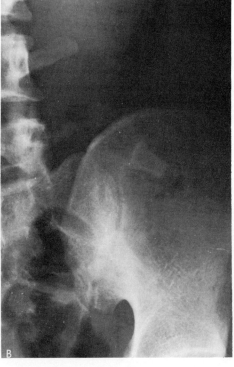

Figure 9–25. Two examples of opacities purposefully placed in the abdominal wall. *A*, Subcutaneous acupuncture wires. *B*, Phalanx "banked" in the abdominal wall for future reimplantation.

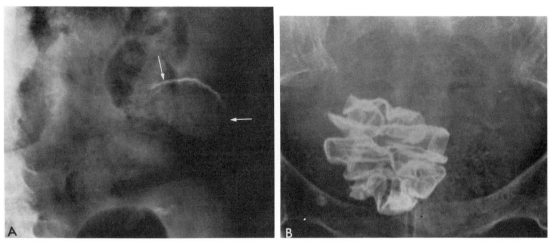

Figure 9–27. Opacification of surgical sponges. *A*, Radiodense threads woven into the sponge (arrows). *B*, Calcification of a sponge within the pelvis.

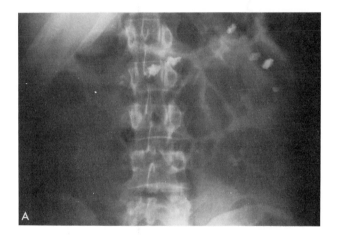

Figure 9–28. Accidental placement of radiopacities. *A*, Opaque pebbles affixed to the skin following trauma. They resemble calcified nodes. *B*, Extravasated contrast material following myelogram extending into the muscle planes of the back and buttocks.

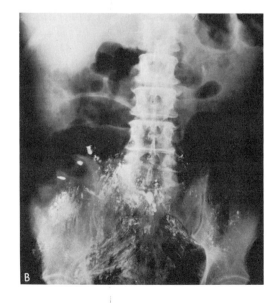

on the skin, within wounds, or in muscles and can be misinterpreted as an intra-abdominal calcification on a single supine film if no history is available (Fig. 9–28).

REFERENCES

1. Morson BC: The Peritoneum, *in* Systemic Pathology by Thirty-Eight Authors, 2nd Edition. Edinburgh, Churchill Livingstone, 1978, pp 1179–1198.
2. Frank LW: Tuberculous peritonitis. Am Rev Tuberc 36:279–282, 1937.
3. Burack WR, Hollister RM: Tuberculous peritonitis. Am J Med 28:510–523, 1960.
4. Stassa G: Tuberculous peritonitis. Am J Roentgenol 101:409–413, 1967.
5. McCort JJ: Roentgen features of chronic tuberculous peritonitis. Arch Surg 49:91–99, 1944.
6. Auerbach O: Pleural, peritoneal and pericardial tuberculosis. Am Rev Tuberc 61:845–861, 1950.
7. Webster AJ, Semple T: Calcification of the peritoneum. Brit Med J 2:1069–1070, 1951.
8. Steinberg B: Infections of the Peritoneum. New York, Paul B. Hoeber, Inc., 1944, pp 253–260.
9. Banner MP, Gohel VK: Peritoneal mesothelioma. Radiology 129:637–640, 1978.
10. Berlinger L, Redmond P: Calcified papillary tumor of the peritoneum. Brit J Radiol 53:1200–1203, 1980.
11. Pugh DG: A roentgenologic aspect of pseudomyxoma peritoneii. Radiology 39:320–322, 1942.
12. Weig CG, Koenig EC, Culver GH: Pseudomyxoma peritoneii report of a case with unusual roentgen findings. Am J Roentgenol 52:505–509, 1944.
13. Elliott CE: Two cases of pseudomyxoma peritonaeii from myxoma of the appendix. Brit J Surg 45:15, 1957.
14. Whitaker WG Jr, Walker ET, Canipelli J: Lipogranuloma of the peritoneum. JAMA 138:363–365, 1948.
15. Bennett HS, Collins EN: Oil granuloma of the peritoneum. Gastroenterology 20:485–491, 1952.
16. Morales O: Calcified appendices epiploicae as freely mobile bodies in the abdominal cavity. Acta Radiol 25:653–661, 1944.
17. Harrigan AH: Torsion and inflammation of the appendices epiploicae. Ann Surg 66:467–478, 1917.
18. Klingenstein P: Some phases of the pathology of the appendices epiploicae. Surg Gynecol Obst 38:376–382, 1924.
19. Borg SE, Whitehouse GH, Griffiths GJ: A mobile calcified amputated appendix epiploica. Am J Roentgenol 127:349–350, 1976.
20. Morson BC: The Large Intestine, *in* Systemic Pathology by Thirty-Eight Authors, 2nd Edition. Edinburgh, Churchill Livingstone, 1978, pp 1099–1152.
21. Patterson DC: Appendices epiploicae. N Engl J Med 209:1255–1259, 1933.
22. Barder RP: Calcified epiploic appendages: a radiological curiosity. Radiology 33:768–769, 1939.
23. Mittelstaedt C: Ultrasonic diagnosis of omental cysts. Radiology 117:673–676, 1975.
24. Teplick JG, Haskin ME: Surgical Radiology. Philadelphia, W. B. Saunders, 1981, p 267.
25. Cockshott WP, Thompson GT, Howlett LJ, et al: Intramuscular or intralipomatous injections? N Engl J Med 307:356–359, 1982.
26. Rose CB: The diagnosis of unusual calcareous shadows found on x-ray films of the abdomen. Radiology 32:600–608, 1939.
27. Leeser F: Uber Gewebsveränderungen nach Salversan und Bismutinjektionen im Röntgenbilde. Fortschr d Roentgenstr. 37:486–491, 1927.
28. Brown JS: Soft tissue calcification secondary to therapeutic quinine injection. Brit J Radiol 18:183–184, 1945.
29. McAfee JB, Donner MW: Differential diagnosis of calcifications encountered in abdominal radiographs. Am J Med Sci 243:609–650, 1962.
30. Katz I, Levine M: Bone formation in laparotomy scars. Am J Roentgenol 84:248–261, 1960.
31. Silver PG: Ossification in a laparotomy wound. Canad Med Assoc J 24:414–416, 1931.
32. Pearson J, Clark OH: Heterotopic calcification in abdominal wounds. Surg Gynecol Obst 146:371–374, 1978.
33. Trafford HS: Rupture of rectus abdominis muscle. Brit Med J 2:1130–1131, 1951.
34. Teske JM: Hematoma of the rectus abdominis muscle. Am J Surg 71:689–695, 1946.
35. Wu KT, Gomez JL: Heterotopic calcification within rectus sheath following laparotomy. NY State J Med 76:84–86, 1976.
36. Hildreth DH: Anticoagulant therapy and rectus sheath hematoma. Am J Surg 124:80–86, 1972.
37. Goldstein HH: Myositis ossificans following suprapubic prostatectomy. J Urol 24:211–216, 1930.
38. Vas W, Cockshott WP, Martin RF, Pai MK, et al: Myositis ossificans in hemophilia. Skel Radiol 7:27–31, 1981.
39. Hutcheson J: Peripelvic new bone formation in hemophilia. Radiology 109:529–530, 1973.
40. Graves VB, Schreiber MH: Tuberculous psoas muscle abscess. J Canad Assoc Radiol 24:268–271, 1973.
41. Blumenthal DH, Morin ME, Tan A, et al: Intestinal penetration by tuberculous psoas abscess. Am J Roentgenol 136:995–997, 1981.
42. Lynch AF: Tuberculosis of the greater trochanter. J Bone Joint Surg 64B:185–188, 1982.
43. Gray ED, Patton JT: The Soft Tissues, *in* A Text-Book of X-ray Diagnosis, Vol. VI, 4th Edition, S. Cochrane Shanks and Peter Kerley (Eds.) Philadelphia, WB Saunders, 1971, pp 772–777.
44. Middlemiss H: Tropical Radiology. London, Heinemann Books, 1961, pp 121–123.
45. Lesoff MJ, Shulman S: An unusual case of calcified bodies in the musculature of the entire body. Radiology 27:491–493, 1936.
46. Chartres JC: Radiological manifestations of parasitism by the tongue worms, flat worms and the round worms more commonly seen in the tropics. Brit J Radiol 38:503–511, 1965.
47. Warner RS, Kallet S, Rowan R, et al: Calcified parasite in retroperitoneum. Urology 7:214–215, 1976.
48. Samuel E: Roentgenology of parasitic calcification. Am J Roentgenol 63:512–522, 1950.
49. Reddy CRRM, Sivaprasad MD, Parvathi G, Chari PS: Calcified guinea worm: Clinical, radiological and pathological study. Ann Trop Med 62:399–406, 1968.
50. Carayon A, Camain R, Guiraud R, et al: Migrations habituelles, aberrants ou manquées de la filaire de médine. Presse Med 69:1599–1600, 1961.
51. Khajavi A: Guinea worm calcification: A report of 83 cases. Clin Radiol 19:433–435, 1968.
52. Williams I: Calcification in loiasis. J Faculty Radiol 6:142–144, 1954.
53. Johnstone RDC: Loiasis. Lancet 1:250–253, 1947.
54. Browne SG: Calcinosis circumscripta of the scrotal wall:

The etiological role of onchocerca volvulus. Brit J Dermatol 74:136–140, 1962.

55. Garland LH: Tropical diseases of interest to the radiologist. Radiology 44:1–13, 1945.

56. O'Connor FW, Golden R, Auchincloss H: The roentgen demonstration of calcified filaria bancrofti in human tissues. Am J Roentgenol 23:494–502, 1930.

57. Widmann BP, Ostrum HW, Freed H: Practical aspects of calcification and ossification in the various body tissues. Radiology 30:598–609, 1938.

58. Hilbrish TF, Bartter FC: Roentgen findings in abnormal deposition of calcium in tissues. Am J Roentgenol 87:1128–1139, 1962.

59. Gayler BW, Brogdon BG: Soft tissue calcifications in the extremities in systemic disease. Am J Med Sci 249:590–605, 1965.

60. Wheeler CE, Curtis AC, Cawley EP, et al, Zheutlin B: Soft tissue calcification with special reference to its occurrence in the "collagen diseases." Ann Intern Med 36:1050–1075, 1952.

61. Connor SK: Calcinosis and collagen diseases. Arizona Med 12:277–280, 1955.

62. Muller SA, Brunsting LA, Winkelmann RK: Calcinosis cutis: Its relationship to scleroderma. AMA Arch Derm 80:15–21, 1959.

63. Muller SA, Winkelmann RK, Brunsting LA: Calcinosis in dermatomyositis. AMA Arch Dermatol 79:669–673, 1959.

64. Ozonoff MB, Flynn FJ Jr: Roentgenologic features of der-matomyositis of childhood. Am J Roentgenol 118:206–212, 1973.

65. Herrington JL, Edwards WH, Grossman LA: Mesenteric manifestations of Weber-Christian disease. Ann Surg 154:949–955, 1961.

66. Anderson DC, Stewart WK, Piercy DM: Calcifying panniculitis with fat and skin necrosis in a case of uraemia with autonomous hyperparathyroidism. Lancet 2:323–325, 1968.

67. Salzman E: Lung Calcifications. Springfield, Illinois, Charles C Thomas, 1968, p 87.

68. Elkeles A: Sex differences in the calcification of costal cartilages. J Am Geriatr Soc 14:456–462, 1966.

69. Sanders CF: Sexing by costal cartilage calcification. Brit J Radiol 39:233, 1966.

70. Navani S, Shah JR, Levy PS: Determination of sex by costal cartilage calcification. Am J Roentgenol 108:771–774, 1970.

71. Imray TJ, Hiramatsu Y: Radiographic manifestations of Japanese acupuncture. Radiology 115:625–626, 1975.

72. Lam CR, Szilagyi DE, Puppendahl M: Tantalum gauze in the repair of large postoperative ventral hernias. Arch Surg 57:234–244, 1948.

73. Flynn WJ, Brant AE, Nelson GG: A four and one-half year analysis of tantalum gauze used in the repair of ventral hernia. Ann Surg 134:1027–1034, 1951.

74. Douglas DM: Repair of large herniae with tantalum gauze. Lancet 2:936–939, 1948.

Chapter 10

PEDIATRIC ABDOMINAL CALCIFICATIONS

DuRee Eaton, M.D., and
Harris Cohen, M.D.

Abdominal radiodensities encountered in infants and children can be divided into two groups: opacities similar in appearance to those seen later in life and opacities that occur most frequently or exclusively in the young. Greater emphasis in this chapter will be placed on the latter group. Also, since there are many calcific entities that are found only in newborns, there will be separate discussions of calcification in neonates and in older children.

NEONATAL CALCIFICATION

Peritoneal Calcification

Perforation of the bowel before birth allows sterile meconium to escape into the peritoneum where it may incite an intense inflammatory reaction. Often within 24 hours, calcium salts are deposited in the extruded meconium.[1] In most cases there is intestinal obstruction as a consequence of atresia or volvulus of the bowel.[2,3] Newborns with calcified meconium should have a sweat test since approximately 25 percent of babies with atresias have cystic fibrosis. Rarely, there will be no demonstrable intestinal obstruction and the mechanism for passage of meconium into the peritoneum may be obscure.

On plain radiographs, calcified intraperitoneal meconium appears as clumps, streaks, or irregular dense clusters. Calcification is often situated in the periphery of the peritoneum: in the colonic gutters, anterior to the liver or just below the diaphragm (Fig. 10–1). If the processus vaginalis is patent, calcified masses may also be found in the scrotum (Fig. 10–2). When the obstruction is relieved, peritoneal calcifications will gradually resolve, although it may take several years for scrotal densities to disappear.[4]

Barium peritonitis results from the leakage of mixtures of barium and water through a perforation in the bowel. This is usually due to the excessively forceful introduction of a stiff catheter into the rectum or to the overexpansion of a balloon above the rectal ampulla.[5] The radiographic appearance of

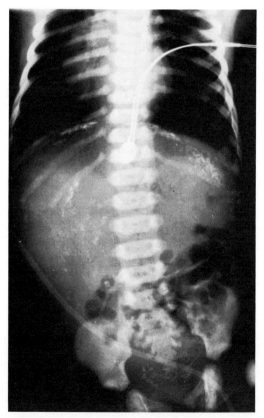

Figure 10–1. Meconium peritonitis. There is streaky and flocculent calcification scattered throughout the peritoneal cavity in this newborn child. (Courtesy of Dr. Jack O. Haller, Downstate Medical Center, Brooklyn, New York.)

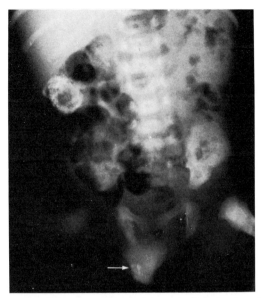

Figure 10–2. In a patient with cystic fibrosis, there is meconium peritonitis with a large conglomeration of calcium in the right midabdomen. There is also a small collection of calcification in the scrotum (arrow).

barium peritonitis is similar to that of meconium peritonitis, with streaks, patches, and clumps of barium scattered throughout the peritoneum (Fig. 10–3).

A much rarer cause of generalized peritoneal calcification in the newborn is plastic peritonitis from

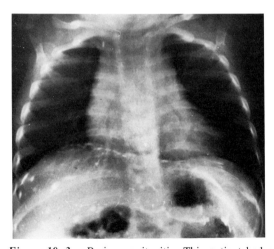

Figure 10–3. Barium peritonitis. This patient had a barium enema in the neonatal period and had a clinically silent colonic perforation. Prior to the study the abdomen was clear. Several months later, a film of the chest and upper abdomen shows plaques and streaks of barium within the peritoneal cavity. (Courtesy of Dr. William J. McSweeny, Children's Hospital National Medical Center, Washington, D.C.)

neonatal hydrometrocolpos. Most often there is an atretic vagina and the only egress of genital tract secretions is into the Fallopian tubes. From here they gain entry into the peritoneum and stimulate an inflammatory reaction, resulting in calcification identical to that seen in meconium peritonitis.[6]

Gastrointestinal Tract Calcifications

Calcification within the gastrointestinal tract in the newborn spans a broad spectrum of entities, all of which are very rare. Both intraluminal and intramural calcifications occur (Table 10–1).

Intraluminal calcification in the first few weeks of life is found most frequently in babies with distal intestinal obstruction. Nearly always males are affected, and in the majority of cases there is an imperforate anus[7] and a rectourinary fistula.[8] Typically, there is no perforation and no peritoneal inflammation. Calcification appears as ill-defined densities or as clusters of discrete concretions. Precipitation of calcium occurs in sites of prolonged stasis and may be promoted by the mixing of urine and meconium in utero. However, intraluminal densities have been reported in newborns with imperforate anus but without fistula.[9] Calcification usually occurs just proximal to a stenotic or atretic ileum but may be present in scattered locations in the bowel in patients with hereditary multiple gastrointestinal atresias.[10,11] Another infrequent cause for small bowel intraluminal calcification is total colonic aganglionosis[12] (Fig. 10–4).

Ten percent of patients with cystic fibrosis have meconium ileus and half of these have intestinal volvulus.[13] If the bowel twists early in pregnancy, atresia results and the devitalized loops are reabsorbed. However, if volvulus takes place in the middle or last trimester, a pseudocyst composed of dilated bowel may form and calcium may be laid down in its walls. Hence, intramural calcification appears as a cystic density with thin smooth streaks of calcification delineating the bowel[14] (Fig. 10–5). If the intestine is not markedly dilated, in-

Table 10–1. Conditions Associated with Intestinal Calcification in the Newborn

I. Intraluminal Calcifications
   A. Imperforate anus and rectourinary fistula
   B. Imperforate anus and no fistula
   C. Total colonic aganglionosis
   D. Ileal stenosis
   E. Hereditary multiple atresias

II. Intramural Calcification
   A. Meconium ileus with intestinal volvulus
   B. Calcification in duplication cyst
   C. Idiopathic—no tumor or volvulus

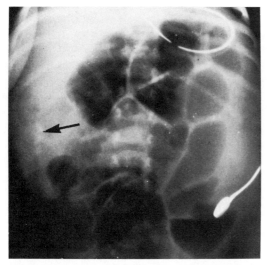

Figure 10–4. Amorphous globular calcifications are seen in the right abdomen (arrow). These were found to be intraluminal calcifications in a child with total colonic aganglionosis. (Courtesy of Dr. Jack O. Haller, Downstate Medical Center, Brooklyn, New York.)

tramural calcification may be seen as parallel tracks when the bowel wall is in profile or as multiple rings of density if the small intestine is en face.[15] Seldom, intramural calcification occurs without obstruction[16,17] (Fig. 10–6).

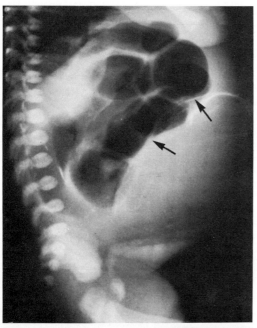

Figure 10–5. A lateral film of the abdomen in a newborn with meconium ileus and intestinal volvulus. Curvilinear calcification is seen within the bowel wall (arrows). (Courtesy of Dr. David H. Baker, Babies Hospital–Columbia Presbyterian Medical Center, New York, N.Y.)

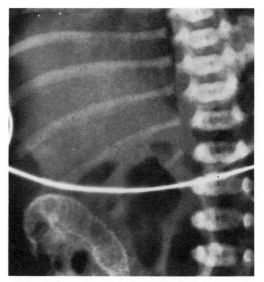

Figure 10–6. A supine radiograph of a newborn on the first day of life shows calcification within the wall of a loop of small bowel in the right abdomen. This was an incidental finding on radiographs taken for mild respiratory distress. There was no evidence of intestinal obstruction or peritonitis. (Courtesy of Dr. Paula W. Brill and Dr. Patricia Winchester, New York Hospital–Cornell Medical Center, New York, N.Y. Reprinted with permission from the American Journal of Roentgenology, 136:826–827, 1981.)

In the stomach, transient mural calcifications may be a result of the oral administration of calcium chloride. High concentration of this salt is toxic to the gastric epithelium and often leads to both mucosal calcification and necrosis.[18] Radiologically detectable calcification in gastrointestinal tumors in newborns is exceedingly rare. An amorphous solid density in the left upper quadrant is characteristic for a gastric teratoma. These tumors are either intramural or exogastric and can become very large. Unlike teratomas elsewhere, recognizable teeth or bones are not seen.[19] Curvilinear or stippled calcification can also occur in ileal duplications in the newborn.[20]

Liver Calcification

In infants and children, primary malignant tumors of the liver have two peaks of incidence. Under three years of age, hepatoblastomas are most frequent, and between the ages of 12 and 15 years hepatocellular carcinomas are most common. Approximately 3 percent of children dying from a primary hepatic malignancy develop the tumor in the first month of life.[21] Calcifications in hepatoblastomas are of the solid mass type and can vary from faint to very dense. A lateral film may be helpful

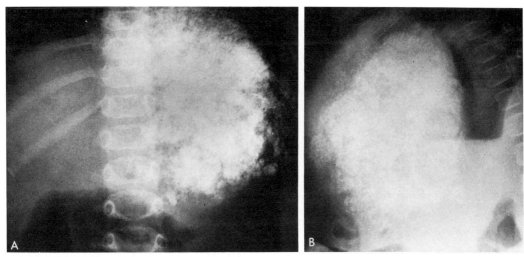

Figure 10–7, A and B. Hepatoblastoma. Supine (*A*) and upright lateral (*B*) radiographs of the abdomen show dense conglomerate calcification in the left lobe of the liver. (Courtesy of Dr. John A. Kirkpatrick, Children's Hospital Medical Center, Boston, Massachusetts.)

in distinguishing hepatic calcifications from opacities in more posterior organs and may reveal subtle intrahepatic densities obscured on frontal projections (Fig. 10–7). Other tumors that calcify in the liver of the newborn and may look exactly like hepatoblastomas are giant hemangiomas, hamartomas, and metastatic neuroblastomas.[22–24]

A diverse list of nontumorous conditions may cause calcification in the liver in neonates. Transplacentally acquired viral infections caused by either herpes simplex or toxoplasmosis can produce nodular calcifications throughout the hepatic parenchyma.[25] Calcium deposited in clots in patients with portal vein thromboemboli appears as a branching or zigzag pattern of increased density within the liver. When multiple portal vein branches in subcapsular locations contain calcified emboli, the radiographic appearance may resemble meconium peritonitis.[26] If the patient survives, these densities will resolve over several months.[27] Calcium salts can also precipitate in clots affixed to indwelling umbilical vein catheters. In both neonates and older children, inferior vena cava thrombosis calcification will often occur without a precipitating illness and can be recognized by its characteristic bullet-shaped appearance.[28]

Adrenal Calcification

In a large autopsy series of young children there was a 1 percent incidence of bleeding into the adrenal glands, in about 20 percent of whom calcification was found within the site of hemorrhage.[29] The majority of newborns with adrenal hemorrhage are asymptomatic, and calcification is usually noted later on as an incidental finding. Forceps delivery, prematurity, breech presentation, and a birth weight greater than nine pounds are predisposing factors.[30] Calcification has been observed as early as eight to 12 days after birth and appears as mottled, punctate, or well-defined triangular densities above the kidney.[31,32] Extensive calcification is usually confined to a gland of normal size, but rarely there may be calcification of cystic type in the margin of a large adrenal hematoma[33] (Fig. 10–8).

Another cause of a calcified suprarenal mass in the neonate is a neuroblastoma arising from the adrenal gland. Although it is the most common pediatric paravertebral mass, neuroblastoma is rare in newborns. Usually, it is seen as a poorly demarcated tumor containing stippled or punctate calcifications.[24]

Wolman's disease is a rare lethal disorder with an autosomal recessive mode of inheritance. Accumulations of cholesterol esters lead to enlargement of the liver, spleen, and adrenals.[34,35] In the acute infantile form, which inexorably leads to death within six months, there is progressive failure to thrive, nausea, vomiting, anemia, and abdominal distension. A hallmark of the disease is bilateral and symmetrical punctate calcification in enlarged adrenal glands[36] (Fig. 10–9). Wolman's disease should not be confused with calcified neuroblastomas, which are rarely bilateral and never symmetrical. Several older lists of adrenal calcification have included Niemann-Pick's disease. Reevaluation of case reports suggests that what had been called Niemann-Pick's disease is, in fact,

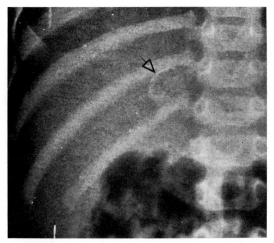

Figure 10–8. Calcification in adrenal hemorrhage. At 16 days of age, a large adrenal mass was seen on intravenous urography to be depressing and flattening the upper pole of the right kidney. On this film taken at eight months, there is a rim of residual calcification in the hematoma (arrow), which had become smaller. (Courtesy of Dr. Paula W. Brill and Dr. Patricia Winchester, New York Hospital–Cornell Medical Center, New York, N.Y. Reprinted with permission from the American Journal of Roentgenology, 127:289–291, 1976.)

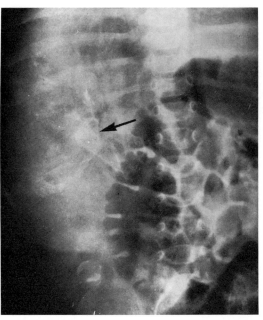

Figure 10–10. Large retroperitoneal teratoma in a young child. The mass is deviating the colon medially and contains bone (arrow).

Wolman's disease.[37] Roentgenographically demonstrable calcifications in Niemann-Pick's disease probably do not occur.

Retroperitoneum

A teratoma is a tumor composed of multiple tissues of kinds that are normally not found in the organ or site in which it arises. The most common components of teratomas are immature skin, bone, nervous tissue, and respiratory and alimentary mucosa. In newborns teratomas are most frequent in the retroperitoneum and sacrococcygeal region. Retroperitoneal teratomas can become very large and often contain roentgenographically detectable bones or teeth (Fig. 10–10). Approximately 10 percent are malignant.[38] An uncommon form of retroperitoneal tumor is a fetus in fetu. Otherwise known as the "included twin," fetus in

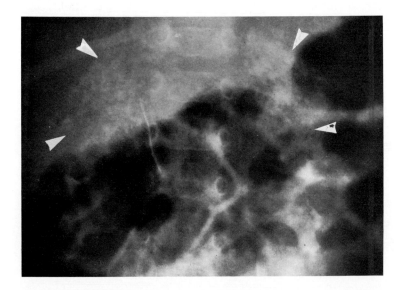

Figure 10–9. Wolman's disease. A film from an intravenous urography shows the typical appearance of faint bilateral amorphous calcification in enlarged adrenal glands (arrowheads). (Courtesy of Dr. John A. Kirkpatrick, Children's Hospital Medical Center, Boston, Massachusetts.)

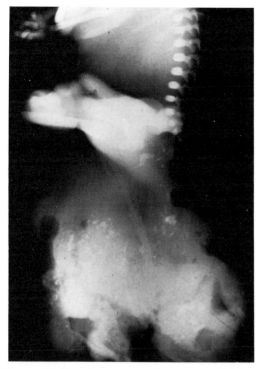

Figure 10–11. Sacrococcygeal teratoma. Flecks of calcifications are scattered throughout a large sacrococcygeal teratoma extending from the sacrum of a stillborn infant. (Courtesy of Dr. Shelley Weiner, Albert Einstein College of Medicine Hospital, Bronx, New York.)

fetu refers to the presence of a genetically identical tumor containing well-defined organs within a fully developed child. To make the diagnosis of fetus in fetu radiographically, the vertebral column of the included twin must be present. Lacking that finding, a definitive diagnosis will be made only at surgery.[39,40]

Four-fifths of sacrococcygeal teratomas occur in females.[41] The overall rate of malignancy is 33 percent, but this depends a great deal on the age of the child when the tumor is detected.[42] At birth only 10 percent are malignant, but a teratoma newly discovered at two months has a malignancy rate of 80 percent.[42] These tumors may arise either anterior or posterior to the sacrum and often protrude from the lower abdomen (Fig. 10–11). Plain films of the sacrococcygeal area will show calcification or ossification in 50 percent of cases.[43]

Calcifications in the Urinary Tract in Neonates

While a great many diseases involve the genitourinary tract in newborns, calcification is rarely observed at this age in the kidneys, ureters, or bladder. There are scattered case reports of calcification in renal cortical necrosis in young children. Characteristically, there is bilateral and symmetrical deposition of calcium in the renal cortex. Calcification may be extensive or involve limited areas of the kidney.[44] Usually calcifications do not appear until several weeks after the onset of renal failure.

Renal vein thrombosis in neonates affects males and females equally. Generally, there are no abnormalities seen on plain films, but occasionally calcification in clots in the renal veins may occur. In the first few weeks of life calcification in the ureters and bladder are exceedingly uncommon.[45,46] In two patients with the prune belly syndrome, consisting of the triad of absent abdominal musculature, undescended testicles, and an abnormal urinary system, calcifications were seen in the pelvis, one in a urachal cyst and the other in the dome of the bladder.[47]

Abdominal Wall Calcification

Calcification in muscles and other soft tissues of the abdominal wall is rare and has diverse etiologies. Hypercalcemia, anoxia, and hypothermia may cause subcutaneous fat necrosis with calcification.[48–50] Hematomas forming after birth trauma or surgical procedures may calcify (Fig. 10–12).

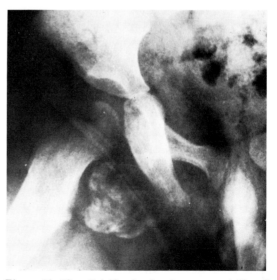

Figure 10–12. Calcification in a hematoma. A film of the right hip of an infant demonstrates calcification in a hematoma that was the result of a femoral vein puncture. (Courtesy of Dr. Irwin Bluth, Brookdale Hospital Medical Center, Brooklyn, New York.)

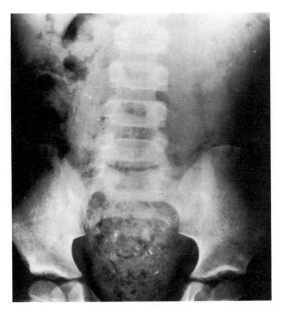

Figure 10–13. Lead chips in the abdomen. Scattered flecks of metallic radiodensity are present in the rectum of a four-year-old patient with lead ingestion. (Courtesy of Dr. Irwin Bluth, Brookdale Hospital Medical Center, Brooklyn, New York.)

Extravascular accumulations of injected calcium gluconate appear on plain films as focal deposits of radiodensity which tend to resolve slowly. However, calcium gluconate in subcutaneous tissue is highly irritative and may lead to extensive necrosis and sloughing of the skin.[51,52]

CALCIFICATIONS IN OLDER CHILDREN

Gastrointestinal Tract

Most radiodensities in the gastrointestinal tract observed on plain films in children are within the lumen of the bowel or stomach. The gamut of substances and objects that pass through the intestines is vast, ranging from radiopaque dirt (Fig. 4–8) to large easily recognizable foreign bodies.[53] In children who ingest particles of lead-containing paint, abdominal radiographs show multiple punctate metallic densities in the intestinal tract, especially in the colon (Fig. 10–13). A similar appearance results from radiopaque amalgam inadvertently swallowed during dental procedures (Fig. 10–14). When a tooth is swallowed, it will almost always pass through the gastrointestinal tract without incident. However, if a plain film is obtained when the tooth is in the ileum or distal large bowel it may be misinterpreted as a tooth in an ovarian cystic teratoma (Fig. 10–15). The presence of ingested materials remaining in the bowel for several days suggests that their progress may be impeded by a paralytic ileus or stenosis or obstruction of the bowel. Occasionally small objects lodge in a diverticulum (Fig. 10–16).

Foreign substances of any density may become trapped in the appendix and form the nidus of an appendicolith.[54] The recognition of an appendiceal stone in children is of clinical importance because

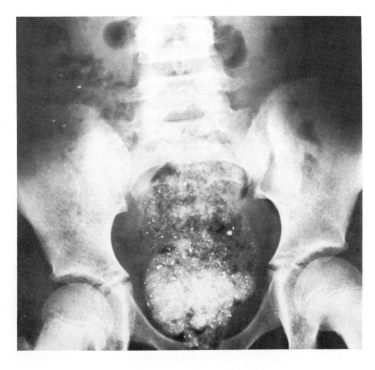

Figure 10–14. Dental amalgam in the colon. There are scattered intraluminal metallic densities in the rectum and sigmoid. They resulted from the swallowing of dental amalgam.

Figure 10–15. An angulated density is seen in the pelvis (arrow) in a film from an intravenous urography. This is a swallowed tooth in the colon, not a tooth in an ovarian teratoma.

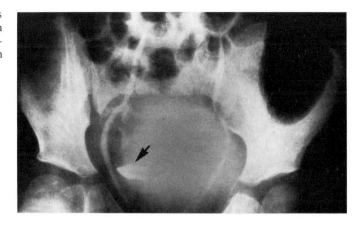

it is almost always associated with appendicitis and its presence increases the probability of an appendiceal rupture.[35] Mostly these calculi consist of laminations of calcium phosphate laid down on a central core of fecal material or foreign matter. Usually they are located in the right lower quadrant or the right side of the pelvis (Fig. 10–17). An ectopic location suggests a very long appendix with a stone at its tip, a mobile cecum, malrotation of the bowel, or perforation of the appendix with the

calculus lying free in the peritoneal cavity. Appendiceal stones may be simulated by gallbladder calculi or by rarer entities, such as a calculus in a Meckel's diverticulum or in a urachal cyst.

Calcification within the wall of hollow organs in the gastrointestinal tract is very rarely noted in children. Curvilinear calcifications have been observed in gastric duplications.[56] Both solid and annular calcifications may occur in ileal duplications.[57]

Calcifications of the Gallbladder

In both children and adults single large rounded stones or multiple faceted calculi may calcify.

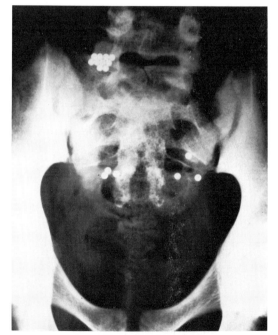

Figure 10–16. Circular metallic radiodensities consistent with swallowed BB's are noted in this teen-aged boy. The especially neat array of these densities to the right of the midline at L5–S1 suggests that they are contained in a Meckel's diverticulum. (Courtesy of Dr. William J. McSweeny, Children's Hospital National Medical Center, Washington, D.C.)

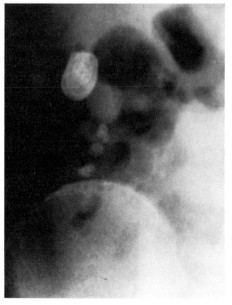

Figure 10–17. Appendicoliths. A three-year-old boy has four appendicoliths, including a large laminated one; they were removed at surgery.

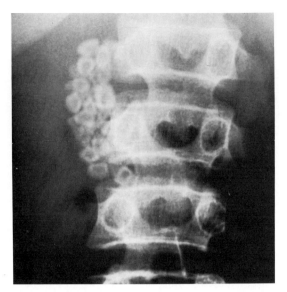

Figure 10–18. Multiple faceted calculi in the gallbladder of a 16-year-old patient with sickle cell anemia.

While only 15 percent of gallbladder calculi in adults are radiopaque, approximately 30 percent of stones are calcified in children. Hence, the plain film plays an important role in detecting gallstones in the young.[58]

There is a high incidence of stones in patients with hemolytic disease, as accelerated red blood cell destruction causes increased bilirubin concentrations in serum and bile. Incorporation of calcium within and at the margin of stones renders them opaque. Calculi are found in approximately 40 percent of patients with sickle cell anemia (Fig. 10–18) and have been noted in up to 66 percent of children with hereditary spherocytosis. The incidence of calculi also increases in patients undergoing repeated transfusions.[59]

Although there is a greater likelihood of calculi in patients with hemolytic anemias, the majority of radiodense stones in children are in patients with no hematologic abnormalities. In a study of childhood cholelithiasis from Sweden, of 56 cases only three had blood dyscrasias and three others had anomalies of the cystic duct. Most of those with gallstone were overweight and 60 percent were female. Patients ranged in age from three months to 14 years at the time of detection of the calculi.[58]

Stone formation may be promoted by biliary stagnation. Sometimes mechanical factors such as choledochal cyst or ductal stenosis retard the flow of bile. Usually physiological derangements, including dehydration, pneumonia, gastroenteritis, and thickened secretions in cystic fibrosis, are the precipitating factors for stone formation.[60] While the signs and symptoms of cholelithiasis in children are similar to those in the adult, there is often a delay in diagnosis owing to failure to suspect the disease.

Liver Calcification

Primary liver tumors are one-tenth as frequent as neuroblastomas or Wilms' tumors in children.[61] Most malignancies derive from hepatocytes, and the two most common tumors that calcify are hepatoblastoma and hepatocellular carcinoma. As mentioned previously, hepatoblastomas occur predominantly in children under three years of age, and approximately 10 percent calcify[62] (Fig. 10–7). Hepatocellular carcinomas are found more often in older children and calcify uncommonly. Characteristically, they will contain faint, scattered irregular densities which may be seen only in oblique and lateral films[63–65] (Fig. 10–19). Other rare tumors that may calcify are hemangioendotheliomas and primary hepatic teratomas.[66]

Metastases from neuroblastoma and Wilms' tumor may calcify in the liver; in such cases calcium is also often present in the primary lesion.[67]. The typical pattern in the liver is mottled densities indistinguishable from those seen in hepatocellular carcinoma or hepatoblastoma.

Chronic granulomatous disease in childhood is a condition in which leukocytes have diminished bactericidal activity. Males are primarily affected, and they may suffer from protracted multiple infections most commonly caused by staphylococci.

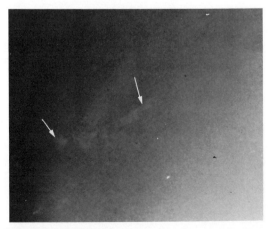

Figure 10–19. A film of the right upper quadrant shows punctate, barely visible calcifications in the liver in a child with a hepatoma. The arrows point to foci of denser calcification within the tumor. (Courtesy of Dr. John A. Kirkpatrick, Children's Hospital Medical Center, Boston, Massachusetts.)

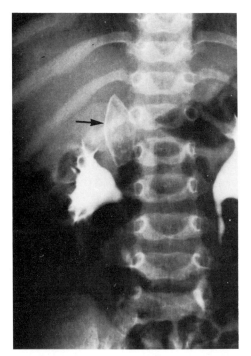

Figure 10–20. Typical bullet-shaped calcification (arrow) of a thrombus in the inferior vena cava in a three-year-old child. (Courtesy of Dr. Jack O. Haller, Downstate Medical Center, Brooklyn, New York.)

sickle cell anemia may develop opacities in the spleen, which are due to deposition of calcium salts and incrustations of iron in the splenic parenchyma.[71,72] Calcification begins early in the second decade, and as the patient grows older the spleen decreases in size and becomes more dense (Fig. 3–32).

Pancreas

The most common cause of pancreatic calcification in children is nutritional pancreatitis, which occurs predominantly in less developed countries in Asia, Africa, and Latin America. Patients frequently present with diabetes or steatorrhea, and in severe cases there is parotid enlargement, changes in hair color, and alopecia. On plain films, calcified stones are often seen scattered throughout the substance of the pancreas[73] (Fig. 10–21). In the United States, pancreatic calcification in childhood is very rare. Occasionally, in cystic fibrosis, plain films reveal granular opacities fainter and smaller than the multiple stones observed in chronic calcifying pancreatitis in adults[74] (Fig. 10–22). Hereditary chronic pancreatitis has been reported in several Caucasian kinships in Appalachia. Typically,

Intrahepatic abscesses can occasionally calcify and present as numerous irregularly marginated discrete nodules within the liver substance.[68] As in the adult, calcification occurs in tuberculosis or histoplasmosis as multiple punctate densities scattered throughout the liver. Single or several calcified intrahepatic cysts suggest *Echinococcus granulosus* infestation.

In the younger child, a calcified thrombus within the intrahepatic portion of the inferior vena cava has the pathognomonic configuration of a bullet-shaped density in the right upper quadrant just anterior and to the right of the thoracolumbar spine (Fig. 10–20). There may be partial or complete obstruction of the vein, but even then patients usually do not have symptoms of venous obstruction or an abundance of retroperitoneal collaterals. Rarely, however, inferior vena cava calcification may be associated with splenomegaly, peripheral edema, and a rapid downhill course.[69,70]

Spleen

Multiple punctate calcifications in the spleen in children, as in adults, suggests tuberculosis or histoplasmosis. As much as 10 percent of patients with

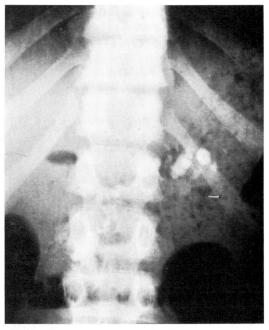

Figure 10–21. Multiple calcifications of varying sizes are noted throughout the pancreas in a 15-year-old Haitian female with a history of poor nutrition. (Courtesy of Dr. William J. McSweeny, Children's Hospital National Medical Center, Washington, D.C.)

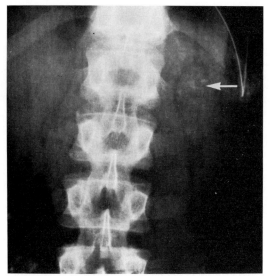

Figure 10–22. Finely granular flecks of calcification are present in the tail of the pancreas (arrow) in a patient with cystic fibrosis. (Courtesy of Dr. William J. Mc-Sweeny, Children's Hospital National Medical Center, Washington, D.C.)

affected individuals have coarse calcific concretions. Opaque stones usually do not appear before the third decade, but they are seen occasionally in teenagers. Patients with hereditary chronic pancreatitis are at a greater risk for the later development of pancreatic carcinoma.[75]

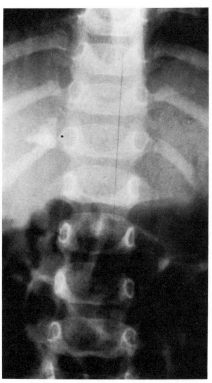

Figure 10–23. The triangular density in the right adrenal gland of this two-and-a-half-year-old child is typical of residual calcification from an unrecognized adrenal hemorrhage occurring in the newborn. (Courtesy of Dr. Jack O. Haller, Downstate Medical Center, Brooklyn, New York.)

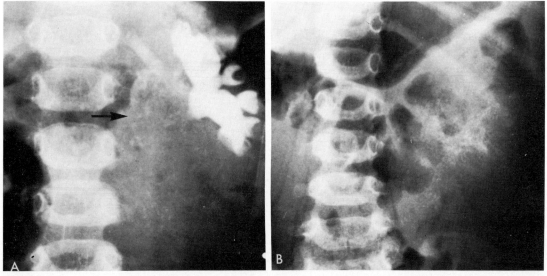

Figure 10–24, A and B. Two examples of neuroblastoma. *A,* In a 16-month-old boy there is a large retroperitoneal mass containing linear and stippled calcifications (arrow), which deviate the kidney laterally. *B,* In an 18-month-old boy, stippled calcifications are seen overlying the left kidney. Subsequent urography showed the kidney to be displaced superiorly.

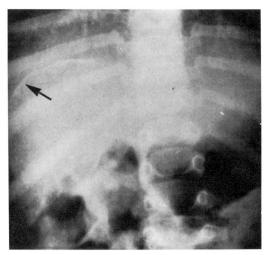

Figure 10–25. Curvilinear calcification (arrow) in a large neuroblastoma arising from the right adrenal gland in an 11-month-old child. (Courtesy of Dr. William J. McSweeny, Children's Hospital National Medical Center, Washington, D.C.)

Adrenal Gland and Retroperitoneum

Adrenal calcification resulting from neonatal hemorrhage may persist into adulthood and will come to attention as an incidental finding on plain films in children. Tuberculosis produces adrenal calcifications that are radiographically indistinguishable from calcified neonatal hemorrhage. Usually the adrenal gland is not enlarged, and it contains mottled or homogeneously dense radiopacities[76] (Fig. 10–23).

The most common tumors in the adrenal in the first decade of life are malignant neuroblastomas and benign ganglioneuromas. Approximately half of neuroblastomas contain calcification that may be detected on plain films. These tumors can arise not only in the adrenal but also in ganglia in the retroperitoneum and in the mediastinum. While adrenal neuroblastomas may depress the kidney, retroperitoneal neuroblastomas can be medial or inferior to the kidney and can move it laterally or superiorly (Fig. 10–24). Most neuroblastomas are solid masses and appear with stippled or mottled calcifications, but occasionally an annular rim of calcium will be seen (Fig. 10–25). Benign ganglioneuromas have an identical plain film appearance, and only histologic examination can differentiate between the two[36] (Fig. 10–26).

Both adenomas and carcinomas of the adrenal cortex occur in children. Either tumor must be considered when a young patient develops signs of virilization or hypercorticism. Adenoma cannot be differentiated from carcinoma by plain film criteria since both may be cystic or solid and either can attain a large size. Sometimes biopsy may not be conclusive, the final diagnosis resting on the biologic behavior of the tumor[77,78] (Fig. 10–27).

Pheochromocytoma is a rare tumor of the adrenal medulla and sympathetic chain. On plain films amorphous densities or streaks of calcification can indicate the lesion, but less frequently calcification of the cystic type occurs[79,80] (Fig. 10–28). Adrenal teratomas, while often very large, are usually benign and almost always contain all three germ layers. Characteristically, there is a large soft tissue mass containing well-defined bone and clearly discernible teeth (Fig. 10–29). However, it is sometimes not possible to determine if a large teratoma in the upper abdomen arises from the adrenal or from other retroperitoneal tissues.

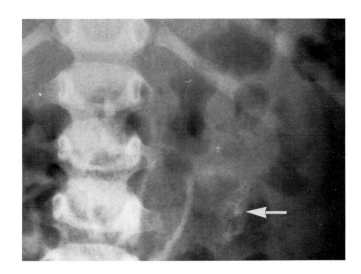

Figure 10–26. Calcification in a ganglioneuroma. A three-year-old boy with a retroperitoneal mass containing stippled calcification (arrow). Histologic evaluation disclosed a benign ganglioneuroma.

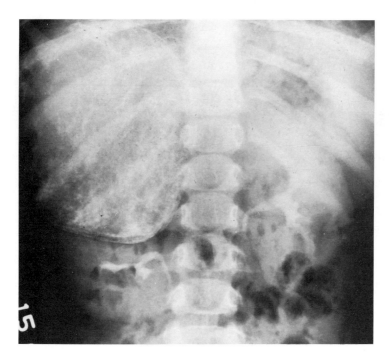

Figure 10–27. Large adrenal adenoma. Dense calcification is seen at the margins and within the substance of a large adrenal mass which is depressing the right kidney. At operation, an adrenal adenoma was found. (Courtesy of Dr. David H. Baker, Babies Hospital–Columbia Presbyterian Medical Center, New York, New York.)

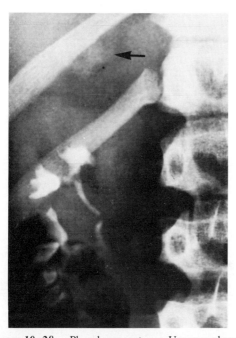

Figure 10–28. Pheochromocytoma. Urogram shows a faint amorphous calcification in a mass in the right adrenal gland (arrow). The superior pole of the kidney is flattened by the mass. At operation, a pheochromocytoma was found. (Courtesy of Dr. William J. McSweeny, Children's Hospital National Medical Center, Washington, D.C.)

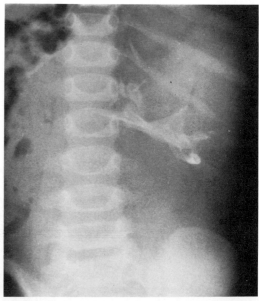

Figure 10–29. This one-year-old child has a large, benign left-sided retroperitoneal teratoma containing clearly defined bones and a tooth. (Courtesy of Dr. Irwin Bluth, Brookdale Medical Center Hospital, Brooklyn, New York.)

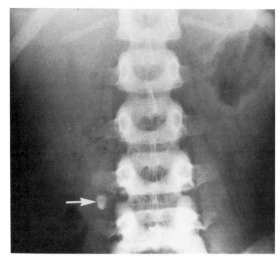

Figure 10–30. A six-year-old boy with intermittent hematuria for one year has a calcific right ureteral stone. The patient has primary oxaluria.

Kidney

Urinary calculi may occur in children of any age. Infection and obstruction of the genitourinary tract are prime predisposing causes. Metabolic abnormalities which promote calculus formation include hyperparathyroidism, renal tubular acidosis, cystinuria, Wilson's disease, idiopathic hypercalciuria and hypercalcemia, and primary oxaluria (Fig. 10–30). In patients with medullary sponge kidney, concretions originating in ectatic collecting tubules may ulcerate into the calyceal system. Stones are also more frequent in children with milk-alkali syndrome owing to excessive ingestion of calcium.[81,82] Increased absorption of oxalate occurs in Crohn's disease and after bowel resection and may be responsible for the higher frequency of oxalate stones in these conditions.[83] With prolonged immobilization, calcium leaves the bones and enters the urine in greater concentration, thereby enhancing the risk for calculi formation. Calcific stones may range from small concretions which are often multiple to a single staghorn calculus filling the pelvicalyceal system.

The metabolic alterations associated with the development of concretions in the collecting system may also lead to nephrocalcinosis. Diffuse small calculi in the renal parenchyma are found in either the medulla or the cortex. Often calcifications are localized to the renal pyramids, and a conglomeration of innumerable, closely spaced minute concretions will appear on plain films as an irregular marginated density with a mottled internal architecture (Fig. 10–31).

Spasm of intrarenal arteries can cause ischemia in the renal cortex, resulting in a narrow band of necrosis within which calcium salts may precipitate. Severe infections, transfusion incompatibility, and exposure to nephrotoxins have been associated with cortical necrosis.[84] Rarely, linear calcifications in the periphery of the kidney may occur in chronic glomerulonephritis.[85,86]

Wilms' tumor is the most common renal malignancy in childhood. Unlike adrenal neuroblastoma, calcification in Wilms' tumor is uncommon, occurring in 9 percent of cases. Calcifications are predominantly of the solid mass type, with granular, flocculent, and punctate densities scattered throughout the tumor (Fig. 10–32). Often the calcification is faint and may not be seen on frontal projections if there is gas and feces in the bowel overlying the kidney. Oblique projections may then be helpful in revealing the calcified mass. Much less often, the calcification in Wilms' tumor has a

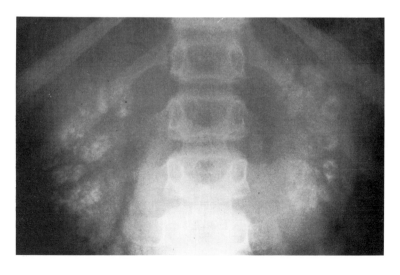

Figure 10–31. Bilateral nephrocalcinosis in a 12-year-old child with Wilson's disease.

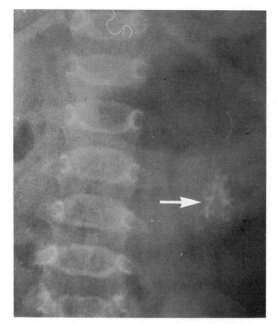

Figure 10–32. Wilms' tumor. A four-month-old infant with flocculent calcification in the lower pole of the left kidney (arrow).

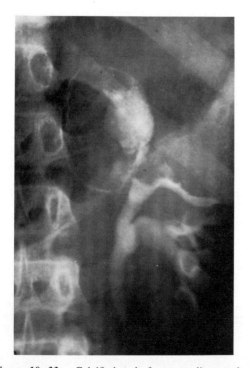

Figure 10–33. Calcified node from an adjacent clear cell adenocarcinoma of the kidney in an adolescent. Calcifications of the cystic type is present above the left kidney. Within it there is a focal area of solid mass calcification. The primary tumor is uncalcified. (Courtesy of Dr. William J. McSweeny, Children's Hospital Medical Center, Washington, D.C.)

cystic configuration. In patients under one year of age calcification identical to that in Wilms' tumor may occur in mesoblastic nephroma, which is a benign tumor.[87]

Renal adenocarcinoma affects older children, with solid mass calcification occurring in 10 percent of cases[88] (Fig. 10–33). Less commonly metastases in lymph nodes may also calcify. An even rarer tumor in childhood is an intrarenal teratoma, which may contain faint punctate densities and, unlike retroperitoneal teratomas, lacks radiographic evidence of teeth or bone.[89]

Bladder

Most calcifications in the lower genitourinary tract are stones. The majority have passed from the kidney, but some may arise in the bladder as a result of infection or obstruction. Bladder calculi can become large and may be single or multiple. Sometimes the stones are only faintly calcified, but almost always they have smooth margins and may have multiple laminations (Fig. 10–34). Calcification in the bladder wall is extremely rare in children and has been noted in chronic infection and after radiation therapy.

Ovarian Calcification

Approximately half of all ovarian tumors in childhood are teratomas.[90] Sometimes calcification may occur as an amorphous density within the mass, but more often teeth or bone are readily vis-

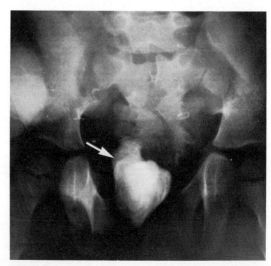

Figure 10–34. A large, roughly triangular laminated bladder stone (arrow). The patient has exstrophy of the bladder and a long history of chronic infection.

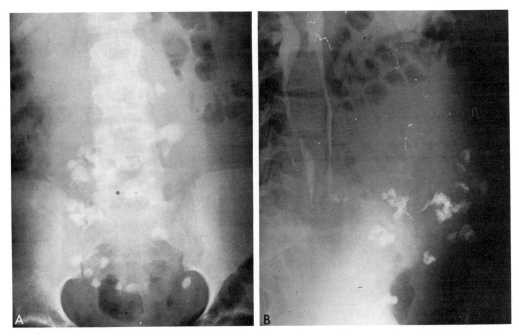

Figure 10–35. Frontal (*A*) and lateral (*B*) projections show a large malignant ovarian teratoma extending superiorly from the pelvis and containing many teeth. At operation, it was a predominantly solid tumor.

ible.[91,92] Almost all (97 percent) are benign, but the risk of malignancy increases if the tumor is solid or if it appears before age five (Fig. 10–35). Usually teratomas present as a silent abdominal mass, but some tumors may cause an acute abdomen as they undergo rupture or torsion.[93] Diffuse punctate calcifications have also been reported in dysgerminomas and gonadoblastomas.[94,95]

REFERENCES

1. Neuhauser EBD: Roentgen diagnosis of fetal meconium peritonitis. Am J Roentgenol 51:421–425, 1944.
2. Tucker AS, Izant RJ Jr.: Problems with meconium. Am J Roentgenol 112:135–142, 1971.
3. Leonidas JC, Berdon WE, Baker DH, et al: Meconium ileus and its complications—A reappraisal of plain film roentgen diagnostic criteria. Am J Roentgenol 108:598–609, 1970.
4. Berdon WE, Baker DH, Becker J, et al: Scrotal masses in healed meconium peritonitis. N Engl J Med 277:585–587, 1967.
5. Caffey J: Pediatric X-Ray Diagnosis, 5th edition. Chicago, Year Book Medical Publishers, 1978, pp 628–629.
6. Ceballos R, Hicks GM: Plastic peritonitis due to neonatal hydrometrocolpos: Radiologic and pathologic observations. J Pediatr Surg 5:63–70, 1970.
7. Selke AC Jr, Cowley CE: Calcified intraluminal meconium in a female infant with imperforate anus. Am J Roentgenol 130:786–788, 1978.
8. Khilnani M, Wolf BS, Arnheim E: Enterolithiasis in the newborn. J Mount Sinai Hospital 22:58–61, 1955.
9. Berdon WE, Baker DH, Wigger HJ, et al: Calcified intraluminal meconium in newborn males with imperforate anus. Am J Roentgenol 125:449–455, 1975.
10. Camp R, Roberts MH: Multiple calcareous deposits in the intestinal tract of the newborn: Report of a case with stenosis of the ileum. Am J Dis Child 78:393–400, 1949.
11. Martin CE, Leonidas JC, Amoury RA: Multiple gastrointestinal atresias with intraluminal calcifications and cystic dilatation of bile ducts. A newly recognized entity resembling "a string of pearls." Pediatrics 57:268–271, 1976.
12. Fletcher BD, Yulish BS: Intraluminal calcification in the small bowel of newborn infants with total colonic aganglionosis. Radiology 126:451–455, 1978.
13. Grossman H, Berdon WE, Baker DH: Gastrointestinal findings in cystic fibrosis. Am J Roentgenol 97:227–238, 1966.
14. Van Buskirk RW, Kurlander GJ, Samter TG: Intraluminal jejunal calcifications in a newborn. Am J Dis Child 110:329–332, 1965.
15. Aharon M, Kleinhous V, Lichtig C: Neonatal intramural jejunal calcifications associated with bowel atresia. Am J Roentgenol 130:999–1000, 1978.
16. Winchester P, Heneghan M, Brill PW, et al: Neonatal intramural bowel calcification without atresia. Am J Roentgenol 136:826–827, 1981.
17. Joshi VV, Winston YE, Kay S: Neonatal enterocolitis. Histologic evidence of healing. Am J Dis Child 126:113–116, 1973.
18. Gryboski J: Gastrointestinal Problems in the Infant. Philadelphia, WB Saunders, 1975, p 154.
19. Atwell JD, Claireoux AE, Nixon HH: Teratoma of the stomach in a newborn. J Pediatr Surg 2:197–204, 1967.
20. Bastable JRG: Intestinal duplication with calcification. Brit J Radiol 37:706–708, 1964.
21. Exelby PR, El-Domeri A, Huvos AG, et al: Primary ma-

lignant tumors of the liver in children. J Pediatr Surg 6:272–276, 1971.

22. Moss AA, Clark RE, Palubinskas AJ, et al: Angiographic appearance of benign and malignant hepatic tumors in infants and children. Am J Roentgenol 113:61–69, 1971.

23. Berdon WE, Baker DH: Giant hepatic hemangioma with cardiac failure in a newborn infant. Value of high-dosage intravenous urography and umbilical angiography. Radiology 92:1523–1528, 1969.

24. Schneider KM, Becker JM, Krasna IH: Neonatal neuroblastoma. Pediatrics 36:359–366, 1965.

25. Shackleford GD, Kirks DR: Neonatal hepatic calcification secondary to transplacental infection. Radiology 122:753–757, 1977.

26. Blanc WA, Berdon WE, Baker DH, et al: Calcified thromboemboli in newborn and stillborn infants. Radiology 88:287–292, 1967.

27. Ablow RC, Effman FL: Hepatic calcification associated with umbilical vein catheterization in a newborn infant. Am J Roentgenol 114:380–385, 1972.

28. Kassner EG, Baumstock MN, Kinkhawala MN, et al: Calcified thrombus in the inferior vena cava in infants and children. Pediat Radio 14:167–171, 1976.

29. Snelling CE, Erb IH: Hemorrhage and subsequent calcification of the suprarenal gland. J Pediatr 6:22–41, 1935.

30. Jarvis JL, Seaman WB: Idiopathic adrenal calcification in infants and children. Am J Roentgenol 82:510–520, 1959.

31. Gabrielle OF, Sheehan WE: Bilateral neonatal adrenal hemorrhage. Am J Roentgenol 91:656–658, 1964.

32. Wagner AC: Bilateral hemorrhagic pseudocyst of the adrenal glands in a newborn. Am J Roentgenol 86:540–544, 1961.

33. Brill PW, Krasna IH, Aaron H: An early rim sign in neonatal adrenal hemorrhage. Am J Roentgenol 127:298–291, 1976.

34. Wolman M, Sterk VV, Gatt S, et al: Primary familial xanthomatosis with involvement and calcification of the adrenal. Report of two more cases in a sibling of a previously described infant. Pediatrics 28:742–757, 1961.

35. Abramov A, Schorr S, Wolman M: Generalized xanthomatosis with calcified adrenals. Am J Dis Child 91:282, 1956.

36. Berdon WE, Baker DH: Radiographic findings in adrenal disease in infants and children. NY State J Med 69:2773–2778, 1969.

37. Crocker AC, Vawter GF, Neuhauser EBD, et al: Wolman's disease: 3 new patients with a recently described lipidosis. Pediatrics 35:627–639, 1965.

38. Engel RM, Elkins RC, Fletcher BD: Retroperitoneal teratoma. Cancer 22:1068–1073, 1968.

39. Lord JM: Intra-abdominal foetus in foetu. J Pathol Bacteriol 72:627–641, 1956.

40. Broghammer BJ, Wolf RS, Geppert CH: The included twin or fetus in fetu—a case report. Radiology 80:844–846, 1963.

41. Lemire LJ, Graham CB, Beckwith JB: Skin covered sacrococcygeal masses in infants and children. J Pediatr 79:948–954, 1971.

42. Donnellan WA, Swenson O: Benign and malignant sacrococcygeal teratomas. Surgery 64:834–846, 1968.

43. Franken EA Jr: Gastrointestinal Radiology in Pediatrics. New York, Harper & Row, 1975, p 246.

44. Leonidas JC: Bilateral renal cortical necrosis in a newborn. J Pediatr 79:623, 1971.

45. Sutton TJ, LeBlanc A, Gauthier N, et al: Radiological manifestations of neonatal renal vein thrombus on follow-up examinations. Radiology 122:435–438, 1977.

46. Nahum H, Gubler JP, Rodier J: Thrombose veineuse rénal unilatérale du nouveau-né. Ann Radiol (Paris) 12:293–307, 1969.

47. Kirks DR, Taybi H: Prune belly syndrome. An unusual case of neonatal abdominal calcification. Am J Roentgenol 123:778–781, 1975.

48. Martin MM, Stevens EM: Subcutaneous fat necrosis of the newborn with calcification of the tissues. Arch Dis Child 32:146–148, 1957.

49. Blake HA, Goyette EM, Lyter CS, et al: Subcutaneous fat necrosis complicating hypothermia. J Pediatr 46:78–80, 1955.

50. Duhn R, Schoen EJ, Siv M: Subcutaneous fat necrosis with extensive calcification after hypothermia in two newborn infants. Pediatrics 41:661–664, 1968.

51. Berger PE, Heidlberger KP, Poznanski AK: Extravasation of calcium gluconate as a cause of soft tissue calcification in infancy. Am J Roentgenol 121:109–117, 1974.

52. Lamm SS: Danger of intramuscular injection of calcium gluconate in infancy. JAMA 129:347–348, 1945.

53. Clayton RS, Goodman PH: The roentgenographic diagnosis of geophagia. Am J Roentgenol 73:203–207, 1955.

54. Carey LS: Lead shot appendicitis in northern native people. J Canad Assoc Radiol 28:171–174, 1977.

55. Faegenburg D: Fecalith of the appendix—incidence and significance. Am J Roentgenol 89:752–759, 1963.

56. Omojoca MF, Hood IC, Stevenson GW: Calcified gastric duplication. Gastrointest Radiol 5:235–238, 1980.

57. Alford BA, Armstrong P, Franken EA Jr, et al: Calcification associated with duodenal duplication in children. Radiology 134:647–648, 1980.

58. Harned RK, Babbitt DP: Cholelithiasis in children. Radiology 117:391–393, 1975.

59. Dewey KW, Grossman H, Canale VC: Cholelithiasis in thalassemia major. Radiology 96:385–388, 1970.

60. Sears HF, Golden GT, Horsley JS III: Cholecystitis in childhood and adolescence. Arch Surg 106:651–653, 1973.

61. Okuda KJ, Peters RL (Eds): Hepatocellular Carcinoma. New York, John Wiley & Sons, 1976, p 216.

62. Sorsdahl OA, Gay BB: Roentgenologic features of a primary carcinoma of the liver in infants and children. Am J Roentgenol 100:117–127, 1967.

63. Ishak KG, Glunz PR: Hepatoblastoma and hepatocarcinoma in infancy and childhood: report of 47 cases. Cancer 20:396–422, 1967.

64. Kattan K, Langer L, Surfrun H: Calcified foci in primary hepatic carcinoma in infancy. A case report—x-ray and pathological study. Israel Med J 18:296–298, 1959.

65. McDonald P: Hepatic tumors in childhood. Clin Radiol 18:74–82, 1967.

66. Selke AC, Cornell SH: Infantile hepatic hemangioendothelioma. Am J Roentgenol 106:200–203, 1969.

67. Ross P: Calcification in liver metastases from neuroblastoma. Radiology 85:1074–1079, 1969.

68. Sutcliff EJ, Chrispin AR: Chronic granulomatous disease. Brit J Radiol 43:110–118, 1970.

69. Singleton EB, Rosenberg HS: Intraluminal calcifications of the inferior vena cava. Am J Roentgenol 86:556–560, 1961.

70. Silverman NR, Borns PF, Goldstein AH: Thrombus calcification in the inferior vena cava. Am J Roentgenol 106:97–102, 1969.

71. Macht SH, Roman PW: Radiologic changes in sickle cell anemia. Radiology 51:697–707, 1948.

72. Jacobson G, Zucherman SD: Roentgenographically demonstrable splenic deposits in sickle cell anemia. Am J Roentgenol 76:47–52, 1956.

73. Soergel KH: The Pancreas, Carey LC (ed). St Louis, C. V. Mosby, 1973, pp 171–173.
74. DiSant'Agnese PA, LePore MG: Involvement of abdominal organs in cystic fibrosis of the pancreas. Gastroenterology 40:64–74, 1961.
75. Kattwinkel J, Lapay A, DiSant'Agnese PA, et al: Hereditary pancreatitis: 3 new kindreds and a critical review of the literature. Pediatrics 51:55–69, 1976.
76. Jarvis JL, Jenkins D, Sosman MC, et al: Roentgenologic observations in Addison disease. A review of 120 cases. Radiology 62:16–29, 1954.
77. Joelson JJ, Persky L, Rose FA: Radiographic diagnosis of tumors of the adrenal gland. Radiology 62:488–495, 1954.
78. Martin JF: Suprarenal calcification. Radiol Clin North Amer 3:129–138, 1965.
79. Stockpole RH, Melicow MM, Uson AC: Pheochromocytoma in children. J Pediatr 63:315–330, 1963.
80. Grainger RG, Lloyd GAS, Williams JL: Egg-shell calcification: A sign of phaeochromocytoma. Clin Radiol 18:282–286, 1967.
81. Belman AD, Kaplan GW: Genitourinary Problems in Pediatrics. Philadelphia, WB Saunders, 1981, pp 309–318.
82. Malek RS, Kelalis PP: Pediatric nephrolithiasis. J Urol 113:545–551, 1975.
83. Bagby RJ, Clements JL, Patrick JW, et al: Genitourinary complications of granulomatous bowel disease. Am J Roentgenol 117:297–306, 1973.
84. McAllister WH, Nedelman SH: Roentgen manifestations of bilateral renal cortical necrosis. Am J Roentgenol 86:129–135, 1961.
85. Cohen HL, Kassner EG, Haller JO: Nephrocalcinosis in chronic glomerulonephritis. Report of the youngest patient. Urol Radiol 2:51–52, 1980.
86. Arons WL, Christensen WR, Sosman MC: Nephrocalcinosis visible by x-ray associated with chronic glomerulonephritis. Ann Intern Med 42:260–282, 1955.
87. Kaufman RA, Holt JH, Heidelberger KP: Calcification in primary and metastatic Wilms' tumor. Am J Roentgenol 130:783–785, 1978.
88. Kelalis PP: Emmett's Clinical Urography, 4th edition, Witten DM, Myers GH Jr, Utz DC (eds). Philadelphia, WB Saunders, 1977, pp 1671–1673.
89. Dehner LP: Intrarenal teratoma occurring in infancy. Report of a case with discussion of extragonadal germ cell tumors in infancy. J Pediatr Surg 8:369–378, 1973.
90. Irons GB Jr, Hoge RH, Salzberg AM: Ovarian teratomas in children. Clin Pediatr 5:151–153, 1966.
91. Wollin E, Ozonoff MB: Serial development of teeth in an ovarian teratoma: a 13-year x-ray record. N Engl J Med 265:897–898, 1961.
92. Hyman RA, Van Micsky LI, Finby N: Ovarian teratoma in childhood. Am J Roentgenol 116:673–675, 1972.
93. Partlow WF, Taybi H: Teratomas in infants and children. Am J Roentgenol 112:155–166, 1971.
94. Nelken RP, Nieburg PL, Bergstrom WH, et al: Dysgerminomas presenting as a calcified abdominal mass with hypercalcemia. Pediatrics 61:791–793, 1978.
95. Cooperman LR, Hamlin J, Ng E: Gonadoblastoma. A rare ovarian tumor related to dysgerminoma with characteristic roentgen appearance. Radiology 90:322–324, 1968.

INDEX

Note: Page numbers in *italics* indicate illustrations; t refers to tables.

Saunders Monographs In Clinical Radiology

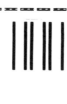

BUSINESS REPLY CARD

FIRST CLASS   PERMIT NO. 101   PHILADELPHIA, PA

POSTAGE WILL BE PAID BY ADDRESSEE

W.B. SAUNDERS COMPANY

West Washington Square
Philadelphia, PA 19105

NO POSTAGE
NECESSARY
IF MAILED
IN THE
UNITED STATES